Orthopedics: Conventional and Modern Approaches

Orthopedics: Conventional and Modern Approaches

Edited by Kingston Hunt

hayle
medical

New York

Hayle Medical,
750 Third Avenue, 9th Floor,
New York, NY 10017, USA

Visit us on the World Wide Web at:
www.haylemedical.com

ISBN: 978-1-63241-711-4

Cataloging-in-Publication Data

Orthopedics : conventional and modern approaches / edited by Kingston Hunt.
   p. cm.
Includes bibliographical references and index.
ISBN 978-1-63241-711-4
1. Orthopedics. 2. Orthopedics--Diagnosis. 3. Orthopedics--Treatment. I. Hunt, Kingston.
RD731 .O786 2019
616.7--dc23

Table of Contents

Preface

Orthopedics refers to the field of surgery which studies the conditions related to the musculoskeletal system. Some common orthopedic conditions include spine disorders, degenerative diseases, congenital disorders, sports injuries, musculoskeletal trauma, tumors and infections. Knee replacement is one of the most common procedures performed by an orthopedic surgeon. It is concerned with the replacement of knee joint to relieve pain and disability. It is usually done to treat patients with osteoarthritis, rheumatoid arthritis, and psoriatic arthritis. The goal of modern orthopedics is to make surgery as minimally invasive as possible. The ever growing need of advanced medical treatments is the reason that has fueled the research in the field of orthopedics in recent times. The various advancements in orthopedics are glanced at in this book and their applications as well as ramifications are looked at in detail. Students, doctors, experts and all associated with orthopedics will benefit alike from this book.

This book unites the global concepts and researches in an organized manner for a comprehensive understanding of the subject. It is a ripe text for all researchers, students, scientists or anyone else who is interested in acquiring a better knowledge of this dynamic field.

I extend my sincere thanks to the contributors for such eloquent research chapters. Finally, I thank my family for being a source of support and help.

Editor

Epiphysiolysis Type Salter I of the Medial Clavicle with Posterior Displacement

C. Siebenmann ⓘ, F. Ramadani, G. Barbier, E. Gautier, and P. Vial

Department of Orthopedic Surgery, HFR Fribourg-Hôpital Cantonal, Switzerland

Correspondence should be addressed to C. Siebenmann; corinne.siebenmann@gmail.com

Academic Editor: Johannes Mayr

Physeal fractures of the medial clavicle with posterior displacement of the metaphysis are very rare injuries, but additional injuries can be life-threatening. Due to the specific clavicular ossification process, skeletally immature patients present usually not true sternoclavicular joint (SCJ) dislocations accordingly to adults but rather displaced physeal fractures. There is no consensus in the current literature on the best treatment of this lesion. Conservative treatment is not resulting in good outcome; closed reduction is often not successful, and open reduction with internal fixation is finally required. Several methods are described for stabilizing these physeal fractures. We treated three osseous immature patients with this lesion. Due to the small dimension of the medial clavicular epiphysis, we performed in one case a transosseous figure-of-eight suture of the clavicular metaphysis towards the sternum, and in the two other cases, a transosseous suture from the clavicular metaphysis on the anterior clavicular periosteum. The latter technique avoids harm to the small epiphysis or the SCJ and minimizes the risk of retrosternal complications.

1. Introduction

Lesions of the sternoclavicular joint (SCJ) including epiphysiolyses type Salter I and II are rare in all age groups, representing less than 5% of all shoulder girdle injuries [1]. Posterior dislocations of the medial end of the clavicle in skeletally immature patients are exceptional. But, potential life-threating complications can occur due to the proximity to the trachea, esophagus, and retrosternal vascular and neural structures. In the literature, severe complications are reported resulting from missed diagnoses like cerebral insult due to vascular lesion [2] and compression of the trachea [3], the subclavian vessels [4], and the brachial plexus [5]; also, fatalities are documented due to a tracheoesophageal fistula [6].

An accurate diagnosis and appropriate treatment are therefore important for a good outcome [7]. Only few case reports or small case series exist in the current literature. These injuries are described as dislocation of the SCJ or epiphysiolysis of the medial end of the clavicle. The mechanism of injury is either a direct force applied to the medial clavicle or an indirect force due to an impact on the posterolateral aspect of the shoulder occurring often during contact sport activities [8].

The SCJ is functionally a saddle joint with a small surface providing only a poor congruence and containment. Therefore, a thick capsule and a strong ligamentous system guarantee joint stability. Spencer et al. showed on a cadaver model that the posterior capsule is the most important restraint for anterior and posterior translation in the SCJ [9]. Anterior dislocations occur nearly three times more often than posterior dislocations [10].

The understanding of the process of clavicular ossification is essential for an appropriate management of injuries around the SCJ in skeletally immature patients. The center of ossification of the medial end of the clavicle appears at the age of 18 to 20 years, and its growth plate fuses at the age of 20 to 25 years [11, 12].

Therefore, the physis of the medial clavicle is the weakest link in the SCJ and it is more likely to sustain a physeal separation than a true SCJ dislocation (Figures 1(a) and 1(b)). The strong ligamentous structures of the SCJ retain the cartilaginous epiphysis in place, and the metaphysis of the clavicle displaces posteriorly towards the retrosternal

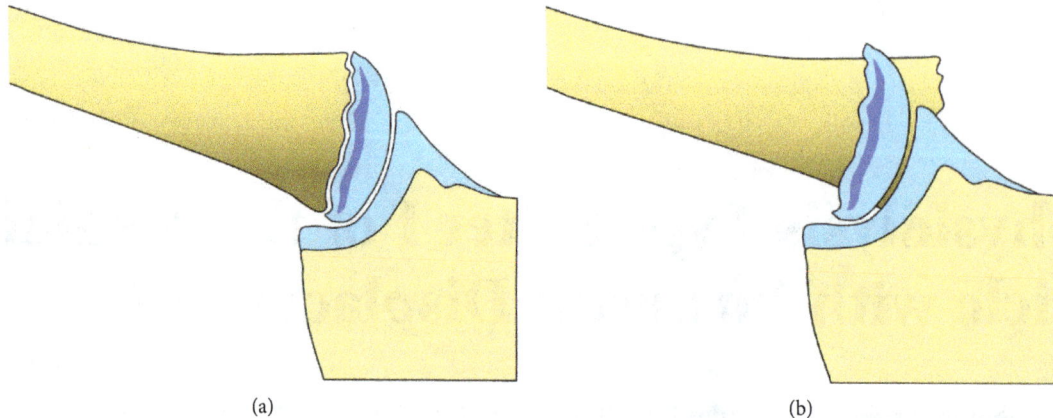

(a)   (b)

FIGURE 1: Sternoclavicular joint of an osseous immature person (a). Typical injury pattern: epiphysiolysis type Salter I with posterior displacement of the clavicular metaphysis (b).

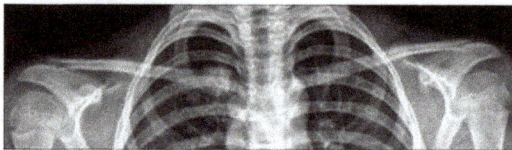

FIGURE 2: Preoperative anteroposterior radiographs revealing an asymmetric position of the medial clavicle on the right side.

space. On standard radiographs, the diagnosis of a SCJ lesion can be missed easily. Therefore, the clinical assessment of local pain and swelling and SCJ instability are important. To confirm the diagnosis and evaluate additional retrosternal injuries, further analysis using a CT scan is mandatory. However, even with a CT scan, discrimination between true SCJ dislocation and displaced epiphysiolysis type Salter I or II can be difficult [13–17]. Often, the final diagnosis is made during surgery [18].

In the current orthopedic literature, there are just a few case reports or small case series reported of the rare entity of epiphysiolysis of the medial clavicle.

Our objective is to propose an appropriate management of epiphysiolysis of the medial end of the clavicle in the skeletally immature patient.

2. Cases

We report on three patients suffering from traumatic epiphysiolysis of the medial clavicle and discuss the surgical management and fixation techniques.

In the first two cases—a 13-year-old boy and an 8-year-old girl, the mechanism of injury consisted in a lateral impact onto the involved shoulder while falling during a soccer play. In the third case of a 16-year-old boy, the mechanism was a direct blow in the anteroposterior direction on the upper thorax while practicing Judo. All three patients suffered from an instant pain in the right SCJ area. Clinically, no neurovascular lesions or dyspnea were present. Standard radiographs revealed an asymmetric position of the medial clavicle with posterior displacement of the medial end on the injured side (Figure 2). CT scan confirmed the diagnosis of epiphysiolysis of the medial clavicular epiphysis (Figures 3(a) and 3(b)). But, due to the absence of the corresponding centers of ossification of the medial clavicular epiphysis, discrimination from a pure posterior dislocation of the SCJ was difficult preoperatively, and final diagnosis was only possible during open surgery.

In the first child, an unsuccessful closed reduction was attempted prior to operation. The operation was performed under general anesthesia with the patient in supine position. A cushion was placed between the scapulae to exert tension on the anterior upper thorax. A 4 cm long skin incision was made in line with the clavicle from its medial end to the sternum. The periosteum, which was found intact anteriorly, was incised over the medial clavicle. The thick periosteal sleeve was disrupted posteriorly allowing posterior displacement of the medial clavicular metaphysis which was locked posterior to the manubrium. The medial clavicular epiphysis remained in place; thus, the lesion was classified as an epiphysiolysis type Salter I.

Reduction of the clavicle back in its periosteal sleeve was performed by gentle traction and the use of a pointed reduction clamp. Stabilization of the medial clavicular metaphysis was performed with a transosseous suture using a Fiber-Tape® in a figure-of-eight fashion from the clavicular metaphysis to the anterior cortex of the sternum.

Due to the experience of the first case in which the clavicular metaphysis was trapped behind the periosteal sleeve, surgical technique was adapted for the second and third children.

The skin incision was shorter, about 2 cm centered on the medial end of the clavicle. The platysma was just fenestrated. In both cases, the periosteal sleeve of the medial clavicle was found to be completely intact in its anterior part. It was incised longitudinally leaving intact the capsule of the SCJ. As seen in the first patient, the medial clavicular epiphysis stayed properly in place and the clavicular metaphysis was displaced retrosternally disrupting the posterior periosteum longitudinally. Open reduction was performed. Three drill

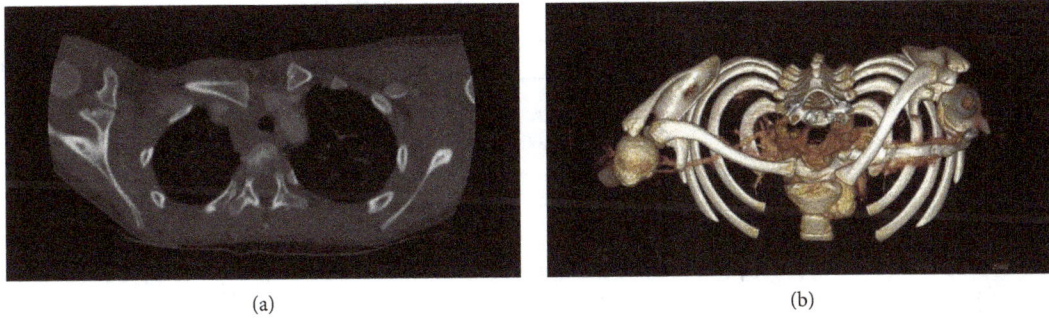

FIGURE 3: Axial (a) and three-dimensional reconstructed (b) computed tomography scans confirm the posteriorly displaced clavicle on the right side. Due to the absence of the corresponding centers of ossification of the medial clavicular epiphysis, discrimination from a pure posterior dislocation of the sternoclavicular joint is difficult.

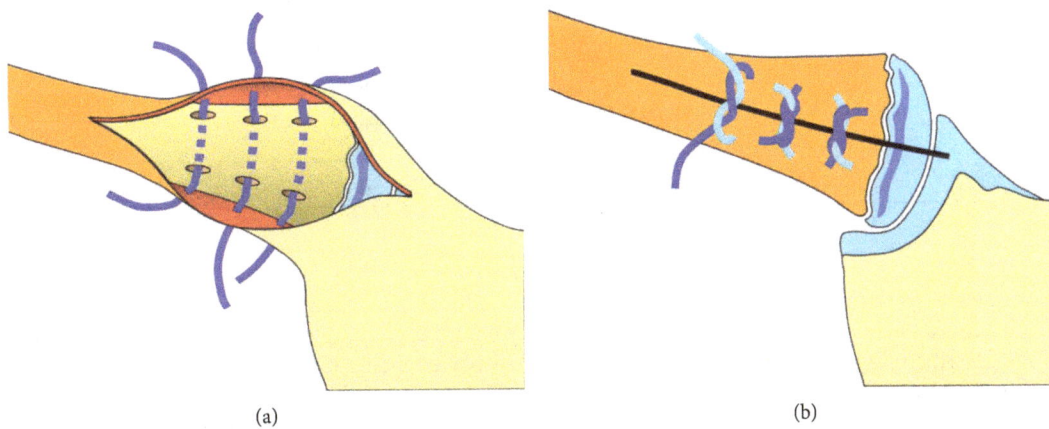

FIGURE 4: Surgical technique: fixation of the reduced clavicular metaphysis with three transosseous sutures (FiberWire®) on the anterior clavicular periosteum (a). The clavicular metaphysis is fixed, and the periosteum is closed by tightening the knots (b).

holes were made in the superior and inferior cortex of the medial clavicular metaphysis avoiding perforation of the posterior cortex. Three FiberWire® were inserted in the holes, and the metaphysis was anchored directly to the strong and solid anterior clavicular periosteum (Figures 4(a) and 4(b)). Closure was completed in layers by additional adaptation of the anterior periosteum and the platysma.

Intraoperatively, in all three children, a good stability was achieved with the proposed suture techniques. No complications occurred during the operation. Facing the rare risk of severe vascular or pulmonal problems especially during the reduction maneuver, we assured backup by a thoracic surgeon in all cases.

Postoperatively, the patients were wearing a posterior figure-of-eight bandage for six weeks and free mobilization of the shoulder was allowed below the horizontal plane. At twelve weeks, all three patients were asymptomatic. The range of shoulder motion was symmetric; the body-cross test negative, and clinically the medial clavicle was stable. Radiographs revealed healing of the epiphysiolysis in correct length of the clavicle and correct position of the medial clavicular metaphysis. Also, at one-year follow-up, the patients remained asymptomatic and without any functional impairment, and all had returned to former sport activities.

3. Discussion

Actually, there is no consensus in the literature concerning the optimal treatment of this physeal fracture. Conservative treatment without anatomical reduction by thinking that the remodeling potential of immature bone would be able to restore correct anatomical position of the medial end of the clavicle is described in the past, but with reported complications like thoracic outlet syndrome by callus formation [19] and pneumothorax [20].

Denham and Dingley published probably one of the first reports of epiphyseal separation of the medial end of the clavicle. He favored an anatomical reduction to improve healing and decrease the number of poor results [21]. Closed reduction was recommended by several authors if there are no additional retrosternal injuries [16, 21–24]. However, the reported success rate was very diverging (Table 1). Often, an open reduction and internal fixation were required after a failed attempt of closed reduction or in case of residual instability [14, 23, 25–27]. Waters et al. [23] reviewed 13 medial clavicle injuries in skeletally immature patients and found 11 physeal fractures. They reported on instability after closed reduction in all cases and recommend immediate open reduction and fixation [23]. Laffosse et al. [14] reported a series of 13 patients with systematic failure of the attempted

TABLE 1: Literature review (since 2000).

Author, year	n	Age	Closed reduction	Definitive treatment
Goldfarb et al., 2001 [25]	6	7–16	6 failed	6 ORIF osteosuture
Waters et al., 2003 [23]	11	13–17	3 failed	11 ORIF osteosuture
Gobet et al., 2004 [16]	3	8–15	1 failed	1 ORIF osteosuture
			2 successful	2 nonoperative
Hofwegen and Wolf, 2008 [26]	2	17–20	1 failed	2 ORIF osteosuture
Laffosse et al., 2010 [14]	13	15–20	5 failed	13 ORIF different techniques
Tennent et al., 2012 [27]	7	14–19	7 failed	7 ORIF osteosuture
Garg et al., 2012 [13]	1	12	1 failed	1 ORIF osteosuture over SCJ
Gil-Albarova et al., 2012 [34]	1	11	1 successful	1 nonoperative
Koch and Wells, 2012 [29]	1	14	0	1 ORIF osteosuture
Lee et al., 2014 [35]	20	13–19	2 failed	18 ORIF osteosuture
			2 successful	2 nonoperative
Ozer et al., 2014 [36]	1	16	1 successful	1 nonoperative
Tepolt et al., 2014 [18]	6	7–17	2 failed	6 osteosuture over SCJ
Perdreau et al., 2014 [37]	1	16	1 failed	1 osteosuture over SCJ
Krantzow, 2015 [38]	1	17	0	1 osteosuture
Kassé et al., 2016 [39]	3	16–19	0	3 osteosuture or cerclage SCJ

closed reduction. They also recommend open reduction with a stabilization procedure [14].

The methods described for stabilizing these physeal fractures are quite different including fixation by Kirschner wires [21], anterior plating [17, 28], or various suture techniques such as costoclavicular cerclage or tenodesis [14], repair of the costoclavicular and sternoclavicular ligaments [13, 23], transosseous fixation in a figure-of-eight manner of the clavicular metaphysis to the intact epiphysis [25, 29], or suturing the clavicle to the manubrium [18, 26, 30, 31]. The use of transarticular Kirschner wires has been abandoned due to the risk of intrathoracic wire migration [32].

Tennent et al. described a new stabilization technique [27]. After open reduction, they sutured the medial clavicle to the anterior periosteum and platysma as a single layer using absorbable sutures, which were passed through drill holes in the medial clavicle. At an average of nine months, their patients presented good functional results. Only one patient had to be reoperated six months after the initial procedure to remove a prominent suture knot and to revise the scar.

We are convinced that it is important to distinguish between a real dislocation of the SCJ and a physeal fracture of the medial end of the clavicle. Osseous immature patients suffer rather from physeal fracture type Salter I or II then from a pure dislocation of the SCJ. Nevertheless, these two entities are not every time properly discriminated in the literature, and in case of successful closed reduction and nonoperative treatment, the exact diagnosis will remain uncertain. We should keep in mind that in epiphysiolysis of the medial clavicle, the strong periosteal sleeve plays an important role. Corresponding to lateral physeal fracture, the clavicle peels off from its physis and periosteal sleeve, which is just disrupted longitudinally [33].

In all our three cases, the medial epiphysis remained anatomically in place, and the clavicular metaphysis was displaced posteriorly to it into the retrosternal space. In all three cases, the periosteal sleeve was only disrupted posteriorly allowing the posterior penetration of the medial clavicular end.

Due to its small dimension, the medial clavicular epiphysis itself does not offer sufficient grip for anchoring sutures. Thus, two different options to restore stability of the medial clavicle are available. The first one consists in a transosseous figure-of-eight suture of the clavicular metaphysis towards the anterior cortex of the sternum. The second one is comparable to the technique described by Tennent et al. [27]. The anteriorly intact periosteal sleeve is incised, the clavicular metaphysis reduced back into its sleeve, and held in place by means of three transosseous sutures from the clavicular metaphysis on the anterior clavicular periosteum. In contrast to the technique described by Tennent et al., we did not include the platysma in the suture allowing a better coverage of the knots by the platysma. In addition, instead of PDS, we used FiberWire®, thus creating less prominent knots.

We attempted a closed reduction in the first patient which failed because the metaphysis was stucked outside the periosteal sleeve posterior to the epiphysis as seen later intraoperatively. This finding agrees with the literature review shown in Table 1, which suggests that a closed reduction is rarely successful. Even if the patients do not present further initial symptoms, in our opinion, an immediate (up to 6 h) open reduction and fixation are indicated to avoid injuries of retrosternal structures by either the instable fragment or callus formation.

In contrast, when physeal fracture of the medial clavicle with anterior displacement occurs, a conservative treatment is often recommended. In this case, the periosteal sleeve is just disrupted anteriorly and stays intact posteriorly, which protects the mediastinal structures.

The advantage of the described methods is that neither the fragile epiphysis nor the SCJ is violated, the retrosternal structures are safe, and there is no hardware irritation. Mechanically, the clavicular metaphysis buttresses against the clavicular epiphysis, and the transosseous sutures into the anterior periosteum prevent the posterior redislocation. The bone is also loaded in compression, and the restored anterior periosteum plays the role of a tension band.

We practiced both stabilization techniques. Both had excellent clinical and radiographical results at one year. Nevertheless, we recommend the second one stabilizing the clavicula on the anterior periosteum, because it is technically simpler and safer referring to possible iatrogenic retrosternal injuries.

Conflicts of Interest

The authors declare that there are no conflicts of interest regarding the publication of this paper.

References

[1] E. F. Cave, *Fractures and Other Injuries*, Year Book Publishers, 1958.

[2] M. S. Marcus and V. Tan, "Cerebrovascular accident in a 19-year-old patient: a case report of posterior sternoclavicular dislocation," *Journal of Shoulder and Elbow Surgery*, vol. 20, no. 7, pp. e1–e4, 2011.

[3] E. Nakayama, T. Tanaka, T. Noguchi, J. Yasuda, and Y. Terada, "Tracheal stenosis caused by retrosternal dislocation of the right clavicle," *The Annals of Thoracic Surgery*, vol. 83, no. 2, pp. 685–687, 2007.

[4] N. W. Emms, A. D. Morris, J. C. Kaye, and S. D. Blair, "Subclavian vein obstruction caused by an unreduced type II Salter Harris injury of the medial clavicular physis," *Journal of Shoulder and Elbow Surgery*, vol. 11, no. 3, pp. 271–273, 2002.

[5] S. Jain, D. Monbaliu, and J. F. Thompson, "Thoracic outlet syndrome caused by chronic retrosternal dislocation of the clavicle. Successful treatment by transaxillary resection of the first rib," *Journal of Bone and Joint Surgery. British Volume (London)*, vol. 84, pp. 16–118, 2002.

[6] M. J. Wasylenko and E. F. Busse, "Posterior dislocation of the clavicle causing fatal tracheoesophageal fistula," *Canadian Journal of Surgery*, vol. 24, pp. 626–627, 1981.

[7] K. D. Carmichael, A. Longo, S. Lick, and L. Swischuk, "Posterior sternoclavicular epiphyseal fracture-dislocation with delayed diagnosis," *Skeletal Radiology*, vol. 35, no. 8, pp. 608–612, 2006.

[8] C. T. Buckerfield and M. E. Castle, "Acute traumatic retrosternal dislocation of the clavicle," *Journal of Bone and Joint Surgery*, vol. 66, no. 3, pp. 379–385, 1984.

[9] E. E. Spencer, J. E. Kuhn, L. J. Huston, J. E. Carpenter, and R. E. Hughes, "Ligamentous restraints to anterior and posterior translation of the sternoclavicular joint," *Journal of Shoulder and Elbow Surgery*, vol. 11, no. 1, pp. 43–47, 2002.

[10] M. S. Bahk, J. E. Kuhn, L. M. Galatz, P. M. Connor, and G. R. Wiliams Jr., "Acromioclavicular and sternoclavicular injuries and clavicular, glenoid, and scapular fractures," *The Journal of Bone and Joint Surgery*, vol. 91-A, pp. 2492–2510, 2009.

[11] C. F. Heinig, "Retrosternal dislocation of the clavicle: early recognition, X-ray diagnosis, and management," *The Journal of Bone and Joint Surgery*, vol. 50-A, p. 830, 1968.

[12] J. Y. Bishop and E. L. Flatow, "Pediatric shoulder trauma," *Clinical Orthopaedics and Related Research*, vol. 432, no. 432, pp. 41–48, 2005.

[13] S. Garg, Z. A. Alshameeri, and W. A. Wallace, "Posterior sternoclavicular joint dislocation in a child: a case report with review of literature," *Journal of Shoulder and Elbow Surgery*, vol. 21, no. 3, pp. e11–e16, 2012.

[14] J. M. Laffosse, A. Espie, N. Bonnevialle et al., "Posterior dislocation of the sternoclavicular joint and epiphyseal disruption of the medial clavicle with posterior displacement in sports participants," *The Journal of Bone and Joint Surgery*, vol. 92-B, no. 1, pp. 103–109, 2010.

[15] F. H. Selesnick, M. Jablon, C. Frank, and M. Post, "Retrosternal dislocation of the clavicle. Report of four cases," *The Journal of Bone and Joint Surgery*, vol. 66, no. 2, pp. 287–291, 1984.

[16] R. Gobet, M. Meuli, S. Altermatt, V. Jenni, and U. V. Willi, "Medial clavicular epiphysiolysis in children: the so-called sterno-clavicular dislocation," *Emergency Radiology*, vol. 10, no. 5, pp. 252–255, 2004.

[17] W. M. Franck, R. M. Siassi, and F. F. Hennig, "Treatment of posterior epiphyseal disruption of the medial clavicle with a modified balser plate," *The Journal of Trauma: Injury, Infection, and Critical Care*, vol. 55, no. 5, pp. 966–968, 2003.

[18] F. Tepolt, P. M. Carry, P. C. Heyn, and N. H. Miller, "Posterior sternoclavicular joint injuries in the adolescent population: a meta-analysis," *The American Journal of Sports Medicine*, vol. 42, no. 10, pp. 2517–2524, 2014.

[19] D. M. Gangahar and T. Flogaites, "Retrosternal dislocation of the clavicle producing thoracic outlet syndrome," *The Journal of Trauma*, vol. 18, no. 5, pp. 369–372, 1978.

[20] L. W. Worman and C. Leagus, "Intrathoracic injury following retrosternal dislocation of the clavicle," *The Journal of Trauma*, vol. 7, no. 3, pp. 416–423, 1967.

[21] R. H. Denham and A. F. Dingley, "Epiphyseal separation of the medial end of the clavicle," *The Journal of Bone & Joint Surgery*, vol. 49, no. 6, pp. 1179–1183, 1967.

[22] J. Yang, H. al-Etani, and M. Letts, "Diagnosis and treatment of posterior sternoclavicular joint dislocations in children," *The American Journal of Orthopedics*, vol. 25, no. 8, pp. 565–569, 1996.

[23] P. M. Waters, D. S. Bae, and R. K. Kadiyala, "Short-term outcomes after surgical treatment of traumatic posterior sternoclavicular fracture-dislocations in children and adolescents," *Journal of Pediatric Orthopedics*, vol. 23, no. 4, pp. 464–469, 2003.

[24] K. R. Zaslav, S. Ray, and C. S. Neer 2nd, "Conservative management of a displaced medial clavicular physeal injury in an adolescent athlete. A case report and literature review," *The American Journal of Sports Medicine*, vol. 17, no. 6, pp. 833–836, 1989.

[25] C. A. Goldfarb, G. S. Bassett, S. Sullivan, and J. E. Gordon, "Retrosternal displacement after physeal fracture of the medial clavicle in children treatment by open reduction and internal fixation," *The Journal of Bone and Joint Surgery*, vol. 83-B, no. 8, pp. 1168–1172, 2001.

[26] C. V. Hofwegen and B. Wolf, "Suture repair of posterior sternoclavicular physeal fractures: a report of two cases," *The Iowa Orthopaedic Journal*, vol. 28, pp. 49–52, 2008.

[27] T. D. Tennent, E. O. Pearse, and D. M. Eastwood, "A new technique for stabilizing adolescent posteriorly displaced physeal medial clavicular fractures," *Journal of Shoulder and Elbow Surgery*, vol. 21, no. 12, pp. 1734–1739, 2012.

[28] H. Asfazadourian and J. F. Kouvalchouk, "Retrosternal luxation of the clavicle. Apropos of 4 cases surgically treated using a temporary screwed anterior plate and review of the literature," *Annales de Chirurgie de la Main*, vol. 16, pp. 152–169, 1997.

[29] M. J. Koch and L. Wells, "Proximal clavicle physeal fracture with posterior displacement: diagnosis, treatment and prevention," *Orthopedics*, vol. 35, pp. e108–e111, 2012.

[30] E. Aydin, T. C. Dülgeroglu, A. Ates, and H. Metineren, "Repair of unstable posterior sternoclavicular dislocation using nonabsorbable tape suture and tension band technique: a case report with good results," *Case Reports in Orthopedics*, vol. 2015, Article ID 750898, 3 pages, 2015.

[31] D. P. Thomas, P. R. Williams, and H. C. Hoddinott, ""A safe" surgical technique for stabilization of the sternoclavicular joint: a cadaveric and clinic study," *Annals of the Royal College of Surgeons*, vol. 82, pp. 432–435, 2000.

[32] N. Venissac, M. Alifano, M. Dahan, and J. Mouroux, "Intrathoracic migration of Kirschner pins," *The Annals of Thoracic Surgery*, vol. 69, no. 6, pp. 1953–1955, 2000.

[33] J. A. Ogden, "Distal clavicular physeal injury," *Clinical Orthopaedics and Related Research*, vol. 188, no. 188, pp. 68–73, 1984.

[34] J. Gil-Albarova, S. Rebollo-González, V. E. Gómez-Palacio, and A. Herrera, "Management of sternoclavicular dislocation in young children: considerations about diagnosis and treatment of four cases," *Musculoskeletal Surgery*, vol. 97, no. 2, pp. 137–143, 2013.

[35] J. T. Lee, A. Y. Nasreddine, E. M. Black, D. S. Bae, and M. S. Kocher, "Posterior sternoclavicular joint injuries in skeletally immature patients," *Journal of Pediatric Orthopedics*, vol. 34, no. 4, pp. 369–375, 2014.

[36] U. E. Ozer, M. B. Yalçin, K. Kanberoglu, and A. E. Bagatur, "Retrosternal displacement of the clavicle after medial physeal fracture in an adolescent: MRI," *Journal of Pediatric Orthopedics B*, vol. 23, no. 4, pp. 375–378, 2014.

[37] A. Perdreau, B. Bingen, L. Gossing, E. Lejeune, and A. Beugnies, "Posterior sternoclavicular epiphyseal fracture-dislocation: case report and review of literature," *Injury Extra*, vol. 45, no. 1, pp. 1–5, 2014.

[38] M. Krantzow, "Medial clavicle physeal fracture: a case report from diagnosis to treatment," *The Orthopod*, vol. 14, 2015.

[39] A. N. Kassé, S. O. Limam, S. Diao, J. C. Sané, B. Thiam, and M. H. Sy, "Fracture-separation of the medial clavicular epiphysis: about 6 cases and review of the literature," *The Pan African Medical Journal*, vol. 25, p. 19, 2016.

Double-Tension Wire Management of Nonunion Patella with Severe Quadriceps Contracture

Rohan Bhimani(ID),[1] **Preeti Singh**(ID),[2] **and Fardeen Bhimani**(ID)[3]

[1]*Department of Orthopaedics, 11th Road, Khar (West), Hinduja Healthcare Surgical, Mumbai 400052, India*
[2]*Department of Orthopaedics, Osmania General Hospital, Hyderabad 500012, India*
[3]*Department of Orthopaedics, Bharati Hospital, Pune 411043, India*

Correspondence should be addressed to Rohan Bhimani; dr.rohanbhimani@gmail.com

Academic Editor: George Mouzopoulos

Introduction. Nonunion patella with quadriceps contracture is an unusual orthopaedic finding. Very few cases have been recorded in the past with this complication. We present a case of a 40-year-old male with nonunion patella with quadriceps contracture secondary to trauma. *Case Report.* A 40-year-old male with posttraumatic nonunion patella with quadriceps contracture since 6 months presented with complaints of defect in the left knee with restriction of movements. X-ray of the left knee confirmed our findings. He underwent quadricepsplasty with double-tension band wiring for the patella followed by rigorous physiotherapy to achieve the current level of the knee flexion of 110 degrees. *Conclusion.* We conclude that quadricepsplasty with tension band wiring and neutralization wire is one of the good modalities of treatment for a nonunion patella associated with quadriceps contracture.

1. Introduction

Fractures of the patella contributes to 1% of all skeletal injuries [1]. The anterior subcutaneous location of the patella makes it vulnerable to direct trauma. Transverse fracture pattern of the patella is a common form of presentation in clinical practice. Delayed presentation of displaced fracture of the patella is a common presentation in practice. Majority of the times when such cases present, the fragments are grossly displaced. Furthermore, there are soft tissue contractures like quadriceps, retinaculum, internal ligaments of the knee joint, associated knee joint stiffness, and extensor lag in these patients. The major hurdle is to bring the fracture fragments together and restore the extensor mechanism either by bone to bone or bone to tendon union. It is essential to maintain the length of the contracted tissues by allowing further flexion of the knee. There are three different school of thoughts in terms of the management for such complex fracture presentation. First school of thought is to go for conservative management with knee ROM exercises. The second group recommends single-stage procedure in which mobilization of the proximal fragment, followed by fixing

with the lower fragment using V-Y or Z-plasty and achieving fractional lengthening [2]. The third group opines the use of preoperative traction to the proximal fragment using pins or Ilizarov method to approximate the fragments and then fixing the fragments. Thus, double-stage surgery is carried out [2]. In our case, we used single-stage procedure whose results were encouraging.

2. Case Report

A 40-year-old male presented with complaints of instability and defect in his left knee since 6 months. The patient gave a history of trauma 6 months back and did not take any treatment for this. Clinically, anterior defect was present over the left knee with visibility of intercondylar articulating surfaces of the tibia and femur. Swelling was seen in the anterior aspect of the left distal third thigh, which, on palpation, was the superior part of the patella. The lower pole of the patella was palpable just above the left tibial tuberosity (Figure 1). The X-ray of the left knee confirmed that the superior fragment of the patella was present in the distal third aspect of

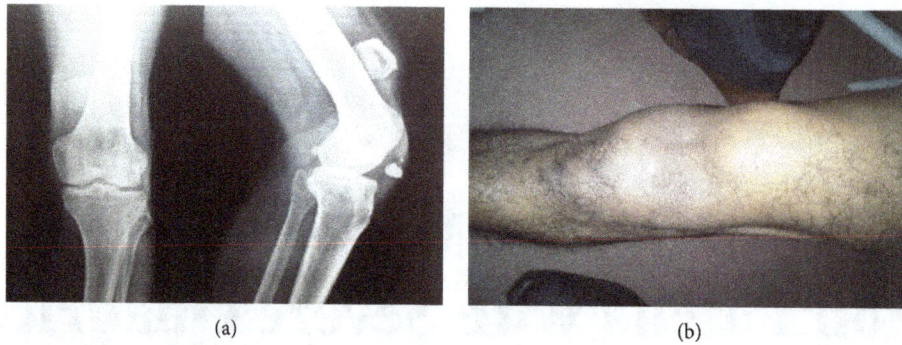

FIGURE 1: Preoperative clinical and radiological images showing proximal fragment in the distal third of the thigh (a, b).

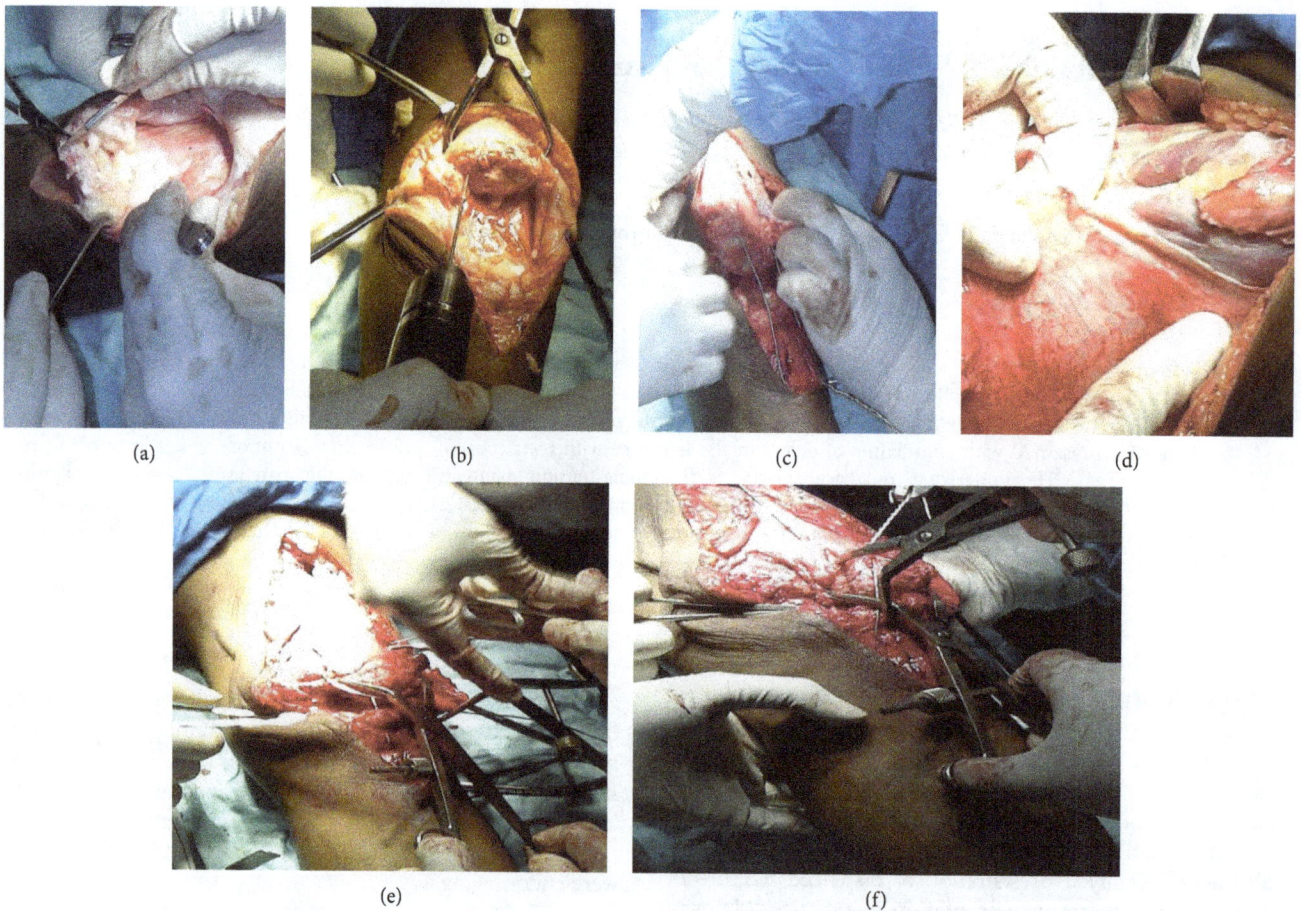

FIGURE 2: Intraoperative images of quadricepsplasty, reduction, and fixation of the patella (a–f).

the thigh and the lower fragment close to the tibial tuberosity (Figure 1).

The patient underwent surgery by anterior approach where quadricepsplasty and tension band wiring for the patella were performed after bringing the superior fragment down (Figure 2). Another tension band wire was passed through the neutralization hole made just posterior to the tibial tuberosity and the retinaculum was repaired.

During the immediate postoperative period, the patient was started on dynamic quadriceps strengthening and active straight-leg-raising exercises. After suture removal,

continuous passive motion for his knee was added. On discharge, the range of knee motion was from 5 degrees of extension lag to 40 degrees of flexion. At 6 weeks of postoperative follow-up, the patient had a 5- to 90-degree knee motion. The range of motion improved to 0–110 degrees at 3 months follow-up (Figure 3).

3. Discussion

The aim of reporting this case is to highlight the double-tension wire management and use of single-stage double-

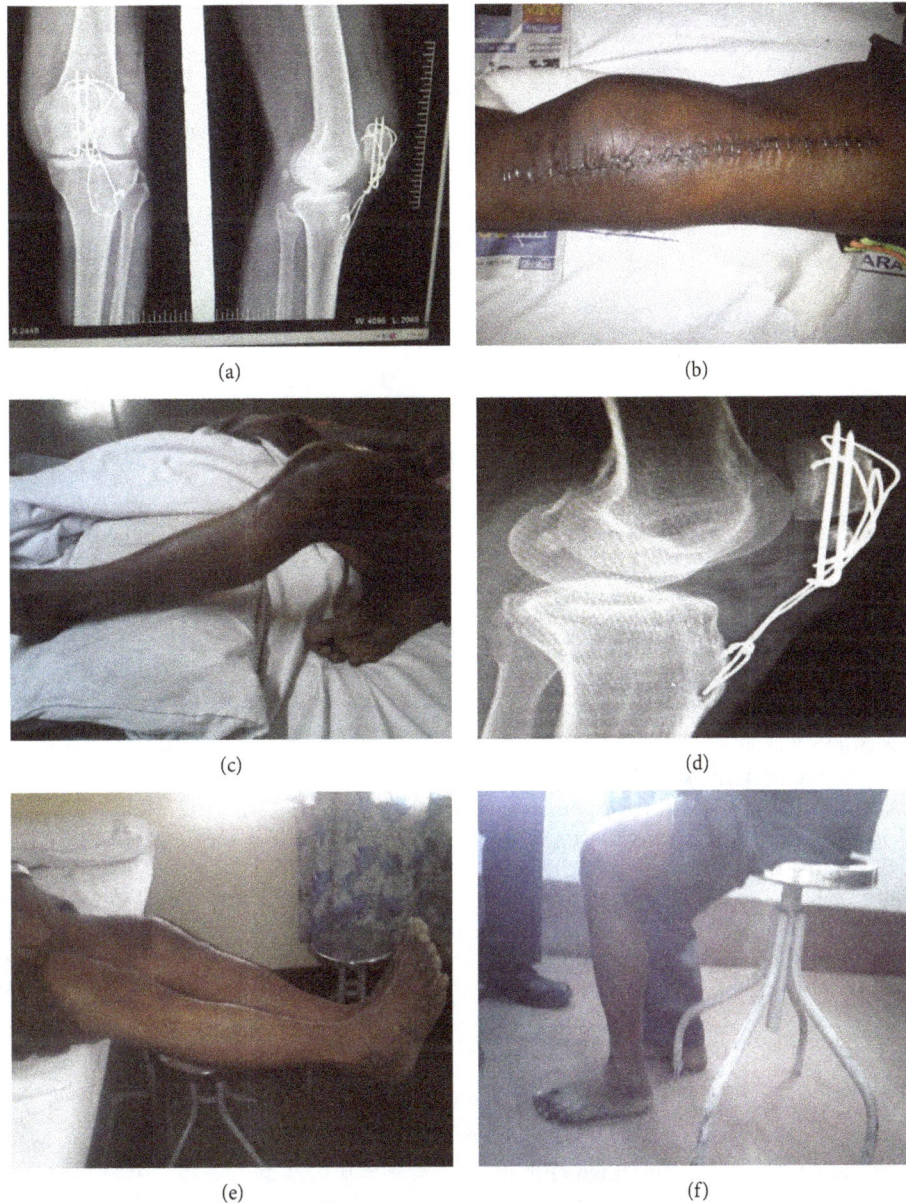

FIGURE 3: Postoperative X-ray, suture line, current X-ray, and present knee range of movement (a–f).

tension wire management of an old neglected nonunion patellar fracture. In the procedure, the proximal fragment was mobilized and fixed with the lower fragment using V-Y plasty and double-tension band wires. The objective during the surgery was to achieve fractional lengthening in order to prevent quadriceps lag in patients of nonunion of patellar fractures with large gaps between the fracture fragments. The rate of nonunion in patellar fractures is about 2.7% [3]. There are few cases reported in the management of such fractures. All of these cases of displaced fracture of the patella required operative intervention. The patients generally land up with a gap nonunion due to ignorance as they walk full-weight-bearing post fracture without surgical intervention. The normal tensile force across a patella is around 3000 N, which increases up to 6000 N in athletes. The generated patellofemoral compressive forces are three times greater than that

of the body weight during routine daily activities and may exceed seven times the body weight while climbing stairs and squatting. These forces only act on the proximal pole in fractures associated with tears in the medial and lateral expansions. The integrity of the medial and lateral expansions along with the anterior fascia lata and Sharpey's fibres allows active extension of the knee after patellar fracture. Unopposed passage of these forces, as in our case, allows a continuous increase in the gap between the fragments leading to the contracture of the proximal quadriceps mechanism. The available supporting literature on such presentation is shown in Table 1.

The problem with double-stage surgeries is that the presence of Ilizarov or skeletal traction poses a mental trauma to the patient along with surgical complications like bone weakening, pin loosening, pin tract infection, and prolonged

TABLE 1: Various studies comparing different modalities of treatment for nonunion patella.

Authors reporting nonunion of patella	Number of cases reported	Number cases treated conservatively	Mean age	Mean duration of delay	Treatment for quadriceps contracture (single-stage or double-stage)	Results (in terms of knee ROM)
Uvaraj et al. [4]	22	—	43 years	3 (range: 2–6.5 months)	No	0 to 110 degrees
Klassen and Trousdale [5]	20	7	38 years	34 months	Yes/single-stage	0 to 109 degrees
Lachiewicz [6]	1	—	67 years	2 years	Yes/single-stage	5 to 80 degrees of flexion
Dhar and Mir [7]	1	—	54 years	1 year	Yes/double-stage	0 to 135 degrees of flexion
Total	44					

duration of treatment. Yet double-stage surgeries have been reported with good results as shown by Dhar and Mir [7].

We opted for single-stage procedure, i.e., proximal fragment mobilization and fixation with the lower fragment/patellar tendon using V-Y/Z-plasty and achieving fractional lengthening. The supplementary fixation with neutralization wire in the region of the patellar tendon not only acted as an internal bracing during the initial rehabilitative period but also as a compressive force that shortens an already contracted patellar tendon. In addition, it also helps in securing the reduction by decreasing the tensile forces, which are exerted by the quadriceps muscle during knee flexion. One major risk with this procedure is overtightening of the neutralization wire resulting in the patella baja. In order to ensure the correct length of the neutralization, an image intensifier should be used intraoperatively to assess and compare the distance of the tibial tuberosity and the distal pole of the patella of the contralateral knee. Moreover, biomechanical assessment of the tension band wire shows that it fails at maximum load of about 695 N after osteosynthesis of the patella. Other methods of treatment like conservative technique and patellectomy are also practiced. In the conservative method, the stability and alignment of fracture fragments are confirmed at 60 degrees of flexion under an image intensifier with no dislocation. The initial restriction of knee flexion is provided by a suitable orthosis, which is gradually increased during the course of treatment. The major risk of conservative management is loss of full extension and stiffness of the knee, which are undesirable especially in a young patient. Patellectomy is another commonly practiced salvage procedure [3, 8]. This results in devastating problems like long periods of rehabilitation, anterior knee pain, restricted range of motion, incidents of giving way, swelling, and substantial reduction in strength of the quadriceps. Patellectomy compromises the length of the lever arm of the external apparatus mechanism, thereby causing excessive stress on the knee joint during extension [9, 10]. This ultimately causes early degenerative changes and is therefore a relative contraindication for young individuals [10]. An ideal management protocol for nonunion patellar fracture does not exist, and little literature is available about the results of different approaches. Of many techniques available, we believe that quadricepsplasty with double-tension band wiring is a superior modality of treatment and should be used for patients with such an unusual presentation.

4. Conclusion

We conclude that quadricepsplasty with double-tension band wire management is a good surgical measure in treatment of nonunion patella with quadriceps contracture.

Conflicts of Interest

The authors declare that there is no conflict of interest regarding the publication of this paper.

References

[1] E. J. Eric, "Fractures do joelho," in *Fractures em adultos*, vol. 1991pp. 1729–1744, Lippincott, Philadelphia, PA, USA, 3rd edition.

[2] R. K. Baruah, "Modified Ilizarov in difficult fracture of the patella. A case report," *Journal of Orthopaedic Case Reports*, vol. 6, no. 1, pp. 26–28, 2016.

[3] C. Gwinner, S. Märdian, P. Schwabe, K. D. Schaser, B. D. Krapohl, and T. M. Jung, "Current concepts review: fractures of the patella," *GMS Interdisciplinary plastic and reconstructive surgery DGPW*, vol. 5, pp. 1–15, 2016.

[4] N. R. Uvaraj, N. Mayil Vahanan, A. Sivaseelam, M. Mohd Sameer, and I. M. Basha, "Surgical management of neglected fractures of the patella," *Injury*, vol. 38, no. 8, pp. 979–983, 2007.

[5] J. F. Klassen and R. T. Trousdale, "Treatment of delayed and nonunion of the patella," *Journal of Orthopaedic Trauma*, vol. 11, no. 3, pp. 188–194, 1997.

[6] P. F. Lachiewicz, "Treatment of a neglected displaced transverse patella fracture," *The Journal of Knee Surgery*, vol. 21, no. 1, pp. 58–61, 2008.

[7] S. A. Dhar and M. R. Mir, "Use of the Illizarov method to reduce quadriceps lag in the management of neglected non union of a patellar fracture," *Journal of Orthopaedics*, vol. 4, p. 12, 2007.

[8] M. Kfuri, R. L. de Freitas, B. B. Batista et al., "Updates in biological therapies for knee injuries: bone," *Current Reviews in Musculoskeletal Medicine*, vol. 7, no. 3, pp. 220–227, 2014.

[9] V. Asopa, C. Willis-Owen, and G. Keene, "Patellectomy for osteoarthritis: a new tension preserving surgical technique to reconstruct the extensor mechanism with retrospective review of long-term follow-up," *Journal of Orthopaedic Surgery and Research*, vol. 10, no. 1, p. 107, 2015.

[10] P. Garg, K. Satyakam, A. Garg, S. Sahoo, D. Biswas, and S. Mitra, "Patellar nonunions: comparison of various surgical methods of treatment," *Indian Journal of Orthopaedics*, vol. 46, no. 3, pp. 304–311, 2012.

3

Patellar Tendon Excision and Repair for Residual Patella Alta after Prior Failed Patellar Tendon Repair: Surgical Decision Making and Outcome

Richard N. Puzzitiello ⓘ, **Avinesh Agarwalla** ⓘ, **Austin Stone, and Brian Forsythe** ⓘ

Midwest Orthopaedics at Rush, Rush University Medical Center, Chicago, IL, USA

Correspondence should be addressed to Brian Forsythe; forsythe.research@rushortho.com

Academic Editor: John Nyland

Presented in this report is a complex revision case of a patellar tendon repair preceded by excess tendon excision to correct for recurrent patella alta deformity, in a workers' compensation patient. The goal of this procedure was to alleviate this patient's pain, to preserve his ability to function in his activities of daily living, and to allow him to return to work at some capacity. On postoperative radiographs, the revision procedure appeared to have successfully corrected this patient's patella alta deformity. After an extended rehabilitation process, this patient had reached maximal medical improvement at 1-year follow-up. He displayed modest improvements in all PROs, including a clinically significant improvement in his short-form mental component score. Despite his functional capacity being still somewhat limited, this patient reported subjective satisfaction after this complicated salvage procedure.

1. Introduction

Patellar tendon rupture is an uncommon yet disabling injury most frequently seen in active adults under 40 years old. Surgical intervention is necessary to restore extensor mechanism functionality [1]. Several surgical techniques and rehabilitation protocols can be utilized to address this pathology based on the mechanism and chronicity of the injury [1]. Outcomes following patellar tendon repair have shown high levels of patient satisfaction and low rates of complications [2–5]. Patella alta, a common radiographic sign associated with patellar tendon rupture, has previously been reported to persist in isolated cases and is considered a surgical failure [5]. Strategies for a failed patellar tendon repair are limited in the literature.

In this report, we present the case of a workers' compensation patient who received a revision procedure for recurrence of symptoms and evidence of patella alta seven months following primary nonaugmented repair of a patellar tendon rupture with early postoperative mobilization. This patient received a patellar tendon advancement procedure

by excision and repair of the patellar tendon using two PEEK corkscrew anchors fixed to the patella. This is a unique case of a salvage procedure with modest outcomes following a previously undescribed procedure for a known complication after patellar tendon repair.

2. Case Report

A 45-year-old male sustained a traumatic work-related patellar tendon rupture from the inferior pole of the patella while exiting a vehicle. The patient had a past medical history of diabetes mellitus type II. The patient was evaluated within 22 days of his injury and initially treated with primary repair 81 days after the injury. The tendon was repaired with two number 2 nonabsorbable sutures in a Krackow suture configuration throughout the length of the patellar tendon and anchored through bone tunnels in the patella. This patellar height was corrected to an Insall-Salvati Index (ISI) and Caton-Deschamps Index (CDI) of 1.23 and 1.14 (Figure 1) from 1.4 and 1.34, respectively (Figure 2). His knee was immobilized in a locking brace for two weeks, and then

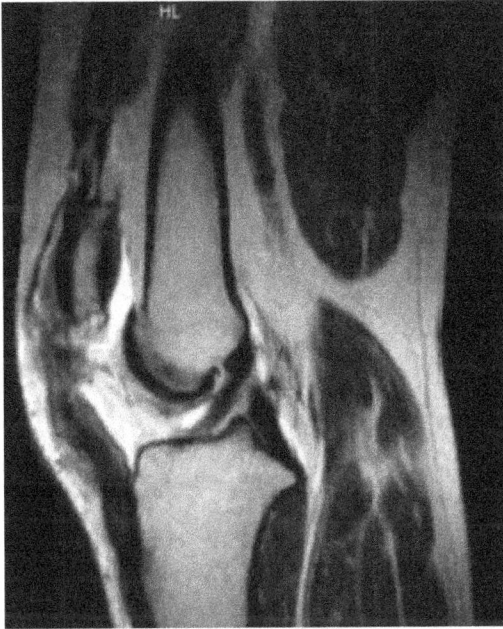

FIGURE 1: T2-weighted MRI of the right knee demonstrating patella alta and a full thickness tear of his proximal patellar tendon, two months following injury and one month prior to this patient's primary procedure. Insall-Salvati Index = 1.4, Caton-Deschamps Index = 1.34.

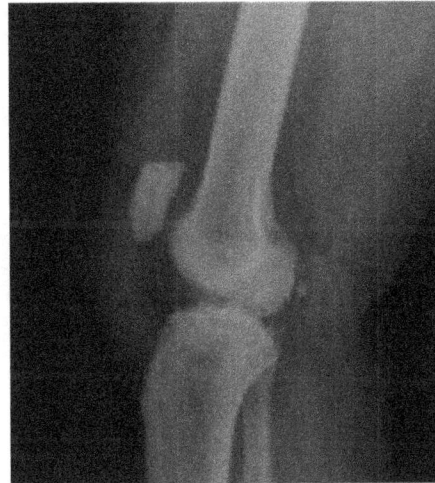

FIGURE 2: Postoperative lateral X-ray of the patient's right knee demonstrating a corrected patella alta deformity immediately following the first procedure. Insall-Salvati Index = 1.23, Caton-Deschamps Index (CDI) = 1.14.

physical therapy was initiated for range of motion at two weeks postoperatively. The patient progressed slowly through physical therapy gaining 100 degrees of active leg flexion but developed significant quadriceps atrophy, patella alta, and 10 degrees of an extensor lag at 7 months following the procedure. The patient was compliant with the standard rehabilitation protocol and had no history of traumatic reinjury. Eleven months after the primary procedure, the patient was referred to our clinic for persistent pain, pain with squatting and kneeling, instability, and stagnation in functional recovery which prevented him from returning to work up to this point. Subjectively, he reported a 4/10 pain level at rest. Clinical examination revealed proximal migration of the patella, 2+ coarse patellar crepitus, full active range of motion, 3+/5 quadriceps strength, and a 10-degree lag with single leg raise. T2-weighted MRI and lateral knee radiograph at 11-month follow-up confirmed patella alta deformity (CDI = 1.51, ISI = 1.55), an intact albeit lax patellar tendon, and cartilage fissuring near the inferior patellar apex (Figure 3). There was no additional ligamentous injury noted on MRI. His preoperative patient-reported outcome scores can be found in Table 1. A collective decision was made with the patient at this time to proceed with revision patellar tendon repair with the goal of returning to work at some capacity and resuming his normal activities of daily living.

The previous midline incision was dissected to visualize and confirm obvious redundancy and thinning of the patellar tendon. A 2 × 4 × 1 cm rectangular block of redundant patellar tendon tissue was outlined and resected to correct the degree of patella alta. The patella was mobilized using blunt dissection. The suture material from the index repair was removed, and the distal patellar footprint was prepared. Two 2.5 PEEK corkscrew anchors (Arthrex, Naples, FL) were anchored 2 cm apart on the distal patellar footprint. Krackow sutures were passed through the midsubstance of the patellar tendon, and with the opposite limb of each stitch, a half hitch was made such that a pulley mechanism was created (Figure 4). The tendon was reapproximated, and final fixation was secured with four mattress anchor knots with five alternating half hitches. The knee was brought to 30 degrees of flexion and the construct was stable. The wound was closed with a standard layered closure. Postoperative lateral knee radiograph displayed a CDI of 1.09 and an ISI of 1.16 (Figure 5), which confirmed that patella alta had been corrected. At 18-month follow-up, the patient had a repeat MRI performed which demonstrated a CDI of 1.35 (Figure 6).

Following the operation, a locked extension brace was applied for full-time use, and he began physical therapy two weeks postoperatively. The patient was compliant with his rehabilitation protocol and did not suffer any setbacks in the postoperative period. At his 1-year follow-up examination, the patient did not appear in acute distress, had no joint effusion, did not have patellar apprehension, demonstrated a nonantalgic gait, showed full active range of motion with no lag (Figure 7), displayed a negative Clarke exam, and had 4/5 quadriceps strength. In addition, the patient had 5 mm of anterior translation bilaterally on KT-1000 arthrometry testing and 20.6 pounds of force on maximal muscle testing of leg extension on the right compared to 21.3 pounds on the left as measured by a handheld dynamometer. The patient reported a pain level of 2/10 with activity, which was a decrease from his preoperative pain level (4/10). He reported occasional use of Tylenol for pain. His PRO scores at 1-year follow-up can be found in Table 1. Despite a relatively benign physical exam (Figure 7) and subjective reporting of satisfaction with the revision procedure and his outcome, the patient reported moderate functional limitations. Permanent work-

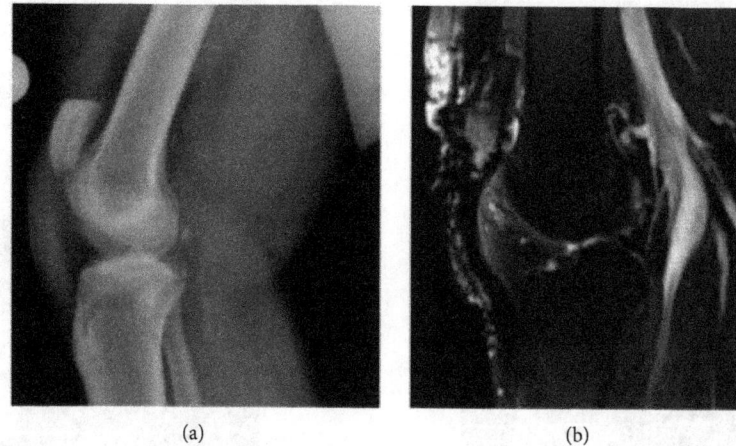

(a)　　　　　　　　(b)

FIGURE 3: Lateral X-ray (a) and T2-weighted MRI (b) of the patient's right knee eleven months following the index procedure showing proximal migration of the patella and a redundant but intact patellar tendon. CDI = 1.51, ISI = 1.55.

TABLE 1: Patient-reported outcomes.

PRO	Preop	Postop	Change
IKDC	27.6	33.3	5.7
KOOS			
Daily living	39.7	57.4	17.7
Pain	33.3	44.4	11.1
Physical symptoms	51.2	48.5	−2.7
Quality of life	12.5	25	12.5
Sports and recreation	5	5	0
Symptoms	35.7	39.3	3.6
JR	36.9	50	13.1
SF-12 mental	44.4	50.9	6.5
SF-12 physical	20	23	3
VR-12 mental	47.1	49.3	2.2
VR-12 physical	19.4	23.9	4.5

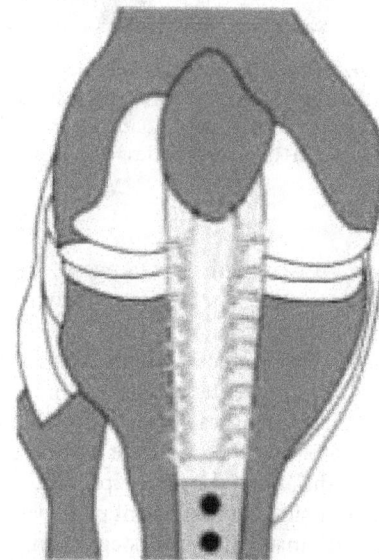

FIGURE 4: Schematic demonstrating the anchor placement and stitching technique used to fixate the patellar tendon repair.

duty restrictions were subsequently outlined as a functional capacity examination, and patient reported outcomes did not permit return to his full occupational capacity.

3. Discussion

Presented in this report is a complex revision case of a patellar tendon repair, with the goal of alleviating this patient's pain and to preserve his ability to function in his activities of daily living. After an extended rehabilitation process, this patient had reached maximal medical improvement resulting in modest improvements in all PROs and ability to return to work albeit with permanent functional restrictions.

Although there are no previously defined values for the minimal clinically important difference (MCID) for PROs after patellar tendon repair, extrapolating the MCIDs for ACL reconstruction [6], this patient demonstrated that he did have an improvement in his SF-12 mental component

score that reached clinical significance. The SF-12 mental component score is a general health-related quality of life which gives an assessment of a patients' well-being and has previously been shown to be reflective of the relative success of surgery [6]. Although this patient had moderate functional limitations at maximal medical improvement, clinically, this patient appreciated a subjective improvement in his general well-being. In addition, this patient had many risk factors predisposing him to worse outcomes including low preoperative functioning, workers' compensation status [7, 8], history of type 2 diabetes [9, 10], and obesity [11] (BMI = 37.5). The only other cases of a revision patellar tendon repair identified in the literature resulted in full functional recoveries; however, these patients were 27 and 28 years old, and both were professional athletes [12, 13].

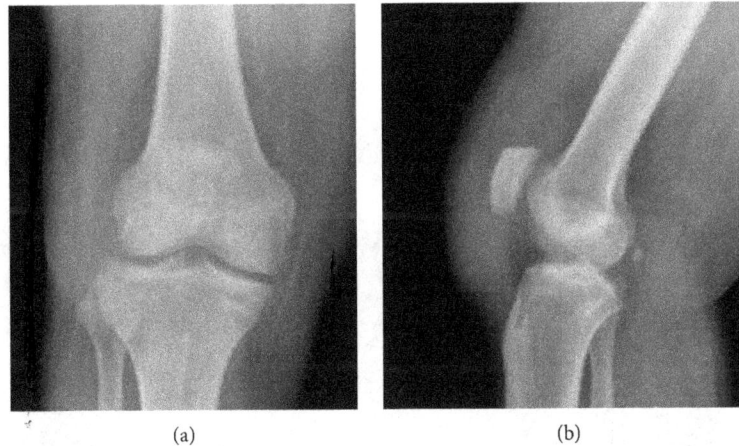

(a)　　　　　　　　　　　　　　　　　　(b)

Figure 5: Postoperative AP (a) and lateral (b) view of the right knee displaying a corrected patellar height after the revision procedure. Caton-Deschamps Index = 1.09, Insall-Salvati Index = 1.16.

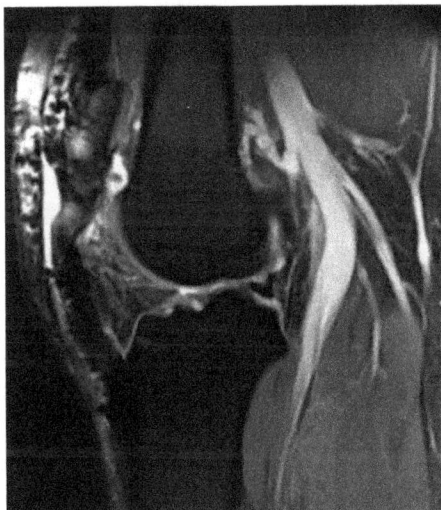

Figure 6: Postoperative MRI of the right knee at 18-month follow-up. Caton-Deschamps = 1.35.

Historically, the treatment of choice for acute patellar tendon rupture has been primary repair augmented with cerclage wire, suture, or grafting to bridge the repair, followed by extended periods (≥6 weeks) of immobilization [2, 3]. However, these techniques have been associated with pain, weakness, patella baja, and decreased mobility with high rates of arthrofibrosis [14, 15]. In addition, augmentation with cables, wires, and Mersilene tape is frequently symptomatic and often requires a second surgery for implant removal [16]. A distinct advantage of primary repair with nonabsorbable suture is that it allows early mobilization and physical therapy initiation within one week of surgery and does not necessitate a second procedure to remove material [15]. Previous reports of primary repair with nonabsorbable suture have shown good functional and objective outcomes, with as much as an 85% return to preinjury level in patients receiving this procedure [14, 15]. For these reasons, primary repair utilizing nonabsorbable sutures to treat this patient's acute patellar tendon injury was decided to be utilized. An important factor taken into consideration was the potential for gap formation with which was previously demonstrated in biomechanical studies of this procedure choice [17, 18]. However, it was ultimately decided that the potential benefits outweighed the risks for this procedure in comparison to the other techniques for patellar tendon repair.

Patella alta, defined as a CDI > 1.2 [19], creates higher patellofemoral contact forces, which causes anterior knee pain and may limit functionality in patients [20]. The primary technique used to correct patella alta is a tibial tubercle osteotomy (TTO) which distalizes the insertion of the tendon [21]. Patella tendon excision and repair has also previously been described to correct patella alta, but only in patients with cerebral palsy who have crouch gait deformity [22]. In this case report, we decided to proceed with the more conservative of these two patellar advancement options for several reasons; a TTO procedure is a particularly aggressive procedure [23] more commonly performed for the indication of patellar instability [21], persistent symptoms are reported in the majority of patients receiving a TTO [21], and it was also believed that this patient's tendon had stretched from the site of the index repair procedure thus compromising the integrity of this tissue. Excision of this portion of tendon followed by primary repair with suture anchors was the most appropriate approach in this case, especially after thinning of the proximal patellar tendon and obvious redundancy were confirmed intraoperatively.

The goals of this revision procedure were to restore functionality so that this patient may achieve his ADLs and return to work at some capacity. This was a very complex case, and the authors contend that the treatment approach was appropriate as it provided him with the greatest opportunity for a positive outcome. This was a salvage procedure, and as such it is satisfactory that he was able to regain ambulatory function with minimal pain. Alternative treatment options that could have been considered include augmentation of the index procedure, prolonged immobilization after the index procedure to prevent tendon lengthening and gap formation, conservative management rather than a revision procedure, or augmentation of the second repair following tendon

(a)

(b)

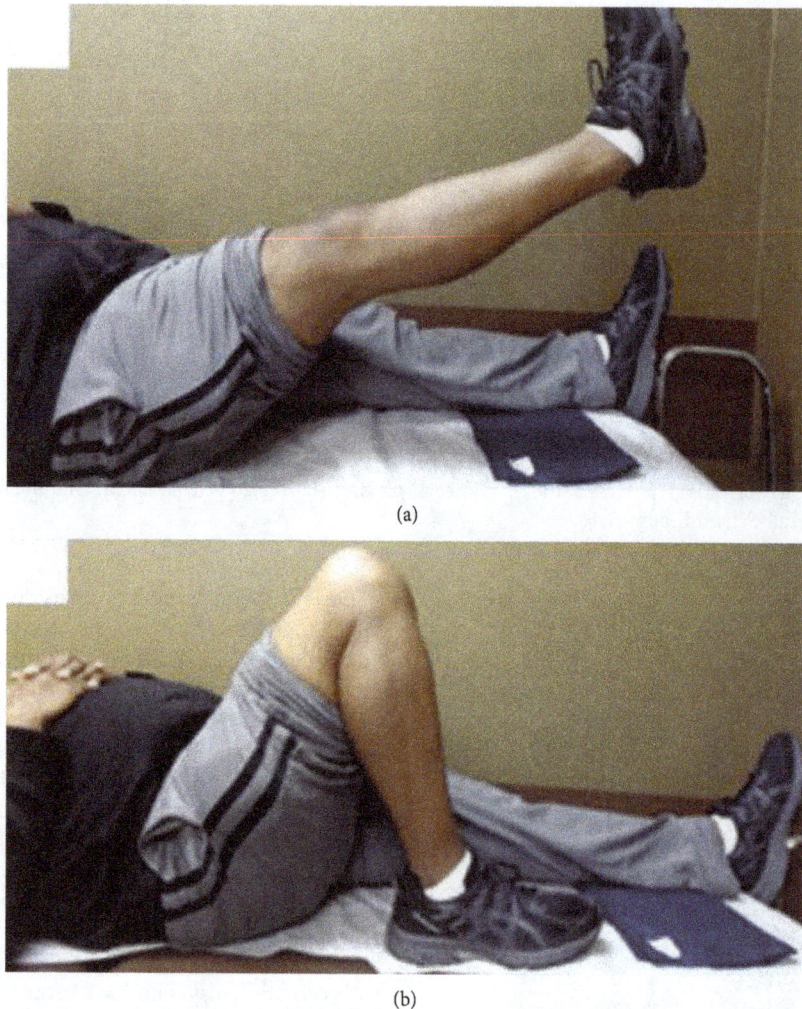

FIGURE 7: Postoperative examination of the patient's active range of motion at 1-year follow-up. (a) Patients' surgical leg in full extension. (b) Patients' leg in 135 degrees of flexion.

resection. Patellar tendon resection followed by primary repair with PEEK corkscrew anchors was able to provide symptomatic relief with modest functional recovery in this patient with a failed patellar tendon repair.

Conflicts of Interest

The authors declare that they have no conflicts of interest.

References

[1] D. Saragaglia, A. Pison, and B. Rubens-Duval, "Acute and old ruptures of the extensor apparatus of the knee in adults (excluding knee replacement)," *Orthopaedics & Traumatology: Surgery & Research*, vol. 99, no. 1, pp. S67–S76, 2013.

[2] J. H. Gilmore, Z. J. Clayton-Smith, M. Aguilar, S. G. Pneumaticos, and P. V. Giannoudis, "Reconstruction techniques and clinical results of patellar tendon ruptures: evidence today," *The Knee*, vol. 22, no. 3, pp. 148–155, 2015.

[3] P. E. Greis, M. C. Holmstrom, and A. Lahav, "Surgical treatment options for patella tendon rupture, part I: acute," *Orthopedics*, vol. 28, no. 7, pp. 672–679, 2005.

[4] D. Lee, D. Stinner, and H. Mir, "Quadriceps and patellar tendon ruptures," *Journal of Knee Surgery*, vol. 26, no. 5, pp. 301–308, 2013.

[5] A. Roudet, M. Boudissa, C. Chaussard, B. Rubens-Duval, and D. Saragaglia, "Acute traumatic patellar tendon rupture: early and late results of surgical treatment of 38 cases," *Orthopaedics & Traumatology: Surgery & Research*, vol. 101, no. 3, pp. 307–311, 2015.

[6] B. U. Nwachukwu, B. Chang, P. B. Voleti et al., "Preoperative short form health survey score is predictive of return to play and minimal clinically important difference at a minimum 2-year follow-up after anterior cruciate ligament reconstruction," *The American Journal of Sports Medicine*, vol. 45, no. 12, pp. 2784–2790, 2017.

[7] V. Y. de Moraes, K. Godin, M. J. S. Tamaoki, F. Faloppa, M. Bhandari, and J. C. Belloti, "Workers' compensation status: does it affect orthopaedic surgery outcomes? A meta-analysis," *PLoS One*, vol. 7, no. 12, article e50251, 2012.

[8] K. I. Gruson, K. Huang, T. Wanich, and A. A. Depalma, "Workers' compensation and outcomes of upper extremity surgery," *Journal of the American Academy of Orthopaedic Surgeons*, vol. 21, no. 2, pp. 67–77, 2013.

[9] K. M. Peters, D. Bucheler, and G. Westerdorf, "Bilateral rupture of the patellar ligament in diabetes mellitus," *Der Unfallchirurg*, vol. 103, no. 2, pp. 164–167, 2000.

[10] M. H. B. Zakaria, W. A. Davis, and T. M. E. Davis, "Incidence and predictors of hospitalization for tendon rupture in type 2 diabetes: the Fremantle Diabetes Study," *Diabetic Medicine*, vol. 31, no. 4, pp. 425–430, 2014.

[11] J. Fairley, J. Toppi, F. M. Cicuttini et al., "Association between obesity and magnetic resonance imaging defined patellar tendinopathy in community-based adults: a cross-sectional study," *BMC Musculoskeletal Disorders*, vol. 15, no. 1, pp. 266–266, 2014.

[12] L. Moretti, G. Vicenti, A. Abate, V. Pesce, and B. Moretti, "Patellar tendon rerupture in a footballer: our personal surgical technique and review of the literature," *Injury*, vol. 45, no. 2, pp. 452–456, 2014.

[13] A. Vadalà, R. Iorio, A. M. Bonifazi, G. Bolle, and A. Ferretti, "Re-revision of a patellar tendon rupture in a young professional martial arts athlete," *Journal of Orthopaedics and Traumatology*, vol. 13, no. 3, pp. 167–170, 2012.

[14] R. A. Marder and L. A. Timmerman, "Primary repair of patellar tendon rupture without augmentation," *The American Journal of Sports Medicine*, vol. 27, no. 3, pp. 304–307, 1999.

[15] J. L. West, J. S. Keene, and L. D. Kaplan, "Early motion after quadriceps and patellar tendon repairs: outcomes with single-suture augmentation," *The American Journal of Sports Medicine*, vol. 36, no. 2, pp. 316–323, 2008.

[16] L. E. Ramseier, C. M. L. Werner, and M. Heinzelmann, "Quadriceps and patellar tendon rupture," *Injury*, vol. 37, no. 6, pp. 516–519, 2006.

[17] J. C. Black, W. M. Ricci, M. J. Gardner et al., "Novel augmentation technique for patellar tendon repair improves strength and decreases gap formation: a cadaveric study," *Clinical Orthopaedics and Related Research®*, vol. 474, no. 12, pp. 2611–2618, 2016.

[18] R. V. Ravalin, A. D. Mazzocca, J. C. Grady-Benson, C. W. Nissen, and D. J. Adams, "Biomechanical comparison of patellar tendon repairs in a cadaver model: an evaluation of gap formation at the repair site with cyclic loading," *The American Journal of Sports Medicine*, vol. 30, no. 4, pp. 469–473, 2002.

[19] H. Dejour, G. Walch, L. Nove-Josserand, and C. Guier, "Factors of patellar instability: an anatomic radiographic study," *Knee Surgery, Sports Traumatology, Arthroscopy*, vol. 2, no. 1, pp. 19–26, 1994.

[20] T. Luyckx, K. Didden, H. Vandenneucker, L. Labey, B. Innocenti, and J. Bellemans, "Is there a biomechanical explanation for anterior knee pain in patients with patella alta?," *The Journal of Bone and Joint Surgery. British volume*, vol. 91-B, no. 3, pp. 344–350, 2009.

[21] R. A. Magnussen, V. De Simone, S. Lustig, P. Neyret, and D. C. Flanigan, "Treatment of patella alta in patients with episodic patellar dislocation: a systematic review," *Knee Surgery, Sports Traumatology, Arthroscopy*, vol. 22, no. 10, pp. 2545–2550, 2014.

[22] A. Seidl, T. Baldini, K. Krughoff et al., "Biomechanical assessment of patellar advancement procedures for patella alta," *Orthopedics*, vol. 39, no. 3, pp. e492–e497, 2016.

[23] D. Wagner, F. Pfalzer, S. Hingelbaum, J. Huth, F. Mauch, and G. Bauer, "The influence of risk factors on clinical outcomes following anatomical medial patellofemoral ligament (MPFL) reconstruction using the gracilis tendon," *Knee Surgery, Sports Traumatology, Arthroscopy*, vol. 21, no. 2, pp. 318–324, 2013.

4

Elbow Posterolateral Rotatory Instability due to Cubitus Varus and Overuse

Juan Martín Patiño ⓘ, **Alejandro Rullan Corna, Alejandro Michelini** ⓘ, **Ignacio Abdon,** and **Alejandro José Ramos Vertiz**

Hospital Militar Central, Buenos Aires, Argentina

Correspondence should be addressed to Juan Martín Patiño; drpatinojm@gmail.com

Academic Editor: Paul E. Di Cesare

A malunion as a complication of distal humerus fractures has been frequently linked with aesthetic problems but less frequently with posterolateral rotatory instability. We report 2 cases of childhood posttraumatic cubitus varus with subsequent posterolateral rotatory instability and their treatment with a minimum of 2 years of follow-up. The etiology of the so-called posterolateral rotatory instability of the elbow is mostly traumatic, but iatrogenic causes have also been described such as the treatment of tennis elbow and less frequently and chronically due to overuse and overload because of distal humerus malunion.

1. Introduction

A malunion as a complication of distal humerus fractures has not only been frequently linked with aesthetic problems but also with instability and dislocation of the ulnar nerve [1], ulnar nerve neuritis [2], medial triceps dislocations [3], recurrence of distal humerus fractures or lateral condyle [4], osteoarthritis [5], and posterior dislocation of the radial head but less frequently with posterolateral rotatory instability [6–11].

The objective of this presentation is the report of 2 cases of childhood posttraumatic cubitus varus with subsequent posterolateral rotatory instability and their treatment with a minimum of 2 years of follow-up.

2. Case Report

2.1. Case 1. A 29-year-old female patient consults for pain and paresthesias in the 4th and 5th fingers with 2 years of evolution with several minor traumas in the past year. The patient had a history of supracondylar elbow fracture at the age of 5, treated nonsurgically. No symptoms were presented until she started with higher activity and physical demand such as bar exercises and push-ups. With the beginning of

these symptoms, she was initially treated at another hospital for epicondylitis with physiotherapy, rest, and 2 corticoid injections without remission of symptoms.

Physical examination showed pain, an evident varus deformity, chair sign positive, and clear pivot shift. In anteroposterior radiograph, varus of 20 degrees and paresthesias in the ulnar nerve territory were observed. Electromyogram reported signs consistent with ulnar nerve entrapment. Her range of motion in flexion extension and supination was complete (grades: 0-145 flexion-extension, 50-50 pronosupination). The MEPI (Mayo Elbow Performance Index) was 60.

2.1.1. Treatment. Valgus osteotomy was performed in the distal humerus through a lateral wedge and ligament reconstruction with tendon graft of the autologus palmaris longus, by tunneling the distal humerus and ulna crest. In rehabilitation, the range of motion was controlled with an articulated splint.

2.1.2. Complications. Postoperative complications were delayed union and radial neuropraxia with spontaneous remission after 3 months.

2.1.3. Result. The osteotomy did not lead to valgus but to a correction of 5 degrees of the varus (previously 20 degrees).

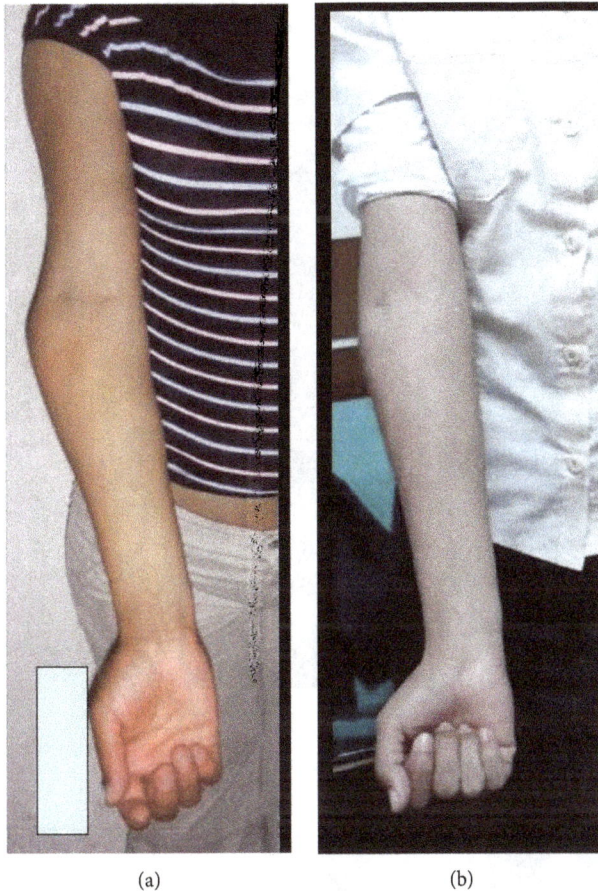

FIGURE 1: Case 1. Clinical appearance: (a) preoperative and (b) postoperative.

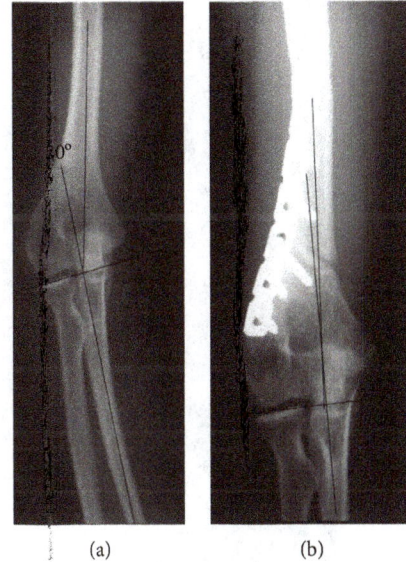

FIGURE 2: Case 1. (a) Preoperative AP radiograph. (b) Postoperative AP radiograph.

In the evaluation, after 4 years of follow-up, partial clinical deformity correction, remission of symptoms of ulnar nerve irritation, and complete range of motion were achieved. However, the patient cannot perform some exercises with high force demand or more than 2 hours of continuous activity. The MEPI was 80 and DASH (Disabilities of the Arm, Shoulder, and Hand) was 13.33 (Figures 1 and 2).

2.2. Case 2. A 19-year-old female patient consults for lateral elbow pain and functional limitation with 3 months of evolution. She mentions a history of elbow fracture when she was 4 years old (apparently lateral condyle) treated nonsurgically. She did not have previous symptoms. These appeared with increased elbow overload because of physical activity when entering the Military Academy. Physical exam showed pain and sign of instability such as positive pivot shift, which had to be confirmed under fluoroscopy; clinical attitude in the elbow varus was less evident than in the first case. In the anteroposterior radiograph, 10-degree varus was observed. MRI informed signs of chondral injuries in the radial head and the lateral collateral ligament, too. The MEPI was 65.

2.2.1. Treatment. A lateral ligament reconstruction with autologous graft of palmaris longus was performed with similar technique of the first case and also capsular plication.

The repair was protected with a transarticular nail for 3 weeks. Then, she began with progressive rehabilitation.

2.2.2. Result. A stable elbow, full flexion and extension range, and full pronosupination were achieved. After 2 years of follow-up, the MEPI is 100 and DASH 0. She was capable of performing all daily life activities (Figures 3–5).

3. Discussion

In the cases presented, improvement was achieved in the stability of the elbow, though with better evolution in case 2 in which the deformity was less marked and the osteotomy was not necessary since the patient was active without limitations.

Bibliography on this subject is scarce. Elbow varus sequelae due to distal humerus fractures and its treatment is mainly related to aesthetic problems and functional issues [12, 13]. We have identified few experiences/publications and these mainly limited to case presentations.

Mondoloni et al. in 1995 [7] published 2 cases of instability in adults with antecedent of elbow supracondylar fractures in which stability and good motion with pain remission were achieved.

Abe et al. in 1997 [6] reported one 16-year-old patient with posterolateral instability, cubitus varus, and a history of distal humerus supracondylar fracture at the age of 5, which had shown no complications until he started playing volleyball with more elbow demand. He underwent ligament reconstruction and external osteotomy and osteosynthesis. He started playing again 5 months later without pain. After 10 months, he showed no instability, same preoperation motion, but with 23 degrees of valgus overcorrection.

O'Driscoll et al. [8] in a multicentric study studied 24 patients with 25 elbows with posterolateral instability and

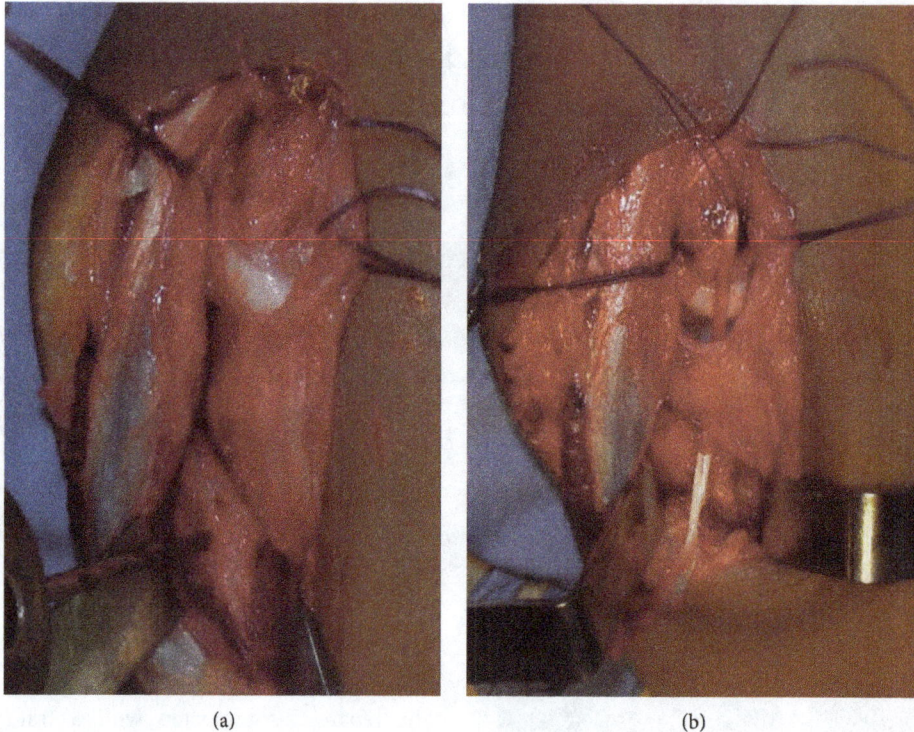

(a)   (b)

FIGURE 3: Case 2. (a, b) Collateral ligament reconstruction.

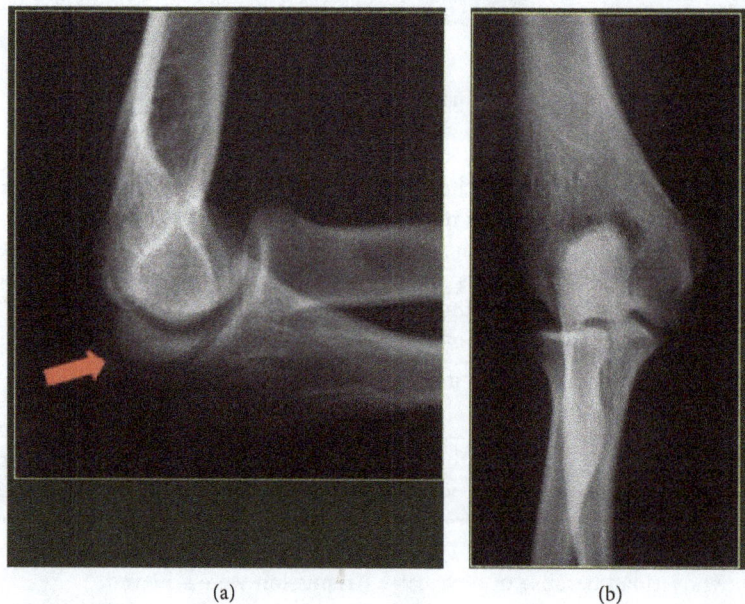

(a)   (b)

FIGURE 4: Case 2. (a, b) L and AP preoperative X-rays.

post fracture cubitus varus in 22 cases and congenital in 3. The instability appeared 2 or 3 decades after the deformity. Besides, all patients presented pain and the varus range was between 15 and 35 degrees. 22 cases underwent surgery: ligament reconstruction and osteotomy in 7 cases, ligament reconstruction as a unique procedure in 10, only osteotomy in 4, and arthroplasty in 1. In 3 cases, the triceps was electrically stimulated in surgery with resistance to extension, and elbow dislocation was observed.

Good or excellent results were achieved in 19 cases; in 3 cases, there was persistent instability. It is concluded that in the cubitus varus, the mechanical axis, the olecranon, and the triceps axis are displayed medially. This causes repetitive cubitus external rotation that can stretch the

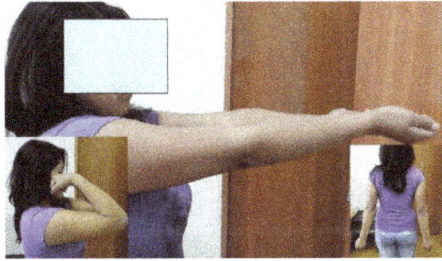

FIGURE 5: Case 2. Final elbow range of motion.

complex lateral ligament and cause posterolateral instability. The secondary cubitus varus malunion does not always imply benign lesion; it may present long-term symptoms, but these can be solved with surgery.

In this publication [8], a physiopathological explanation is proposed where the cubitus varus due to the malunion of the distal humerus causes 2 biomechanical alterations that alter the complex lateral ligament. Firstly, with the varus, the mechanical axis between the shoulder and the wrist moves medially. The repeated varus torque increases the lateral ligament stress especially with axial force on the limb (as it occurs when standing after having been seated on a chair). Secondly, the varus also displaces the medial triceps force vector leading the cubitus to move in this direction and to rotate externally to 90 degrees of flexion. Both are complementary reasons to the previously described explanations for instability [14]. This explanation was confirmed in a cadaveric study in which valgus osteotomies were practiced in 11 elbows, and when exposed to force, an increased lateral tension with larger varus was observed [15].

Ligament reconstruction as a unique procedure is suggested in varus below 15 degrees in the elderly or low force demand (not athletes) patients because without osteotomy, stress on the reconstruction increases.

The valgus osteotomy helps in stabilizing ligamentous laxity. The osteotomy as a unique procedure is feasible in cases with low instability and low demand to the elbow. In larger deformities, it has been suggested to combine osteotomy with the ligament reconstruction, as separately they would be related to a higher failure rate as well as to osteotomies which do not restore the valgus.

Elbow lateral pain is a reason of frequent consultation. Due to the fact that pain often appears as a symptom of instability, we consider that this pathology should be suspected and investigated, especially in cases wherein pain is associated with physical demand and traumatic events in childhood with sequels in the elbow.

Conflicts of Interest

The authors declare that there is no conflict of interest regarding the publication of this article.

References

[1] N. Acciarri, C. Davalli, G. Giuliani, M. Monesi, and M. Poppi, "Delayed paralysis of the anterior ulnar nerve in posttraumatic varus deformity of the elbow," *Archivio "Putti" di Chirurgia degli Organi di Movimento*, vol. 39, no. 1, pp. 115–128, 1991.

[2] M. Abe, T. Ishizu, H. Shirai, M. Okamoto, and T. Onomura, "Tardy ulnar nerve palsy caused by cubitus varus deformity," *The Journal of Hand Surgery*, vol. 20, no. 1, pp. 5–9, 1995.

[3] R. J. Spinner, S. W. O'Driscoll, J. R. Davids, and R. D. Goldner, "Cubitus varus associated with dislocation of both the medial portion of the triceps and the ulnar nerve," *The Journal of Hand Surgery*, vol. 24, no. 4, pp. 718–726, 1999.

[4] M. Takahara, I. Sasaki, T. Kimura, H. Kato, A. Minami, and T. Ogino, "Second fracture of the distal humerus after varus malunion of a supracondylar fracture in children," *Journal of Bone & Joint Surgery*, vol. 80-B, no. 5, pp. 791–797, 1998.

[5] H. Fujioka, Y. Nakabayashi, S. Hirata, G. Go, S. Nish, and K. Mizuno, "Analysis of tardy ulnar nerve palsy associated with cubitus varus deformity after supracondylar fracture of the humerus: a report of four cases," *Journal of Orthopaedic Trauma*, vol. 9, no. 5, pp. 435–440, 1995.

[6] M. Abe, T. Ishizu, and J. Morikawa, "Posterolateral rotatory instability of the elbow after posttraumatic cubitus varus," *Journal of Shoulder and Elbow Surgery*, vol. 6, no. 4, pp. 405–409, 1997.

[7] P. Mondoloni, E. Vandenbussche, P. Peraldi, and B. Augereau, "Instability of the elbow after supracondylar humeral nonunion in cubitus varus rotation. Apropos of 2 cases observed in adults," *Revue de Chirurgie Orthopédique et Réparatrice de l'Appareil Moteur*, vol. 82, no. 8, pp. 757–761, 1996.

[8] S. W. O'Driscoll, R. J. Spinner, M. D. McKee et al., "Tardy posterolateral rotatory instability of the elbow due to cubitus varus," *The Journal of Bone and Joint Surgery-American Volume*, vol. 83, no. 9, pp. 1358–1369, 2001.

[9] V. A. Kontogeorgakos, A. F. Mavrogenis, G. N. Panagopoulos, A. Lagaras, A. Koutalos, and K. N. Malizos, "Cubitus varus complicated by snapping medial triceps and posterolateral rotatory instability," *Journal of Shoulder and Elbow Surgery*, vol. 25, no. 7, pp. e208–e212, 2016.

[10] P. Arrigoni and S. Kamineni, "Uncovered posterolateral rotatory elbow instability with cubitus varus deformity correction," *Orthopedics*, vol. 32, no. 2, p. 130, 2009.

[11] D. Osada, M. Kameda, and K. Tamai, "Persistent posterolateral rotatory subluxation of the elbow in cubitus varus: a case report," *Hand Surgery*, vol. 12, no. 2, pp. 101–105, 2007.

[12] S. G. Seo, H. S. Gong, Y. H. Lee, S. H. Rhee, H. J. Lee, and G. H. Baek, "Posterolateral rotatory instability of the elbow after corrective osteotomy for previously asymptomatic cubitus varus deformity," *Hand Surgery*, vol. 19, no. 2, pp. 163–169, 2014.

[13] Y. Kawanishi, J. Miyake, T. Kataoka et al., "Does cubitus varus cause morphologic and alignment changes in the elbow joint?," *Journal of Shoulder and Elbow Surgery*, vol. 22, no. 7, pp. 915–923, 2013.

[14] S. W. O'Driscoll, B. F. Morrey, S. Korinek, and K. N. An, "Elbow subluxation and dislocation. A spectrum of instability," *Clinical Orthopaedics and Related Research*, vol. 280, pp. 186–197, 1992.

[15] M. J. Beuerlein, J. T. Reid, E. H. Schemitsch, and M. D. McKee, "Effect of distal humeral varus deformity on strain in the lateral ulnar collateral ligament and ulnohumeral joint stability," *The Journal of Bone & Joint Surgery*, vol. 86, no. 10, pp. 2235–2242, 2004.

5

A Type III Monteggia Injury with Ipsilateral Fracture of the Distal Radius and Ulna in a Child

Takeshi Inoue ⓘ**, Makoto Kubota, and Keishi Marumo**

Department of Orthopaedic Surgery, Jikei University School of Medicine, 3-25-8 Nishishinnbashi, Minato-ku, Tokyo 105-8461, Japan

Correspondence should be addressed to Takeshi Inoue; inoue@jikei.ac.jp

Academic Editor: Georg Singer

Bado type III Monteggia injuries complicated by ipsilateral forearm fractures are extremely rare. We report a case of a 6-year-old boy who sustained such an injury after falling from the top of a 3 m climbing pole. He was diagnosed with a Bado type III Monteggia fracture and forearm fractures. Manual reduction was attempted on the day of injury. However, because it was difficult to maintain the reduction of the radial head, open and percutaneous procedures were performed to reduce and fixate the fractures with Kirschner wires. The postoperative course was favorable. Twenty-one years later, the patient, now 27 years old, had no decreased range of joint motion or problems with activities of daily living. The fracture morphology observed in this case is rare, and this is the only case for which long-term follow-up has been carried out to adulthood.

1. Introduction

In pediatric patients, fractures around the elbow and wrist joints are often encountered. However, patients with concomitant fractures of the ipsilateral elbow and wrist joints are rarely seen [1]. Monteggia fracture is a rare fracture that is observed in only 0.4% of all forearm fractures [2]. The condition is named after Giovanni Battista Monteggia, who reported 2 patients with fractures of the proximal third of the ulna with anterior dislocation of the radial head in 1814 [3]. These lesions have most commonly been further classified in accordance with the Bado classification system [4].

Here, we report an extremely rare case of type III Monteggia injury with ipsilateral fracture of the distal radius and ulna in which the patient was followed up for 21 years.

2. Case Presentation

A 6-year-old boy with no pathological history accidentally fell from the top of an approximately 3 m climbing pole and injured his right extended elbow and wrist joint. Due to pain and deformity in the right elbow and wrist joints, he visited our hospital. Swelling and a dinner fork deformity of the right wrist joint and pronounced swelling of the right elbow joint were observed. No skin damage was observed. No findings of nerve injury or arterial injury were obtained in the right upper limb. Radiography revealed lateral dislocation of the radial head, a fracture of the proximal ulnar metaphysis, and mild bending deformation at the fracture site. In addition, fractures of the distal radius and ulna, as well as dorsal displacement of the distal fragment, were seen (Figure 1). Thus, the patient was diagnosed with Bado type III Monteggia injury with ipsilateral fracture of the distal radius and ulna.

Manual reduction under nerve block was attempted on the day of injury. However, because it was difficult to maintain the reduction of the radial head, as shown in Figure 2, open reduction and percutaneous procedures were performed under general anesthesia. A Kirschner wire was inserted, percutaneously, from the olecranon into the ulnar diaphysis. When the Kirschner wire was in place, the dislocation of the radial head immediately showed good reduction. Further, open reduction and fixation of the fractured distal radius and ulna were performed with Kirschner wires (Figure 3). A long-arm cast was used for external fixation with the elbow in 90° flexion and the forearm in an intermediate position.

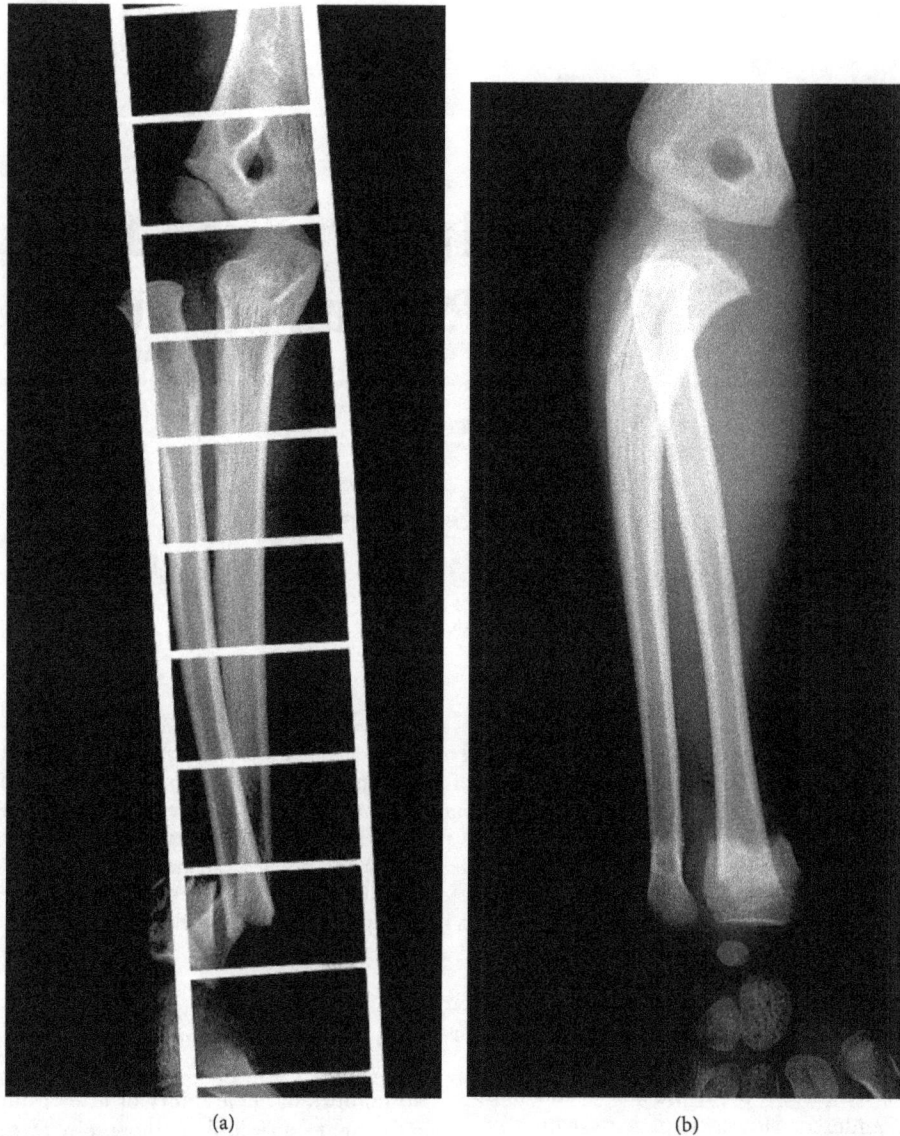

(a)   (b)

FIGURE 1: X-rays at first visit. A Bado type III Monteggia fracture and fractures of the distal radius and ulna were observed on the same side. (a) AP view of the elbow joint. (b) Oblique view of the elbow joint.

Two weeks after surgery, callus formation at the fractured bone was observed. Therefore, the cast was removed, and range of motion (ROM) exercises of the elbow and wrist joints were initiated. Since bone union was achieved at 6 weeks postsurgery, the Kirschner wires were removed. Pain, ROM limitation, and lateral instability were not observed in the elbow or wrist joints at 3 months after surgery. Additionally, plain radiographs taken at the same time showed a radially convex curvature at the proximal portion of the ulna and lateral subluxation of the radial head (Figure 4). However, a gradual correction in the outward displacement of the radial head was observed during the 3-year follow-up.

Twenty-one years after surgery, the patient returned to our hospital for another disorder. At that time, we obtained informed consent to perform an examination and take radiographs of the previous Monteggia injury. Neither spontaneous pain, pain during exercise, tenderness, nor ROM asymmetry were observed (Figure 5). The biocompatibility of the radiocapitellar joint was good, and no malunion was found in the distal radius and ulna (Figure 6). The patient reports that he has been working as a computer programmer and performs weight training as a hobby without limitations.

3. Discussion

Nerve injuries, vascular injuries, compartment syndrome, and ipsilateral fractures of the forearm, in the early stages of the injury, as well as redislocation and malunion of the ulna fracture site, in the late stages, have been reported as complications of Monteggia fractures [5]. Fractures of the forearm, including distal radius fractures [6–8], have rarely been reported in association with Monteggia fractures, as documented by Letts et al. [9] and Olney and Menelaus [5]. They found that only one out of 33 or 2 out of 102

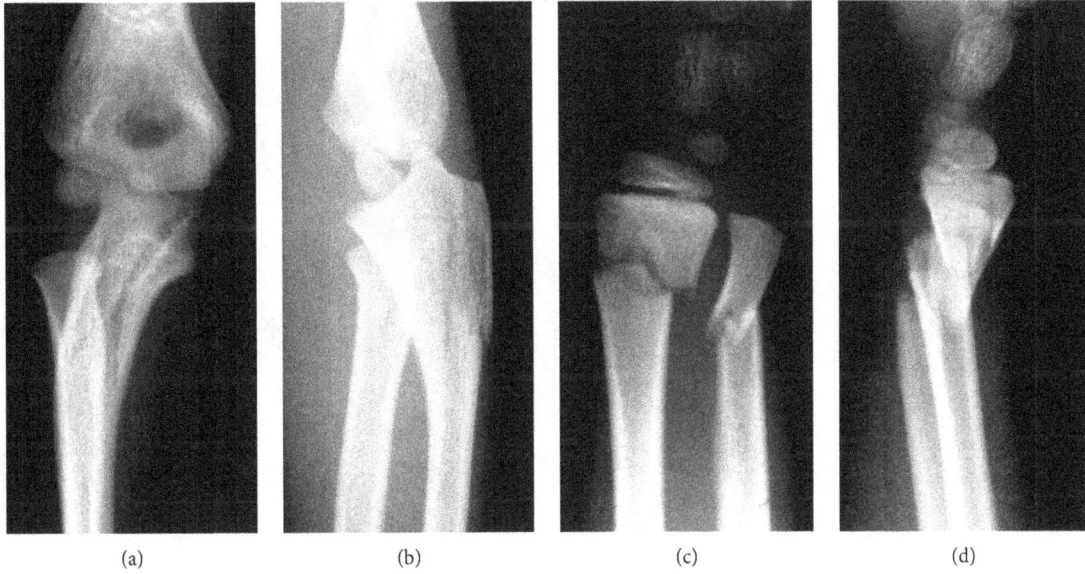

FIGURE 2: X-rays images after manual reduction. (a) AP view of the elbow joint showing subluxation of the radial head. (b) Lateral view of the elbow joint. (c) Front view of the wrist joint showing dislocation of the distal radius. (d) Lateral view of the wrist joint showing dislocation of the distal radius.

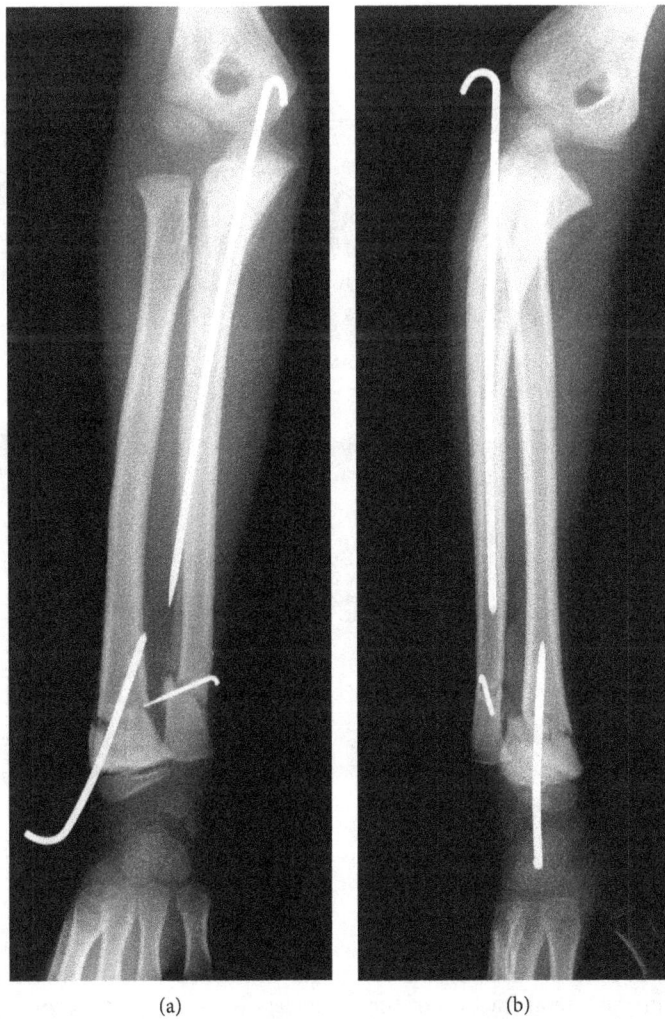

FIGURE 3: X-rays postoperation. (a) AP view. (b) Lateral view.

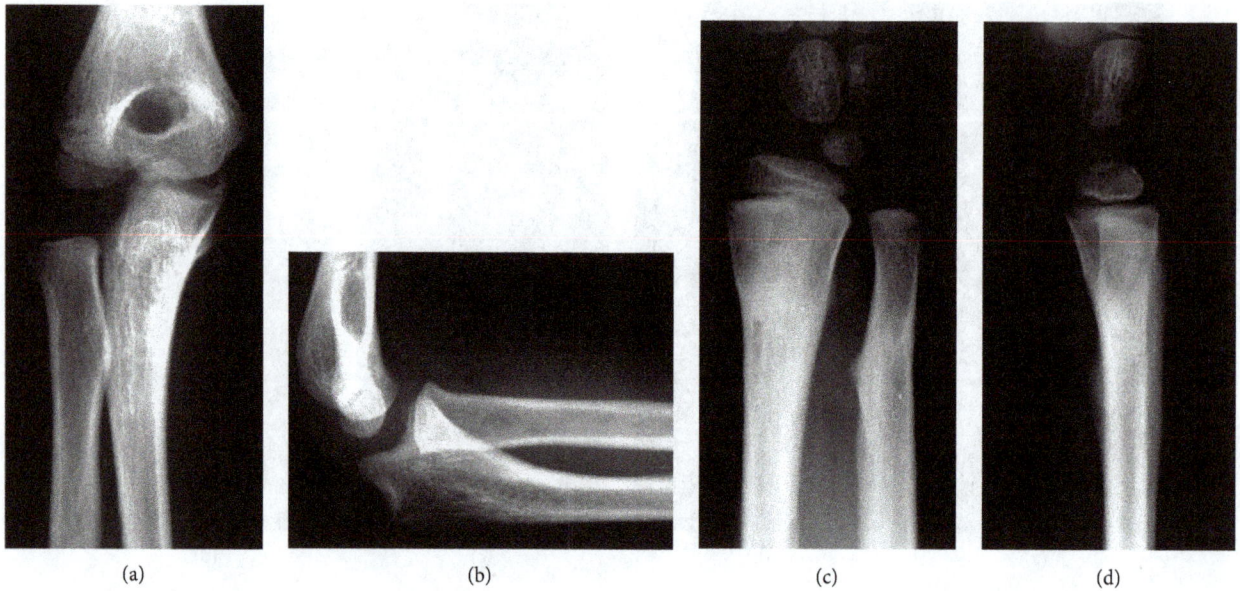

FIGURE 4: X-rays 3 months after surgery. (a) Front view of the elbow joint. (b) Lateral view of the elbow joint. (c) Front view of the wrist joint. (d) Lateral view of the wrist joint.

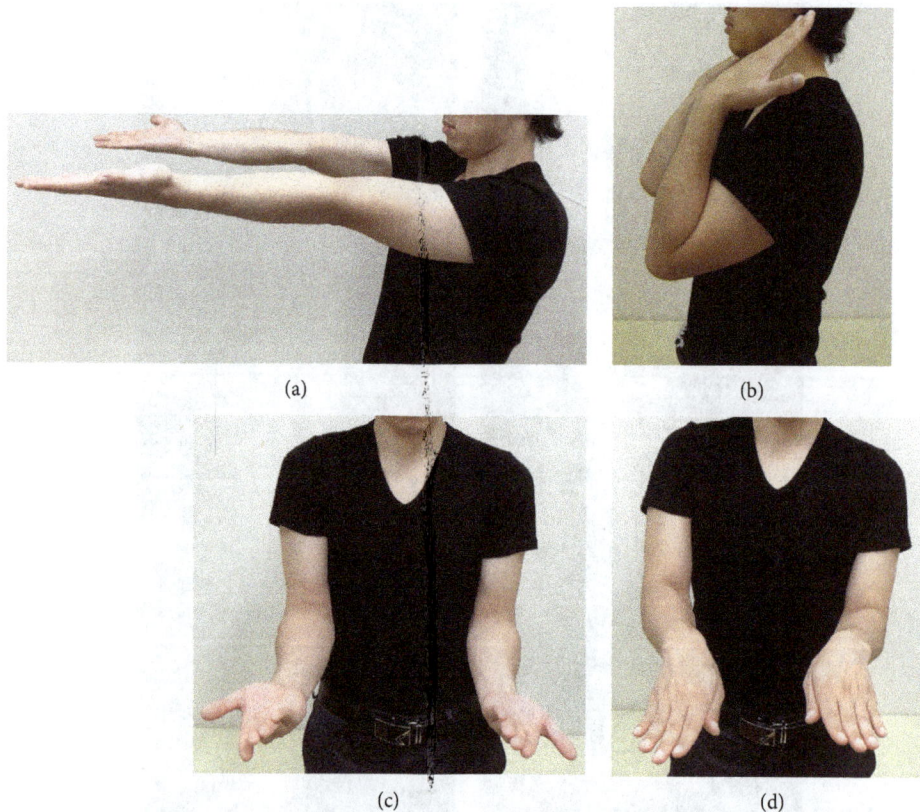

FIGURE 5: Twenty-one years after surgery. (a) Extended elbow. (b) Flexed elbow. (c) Forearm supination. (d) Forearm pronation.

patients with Monteggia fractures exhibit associated fractures [5, 9]. To our knowledge, beyond these cases, only 3 cases of Monteggia fractures with ipsilateral fracture of the distal radius and ulna have been reported, as in the present case [10–12].

The observation period in all previous reports of Monteggia injury with ipsilateral forearm fractures has been 2 years or less [6–8, 10–14], except for a 6-year follow-up reported by Biyani [1]. This is the only case wherein long-term postoperative follow-up evaluation was feasible until adulthood.

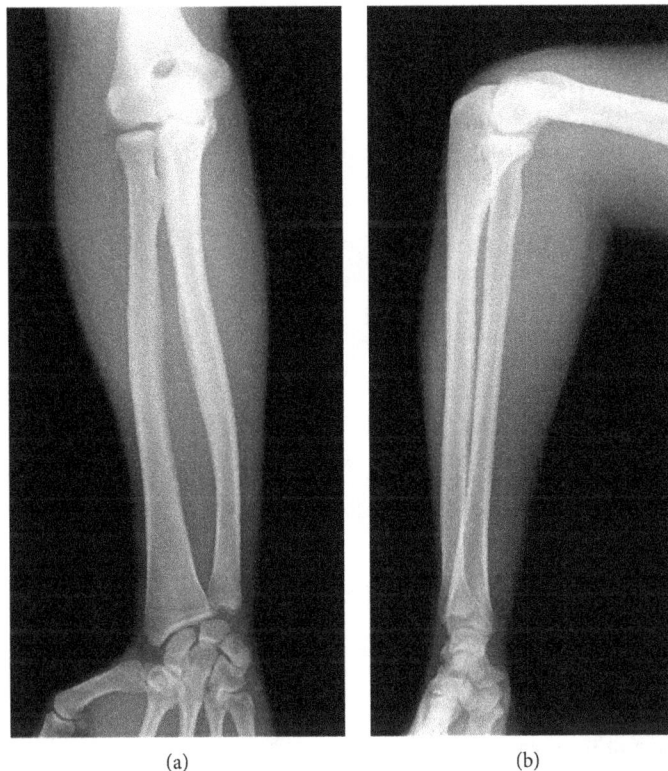

(a)   (b)

FIGURE 6: X-rays 21 years after surgery. (a) Front view. (b) Lateral view. The compatibility of the radiocapitellar joint was good, and no malunion was observed.

There is no established theory of the pathogenesis of Monteggia fracture. In addition, it is difficult to infer the mechanisms of double fractures, as in this case. However, Sinha et al. [12] reported a similar case of an affected child who fell with their forearm pronated and the wrist dorsiflexed, which resulted in distal radius and ulna fractures. The impact from the fall was subsequently transmitted to the elbow, which was in valgus extension, and resulted in dislocation of the radial head and fractures in the proximal end of the ulna [12].

While treating a Monteggia fracture, examination of both the cubital joint and the wrist joint is important because a fracture of the distal forearm may also occur, as in this case [10]. Since a child who has sustained such an injury may be experiencing pain and/or anxiety and therefore unable to sufficiently express himself, the presence or absence of any swelling, deformities, abrasions possibly due to direct force, and ROM limitation should be carefully examined. It is important to perform accurate radiography in 2 planes (i.e., frontal and lateral views) [6, 10]. Since Monteggia fractures in children are mostly incomplete greenstick fractures, reduction and maintenance are easy to perform. Therefore, conservative treatment can often be employed in cases with timely diagnosis [15, 16]. However, since it was difficult to perform manual reduction owing to a double fracture of the ulna, surgery was the only treatment option available in the presented patient. Nevertheless, to obtain good treatment results, it is important to accurately diagnose and promptly treat the condition [15, 16].

Conflicts of Interest

The authors declare that there is no conflict of interest regarding the publication of this article.

References

[1] A. Biyani, "Ipsilateral Monteggia equivalent injury and distal radial and ulnar fracture in a child," *Journal of Orthopaedic Trauma*, vol. 8, no. 5, pp. 431–433, 1994.

[2] A. S. Shah and P. M. Waters, ""Monteggia-fracture dislocation in children," in Rockwood and Wilkins," in *Fractures in Children*, J. M. Flynn, D. L. Skaggs, and P. M. Waters, Eds., pp. 527–563, Wolters Kluwer, Philadelphia, PA, USA, 2015.

[3] G. B. Monteggia, *Instituzione Chirurgiche*, Maspero, Milan, Italy, 2nd edition, 1814.

[4] J. L. Bado, "The Monteggia lesion," *Clinical Orthopaedics and Related Research*, vol. 50, pp. 71–86, 1967.

[5] B. W. Olney and M. B. Menelaus, "Monteggia and equivalent lesions in childhood," *Journal of Pediatric Orthopedics*, vol. 9, no. 2, pp. 219–223, 1989.

[6] S. Deshpande and D. O'Doherty, "Type I Monteggia fracture dislocation associated with ipsilateral distal radial epiphyseal injury," *Journal of Orthopaedic Trauma*, vol. 15, no. 5, pp. 373–375, 2001.

[7] W. B. Rodgers and B. G. Smith, "A type IV Monteggia injury with a distal diaphyseal radius fracture in a child," *Journal of Orthopaedic Trauma*, vol. 7, no. 1, pp. 84–86, 1993.

[8] B. Kristiansen and A. F. Eriksen, "Simultaneous type II Monteggia lesion and fracture-separation of the lower radial epiphysis," *Injury*, vol. 17, no. 1, pp. 51-52, 1986.

[9] M. Letts, R. Locht, and J. Wiens, "Monteggia fracture dislocations in children," *The Journal of Bone and Joint Surgery, British Volume*, vol. 67-B, no. 5, pp. 724–727, 1985.

[10] H. L. Williams, T. R. Madhusudhan, and A. Sinha, "Type III Monteggia injury with ipsilateral type II Salter Harris injury of the distal radius and ulna in a child: a case report," *BMC Research Notes*, vol. 7, no. 1, p. 156, 2014.

[11] N. Peter and S. Myint, "Type I Monteggia lesion and associated fracture of the distal radius and ulna metaphysis in a child," *Canadian Journal of Emergency Medical Care*, vol. 9, no. 5, pp. 383–386, 2007.

[12] S. Sinha, W. R. Chang, A. C. Campbell, and S. M. Hussein, "Type III Monteggia injury with ipsilateral distal radius and ulna fracture," *The Internet Journal of Orthopedic Surgery*, vol. 1, no. 2, 2003.

[13] D. Singh, B. Awasthi, V. Padha, and S. Thakur, "A very rare presentation of type 1 Monteggia equivalent fracture with ipsilateral fracture of distal forearm-approach with outcome: case report," *Journal of Orthopaedic Case Reports*, vol. 6, no. 4, pp. 57–61, 2016.

[14] A. R. Nataraj and T. Sreenivas, "Type III Monteggia fracture with ipsilateral epiphyseal injury of the distal radius," *European Journal of Orthopaedic Surgery and Traumatology*, vol. 21, no. 3, pp. 185–187, 2011.

[15] K. Chin, S. H. Kozin, M. Herman et al., "Pediatric Monteggia fracture dislocations: avoiding problems and managing complications," *Instructional Course Lectures*, vol. 65, pp. 399–410, 2016.

[16] A. Leonidou, J. Pagkalos, P. Lepetsos et al., "Pediatric Monteggia fractures: a single-center study of the management of 40 patients," *Journal of Pediatric Orthopaedics*, vol. 32, no. 4, pp. 352–356, 2012.

6

Arthroscopically Assisted Retrograde Intramedullary Nailing for Periprosthetic Fracture of the Femur after Posterior-Stabilized Total Knee Arthroplasty

Kazuhiko Udagawa,[1] Yasuo Niki ⓘ,[1] Kengo Harato,[1] Shu Kobayashi,[1] and So Nomoto[2]

[1]Department of Orthopaedic Surgery, Keio University School of Medicine, Tokyo, Japan
[2]Department of Orthopaedic Surgery, Yokohama-City Tobu Hospital, Yokohama, Japan

Correspondence should be addressed to Yasuo Niki; y-niki@keio.jp

Academic Editor: John Nyland

Retrograde intramedullary nailing (RIMN) has been used for periprosthetic fracture of the distal femur after total knee arthroplasty (TKA), yielding good fracture union rates and satisfactory outcomes. However, RIMN for posterior-stabilized- (PS-) TKA risks malpositioning the entry point and disturbing the post of the tibial insert, and the surgeon therefore usually requires knee joint arthrotomy. We report a case of a 79-year-old male who was involved in bicycle accident resulting in periprosthetic fracture of the distal femur after PS-TKA. We performed osteosynthesis with arthroscopically assisted RIMN to define an appropriate entry point. RIMN for posterior-stabilized- (PS-) TKA risks malpositioning the entry point and disturbing the post of the tibial insert. Because arthroscopy can directly visualize the entry point and the tibial post without arthrotomy, arthroscopically assisted RIMN offers a useful technical option for periprosthetic fracture of the distal femur after PS-TKA.

1. Introduction

Total knee arthroplasty (TKA) is the gold standard for patients with end-stage knee osteoarthritis and can be helpful to correct deformity, relieve pain, and restore function. With the shift toward an increasingly aging society, the number of TKAs is expected to increase. Incidences of primary and revision TKAs have been reported as 0.6% and 1.7%, respectively [1], suggesting that post-TKA periprosthetic fracture is also increasing. Open reduction and internal fixation with a nonlocked plate or condylar plate has been the standard for post-TKA periprosthetic fracture, but clinical results have been poor, with complication rates up to 53% [2]. For now, both retrograde intramedullary nailing (RIMN) and use of locking compression plates (LCPs) have become common for the treatment of the periprosthetic fracture after TKA, and these techniques have achieved improved union rates and functional outcomes [3]. Although a recent meta-analysis demonstrated similar clinical outcomes between RIMN and the use of LCPs [3], RIMN cannot be indicated for certain designs of the femoral component, such as a stemmed design, posterior-stabilized- (PS-) TKA and closed box design. In addition, the post of the polyethylene insert is at risk of breakage during reaming, regardless of the PS-TKA design. Even for cruciate-retaining- (CR-) TKA or open box PS-TKA, the entry point for RIMN cannot be detected accurately even using fluoroimages, due to overlap with both femoral condyles. Consequently, surgeons inevitably perform knee joint arthrotomy.

Currently, we use arthroscopy to accurately detect the appropriate entry point for RIMN intraoperatively. In this article, we present an arthroscopically assisted RIMN technique for the treatment of periprosthetic fracture after closed box PS-TKA.

2. Case Presentation

A 79-year-old man with right knee osteoarthritis underwent PS-TKA (Vanguard System; Zimmer Biomet, Tokyo, Japan). At 10 months postoperatively, he was involved in a bicycle

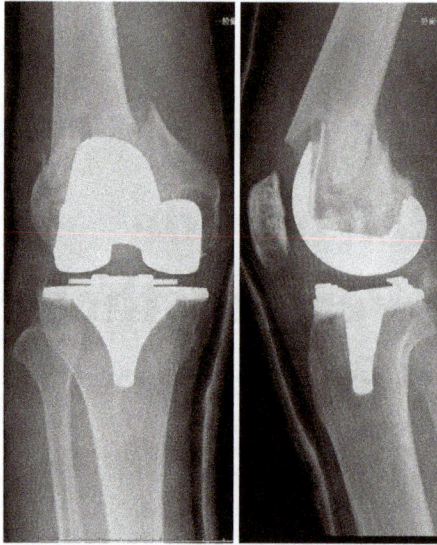

FIGURE 1: Preoperative radiograph.

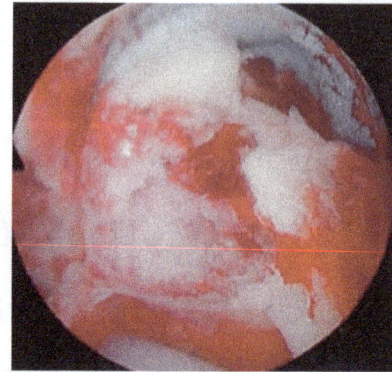

(a)

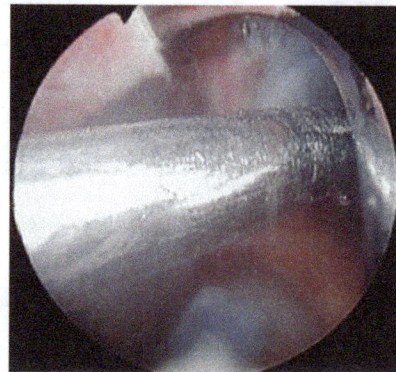

(b)

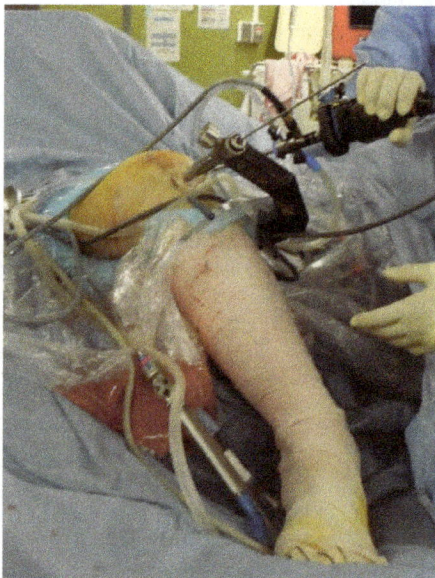

FIGURE 2: Knee joint positioning and set up of image intensifier.

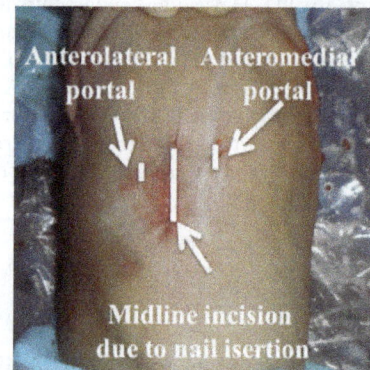

(c)

FIGURE 3: Synovectomy and exposure of insertion point (a). Guide-wire insertion (b). Skin incisions for arthroscopy and nail insertion (c).

accident and visited a local hospital, where he was diagnosed with periprosthetic fracture of the distal femur (Figure 1).

Three days after the accident, he was referred to our hospital, and osteosynthesis with arthroscopically assisted RIMN was performed.

The patient was positioned supine with a standard leg holder, and the knee was flexed to 90° to allow the nail to pass behind the femoral shield on a radiolucent fracture table (Figure 2).

Synovectomy was performed under arthroscopy, and the entry point between the condyles of the femoral component was identified using a standard anterolateral portal and an anteromedial portal (Figure 3(a)). 3 cm midline incision was made and the patellar tendon was split, and then the guide-wire was inserted (Figures 3(b) and 3(c)).

After definitive guide-wire placement, the entry point was reamed without compromising the tibial post, and a ball-tip guide rod was inserted into the canal of the proximal femur (Figure 4).

As the distal fragment was shifted posteriorly, a 3.0 mm Kirschner wire was inserted just posteriorly from the ball-tip guide rod in a proximal fragment as a block pin as reported previously [4]. The intramedullary canal was reamed, and a 12 mm diameter × 170 mm length T2 Supracondylar Nail (Stryker, Schönkirchen, Germany) was then inserted (Figure 5).

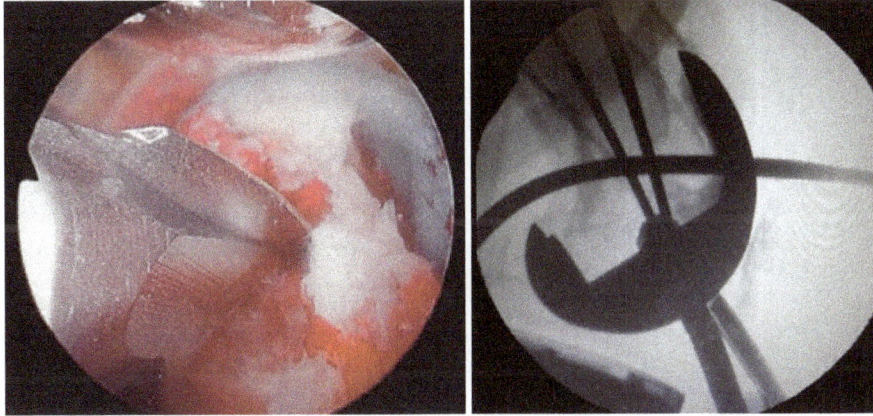

FIGURE 4: Entry point reaming without compromising the tibial post.

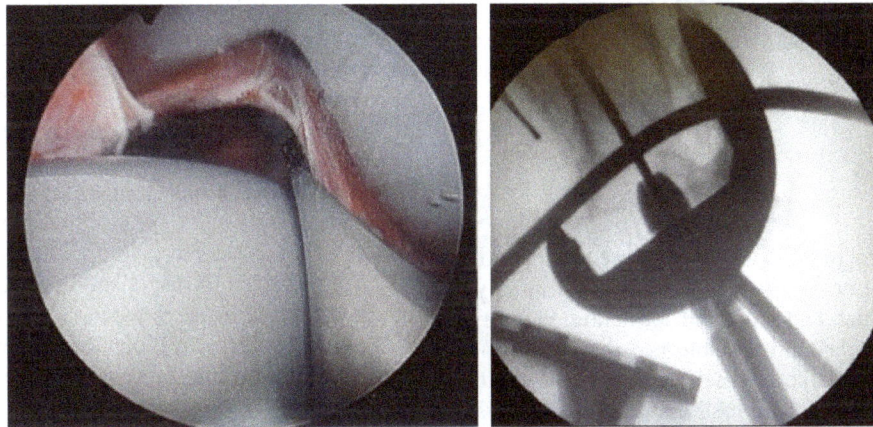

FIGURE 5: Nail insertion.

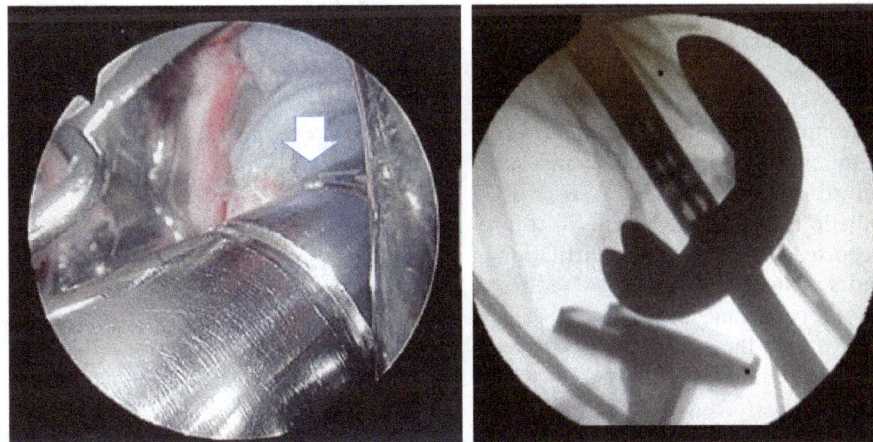

FIGURE 6: White arrow indicates the end of the nail.

To acquire the appropriate positioning of the distal locked screws and prevent the end of the nail from compromising the tibial post after surgery, the depth of the nail should be placed just at the end of the distal femur (Figure 6).

The proximal and distal locked screws were then inserted, followed by removal of the jig. Finally, nail impingement on the tibial post was confirmed using arthroscopy, and the patellar tendon was repaired. Postoperative radiograph indicated good sagittal and coronal alignment of the distal femur (Figure 7).

He exhibited good recovery with knee range of movement from 5° to 120° at 4 weeks postoperatively and successfully returned to preinjury functional activities at 4 months.

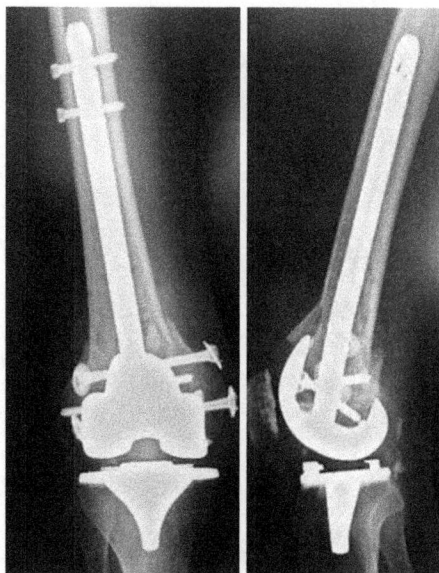

FIGURE 7: Postoperative radiograph.

3. Discussion

Various clinical characteristics are encountered with peri-prosthetic fracture after TKA, such as poor bone quality, delayed fracture healing, and prosthetic loosening. Fracture without displacement around a stable prosthesis may be treated conservatively, while internal fixation is the treatment option for displaced periprosthetic fracture without component loosening. Although the current findings suggested that both RIMN and use of an LCP could be indicated for these fractures [3], the priority of the implant choice remains controversial. The LCP may be applied in nearly all periprosthetic fracture situations without loosening. However, some drawbacks have been identified in the use of LCP. Potential periosteal stripping may violate the periosteal blood supply and interrupt bony union. Hoffmann et al. reported that the nonunion rate reached 22.2%, and hardware failure was observed in 8.3% of their LCP series of 55 consecutive periprosthetic fractures after TKA [5]. Moreover, Johnston et al. reported that an LCP caused irritation of the iliotibial band and soft-tissues of the knee, leading to premature removal in a separate anesthetic session [6].

RIMN is less invasive than the LCP technique, due to greater sparing of the fracture site, with minimal soft-tissue dissection and avoidance of periosteal stripping. However, some authors have advocated postoperative malalignment of RIMN. Lee et al. reported that 16% of procedures developed malalignment, including hyperextension and valgus alignment [7] according to Rorabeck and Taylor criteria [8]. To avoid hyperextension of the femoral component and damage to the tibial post during reaming, accurate identification of the appropriate entry point and direction of nail insertion are paramount. Because the entry point overlaps with the femoral component even under intraoperative fluoroimaging, accurate detection of the entry point and tip of the tibial post intraoperatively is difficult. With the technique we have described here, arthroscopy can directory visualize the entry point and the tibial post.

In cases with a small distal fragment, in order to insert multiple distal locked screws in RIMN, the distal end of the nail should be placed just at the surface of the intercondylar notch. Using arthroscopy, the end of the nail can be positioned as distally as possible, and RIMN is thus indicated for distal periprosthetic fractures with a small distal fragment.

Several contraindications for the present technique should be taken into account. Our technique is not indicated for patients with a stiff knee. If preoperative flexion angle is less than 90°, we cannot insert the nail using arthroscopy. In cases with the femoral component placed in flexion, the appropriate position of the entry point would be obscured. The diameter of medullary canal sometimes becomes a point of discussion. When the canal diameter of the isthmus is smaller than the smallest diameter of retrograde nails, the nail cannot be inserted through the canal of the femur. Thus, the surgeons should pay careful attention to whether the intramedullary canal diameter matches the nail diameter before surgery. Moreover, compatibility of the retrograde nail and TKA prostheses is a more critical issue. Most standard-sized retrograde nails are able to be technically inserted through most TKA prostheses. However, the recent study using sawbones indicated that six of the eight commonly used TKA prostheses scratched the nail or excessive force was needed on insertion [9]. From this perspective, our arthroscopically assisted technique can monitor and prevent the contact between the nail and the prosthesis during insertion.

In conclusion, this arthroscopically assisted technique is less invasive and useful for periprosthetic fracture when considering RIMN for periprosthetic fracture of the distal femur after PS-TKA.

Consent

Written informed consent was obtained from the patient for publication of this case report and accompanying images.

Conflicts of Interest

The authors have no conflicts of interest directly relevant to the content of this article.

References

[1] R. M. Meek, T. Norwood, R. Smith, I. J. Brenkel, and C. R. Howie, "The risk of peri-prosthetic fracture after primary and revision total hip and knee replacement," *Journal of Bone and Joint Surgery*, vol. 93, no. 1, pp. 96–101, 2011.

[2] D. A. Herrera, P. J. Kregor, P. A. Cole, B. A. Levy, A. Jonsson, and M. Zlowodzki, "Treatment of acute distal femur fractures above a total knee arthroplasty: Systematic review of 415 cases (1981–2006)," *Acta Orthopaedica*, vol. 79, no. 1, pp. 22–27, 2008.

[3] Y. S. Shin, H. J. Kim, and D. H. Lee, "Similar outcomes of locking compression plating and retrograde intramedullary nailing for periprosthetic supracondylar femoral fractures

following total knee arthroplasty: a meta-analysis," *Knee Surgery, Sports Traumatology, Arthroscopy*, vol. 25, no. 9, pp. 2921–2928, 2017.

[4] C. Krettek, T. Miclau, P. Schandelmaier, C. Stephan, U. Mohlmann, and H. Tscherne, "The mechanical effect of blocking screws ("Poller screws") in stabilizing tibia fractures with short proximal or distal fragments after insertion of small-diameter intramedullary nails," *Journal of Orthopaedic Trauma*, vol. 13, no. 8, pp. 550–553, 1999.

[5] M. F. Hoffmann, C. B. Jones, D. L. Sietsema, S. J. Koenig, and P. Tornetta III, "Outcome of periprosthetic distal femoral fractures following knee arthroplasty," *Injury*, vol. 43, no. 7, pp. 1084–1089, 2012.

[6] A. T. Johnston, E. Tsiridis, K. S. Eyres, and A. D. Toms, "Periprosthetic fractures in the distal femur following total knee replacement: a review and guide to management," *Knee*, vol. 19, no. 3, pp. 156–162, 2012.

[7] S. S. Lee, S. J. Lim, Y. W. Moon, and J. G. Seo, "Outcomes of long retrograde intramedullary nailing for periprosthetic supracondylar femoral fractures following total knee arthroplasty," *Archives of Orthopaedic and Trauma Surgery*, vol. 134, no. 1, pp. 47–52, 2014.

[8] C. H. Rorabeck and J. W. Taylor, "Classification of periprosthetic fractures complicating total knee arthroplasty," *Orthopedic Clinics of North America*, vol. 30, no. 2, pp. 209–214, 1999.

[9] M. D. Jones, C. Carpenter, S. R. Mitchell, M. Whitehouse, and S. Mehendale, "Retrograde femoral nailing of periprosthetic fractures around total knee replacements," *Injury*, vol. 47, no. 2, pp. 460–464, 2016.

7

Treatment of a Neglected Patellar Tendon Rupture with a Modified Surgical Technique: Ipsilateral Semitendinosus Autograft Reconstruction with Suture Tape Augmentation

Sanjum P. Samagh ⓘ, **Fernando A. Huyke, Lucas Buchler, Michael A. Terry, and Vehniah K. Tjong**

Department of Orthopaedic Surgery, Northwestern University Feinberg School of Medicine, 259 East Erie Street, Suite 1350, Chicago, IL 60611, USA

Correspondence should be addressed to Sanjum P. Samagh; sanjum.samagh@gmail.com

Academic Editor: Johannes Mayr

Patellar tendon ruptures are rare, but debilitating injuries are typically seen in young active males in the third and fourth decades of life. They can occur as a single acute injury or from repetitive microtrauma weakening the tendon. Patients typically present complaining of knee pain, swelling, and an inability to perform a straight leg raise. Most conventionally, these injuries are classified as acute (less than two weeks) or chronic (greater than two weeks) based upon the timing of presentation. In patients with patellar tendon ruptures and inability to perform a straight leg raise, patellar tendon repair is most often recommended. A subset of patients with chronic patellar tendon ruptures, however, presents several months after their initial injuries. These neglected patella tendon ruptures present a particularly challenging clinical scenario in which primary repair is often difficult or not possible. This case report describes a modification to an existing surgical technique for reconstructing the patellar tendon using an ipsilateral semitendinosus tendon autograft with suture tape augmentation.

1. Introduction

Patellar tendon ruptures are rare, but debilitating injuries are typically seen in young active males in the third and fourth decades of life [1]. In older patient populations, these injuries are commonly the result of isolated trauma with a forceful indirect contraction of the quadriceps. In patients under 40, there is often underlying microtrauma from repetitive injury. A force of 17.5 times body weight is estimated to cause a rupture; by comparison, the patellar tendon experiences a force of 3.2 times body weight while ascending stairs. Forces on the patella are greatest at 60 degrees of flexion, and ruptures are most common at the distal pole of the patella as the tensile load is greatest at the insertion site [2].

Various classification systems have been used to describe patellar tendon ruptures. Siwek and Rao divided these injuries into acute (diagnosis and treatment less than two weeks after injury) or chronic (more than two weeks) [1]. Jobe's group later described patellar tendon injuries as transverse, Z-type, or inverted-U based on the tear configuration [3]. Hsu et al. further divided ruptures as distal pole, tendon midsubstance, or tibial tubercle [4]. Currently, the Siwek and Rao classification of patellar tendon ruptures as acute or chronic and the surgical technique for treatment of ruptures seem to be the main perioperative factors that determine patient outcomes postoperatively [5–7].

Neglected patellar tendon ruptures are challenging to manage secondary to the retraction of the patella proximally and scarring of the surrounding tissues. Several surgical techniques have been described for treatment of chronic ruptures, but the ideal approach remains debatable [8, 9]. While studies have demonstrated less favorable outcomes in chronic patellar tendon ruptures compared to acute injuries, augmentation strengthens the construct and allows earlier return to range of motion [10–12]. Options for augmentation include autologous semitendinosus and gracilis

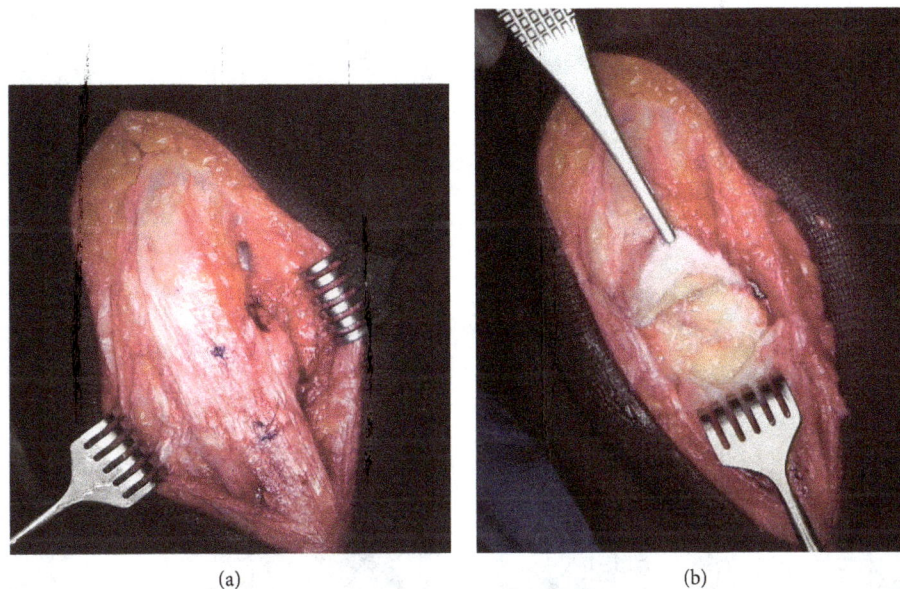

(a)

(b)

FIGURE 1: (a) The peritenon is identified superiorly, and peritendonous flaps are elevated to reveal the chronic, scarred patellar tendon rupture (approximately 3.5 cm in the midsubstance of the tendon). (b) The chronically scarred portion of the tendon is then debrided along with the medial and lateral retinacula. A Cobb elevator is used to release the superficial and deep aspects of the quadriceps tendon from the surrounding tissues.

tendon grafts, contralateral bone-patellar tendon-bone auto-grafts, turndown of the quadriceps tendon, Achilles and extensor mechanism allografts, and artificial materials [13–19]. Recent publications advocate for the use of autologous ipsilateral hamstring tendon graft reconstruction as a surgical option for the management of chronic patellar tendon rupture due to its association with good patient functional recovery and return to preinjury levels of activity [20–22]. The purpose of this case report is to share a modification of this surgical technique for reconstructing a neglected patellar tendon rupture: an autologous ipsilateral hamstring tendon graft reconstruction with additional suture tape augmentation.

2. Patient Presentation and Physical Examination

In delayed presentations of patellar tendon rupture, a patient may complain of difficulty with activities requiring active knee extension such as stair climbing or rising from a seated position. On physical exam, some active extension may be possible, but this is typically weak, and an extensor lag may be present. The patient sometimes presents with no effusion or hemarthrosis of the knee, but some mild swelling is possible. A palpable gap in the tendon may or may not be present as a scar often fills in over time [23].

Plain radiographs of the knee in the lateral plane and comparing this to the contralateral leg often demonstrate patella alta with an Insall-Salvati ratio greater than 1.2 [24]. Ultrasound or an MRI may be useful in qualifying the amount of tendon degeneration and other associated knee injuries in delayed diagnoses.

The patient in this case was a 25-year-old obese male with a past medical history of borderline hypertension and

diabetes well controlled with medication and a moderate level of physical activity that heard a pop in his knee after playing basketball. The patient ignored his knee injury until 5 months later when he presented to a clinic with instability in his knee, inability to fully straighten his leg, and anterior knee pain with flexion. On physical exam, the patient's preoperative range of motion was 10 to 100 degrees. The patient began experiencing anterior knee pain and tightness after 90 degrees of flexion.

3. Surgical Technique

3.1. Patient Positioning. The patient is brought to the operative suite and positioned supine on the operating room table, and general anesthesia is induced. Prior to draping, the contralateral knee is placed in 60 degrees of flexion, and the length of the native patellar tendon is measured (4.5 cm in the case pictured). The operative extremity is prepped and draped to the proximal thigh. A sterile triangle is placed to hold the knee in 60 degrees of flexion. The distance between the inferior pole of the patella and the tibial tubercle is then measured on the injured extremity (8.0 cm). A sterile tourniquet is applied to the thigh but will only be inflated if needed.

3.2. Surgical Approach and Repair. A midline longitudinal incision is made from the superior pole of the patella to the tibial tubercle through the skin and subcutaneous tissue. The underlying fascia is identified and incised longitudinally. The peritenon is identified superiorly, and the peritendonous flaps are elevated to reveal the chronic, scarred patellar tendon rupture (approximately 3.5 cm in the midsubstance of the tendon) (Figure 1(a)). The scarred portion of the tendon is debrided along with any redundancy of the medial and lateral retinacula. A Cobb elevator is used to release the

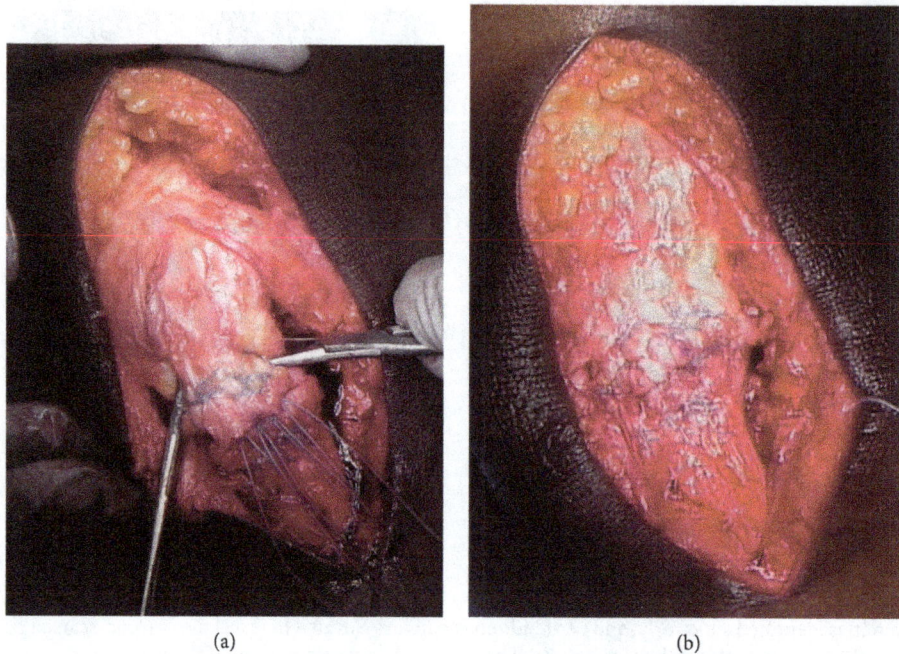

(a)   (b)

FIGURE 2: (a) A four-stranded end-to-end repair is then undertaken using a #5 FiberWire (Arthrex, Naples, FL) in a Krackow fashion. (b) To secure the repair, a #2 FiberWire (Arthrex, Naples, FL) is used in a running-locking fashion to imbricate the elongated medial and lateral retinacula and oversew the tendon repair.

superficial and deep aspects of the quadriceps tendon from the surrounding tissues (Figure 1(b)).

The vastus medialis is left intact, and the surgeon ensures that the patella can be reduced to its native position at 60 degrees of flexion as measured on the contralateral knee preoperatively. A four-stranded end-to-end repair is then undertaken using a #5 FiberWire (Arthrex, Naples, FL) in a Krackow fashion (Figure 2(a)). A #2 FiberWire (Arthrex, Naples, FL) is used in a running-locking fashion to imbricate the elongated medial and lateral retinacula and oversew the tendon repair (Figure 2(b)).

Next, the semitendinosus autograft is harvested. The insertion of the pes anserine is visualized through the same incision, and the semitendinosus tendon is identified and detached from its insertion. Once rid of adhesions, the tendon is harvested in standard fashion with a closed tendon harvester. The graft is prepared on the back table with both ends tied in a Krackow manner using #2 FiberWire sutures and then sized when doubled (6.5 mm).

A tibial bone tunnel is created using an appropriately sized (6.5 mm) cannulated reamer (Arthrex, Naples, FL), 3 cm distal to the tibial tubercle and 2 cm posterior from the anterior tibial crest (6.5 × 40 mm). The graft is passed through the bone tunnel from medial to lateral and courses along the lateral aspect of the native patellar tendon. Small rents are created in the medial and lateral retinacula at the level of the superior pole of the patella, and the graft is woven transversely through the distal quadriceps tendon from lateral to medial. The graft is then brought down along the medial border of the native patellar tendon and passed through the bone tunnel from lateral to medial. The free ends cross in opposite directions within the tibial

bone tunnel and are secured using interference screws (Tenodesis Screw, BioComposite, 6.25 × 15 mm; Arthrex, Naples, FL)—one from medial to lateral and one from lateral to medial (Figure 3(a)).

Finally, an InternalBrace (Arthrex, Naples, FL) is used to augment and protect the reconstruction. Two 4.75 × 15 mm SwiveLock BioComposite suture anchors (Arthrex, Naples, FL) are placed into the distal pole of the patella securing the midpoint of one 2 mm FiberTape suture tape (Arthrex, Naples, FL) each. The free limbs of the FiberTape cross the repair site—one limb straight inferior and the other in an "X" fashion—and are then secured to the tibial tubercle using two 4.75 × 15 mm SwiveLock BioComposite suture anchors (Figure 3(b)). The tension of the InternalBrace is set such that the knee can be passively flexed to 90 degrees. The wounds are thoroughly irrigated, closed, and dressed in the surgeon's usual sterile fashion.

3.3. Postoperative Rehabilitation. The patient was placed in a locked hinged knee brace and instructed to bear weight as tolerated with crutches in extension for 6 weeks. A supervised physical therapy program lasting 4 months was recommended. At 6 weeks, the patient was able to perform passive and active flexion to 90 degrees. At 12 weeks, the patient discontinued the brace and began zero-resistance straight leg raise exercises, as recommended. The patient began quadriceps strengthening at 12 weeks and ultimately should return to impact cardiovascular activity after 20–24 weeks. This current patient has had a six-month follow-up. He has active range of motion from 0–120 degrees with no extensor lag and has returned to sporting activity.

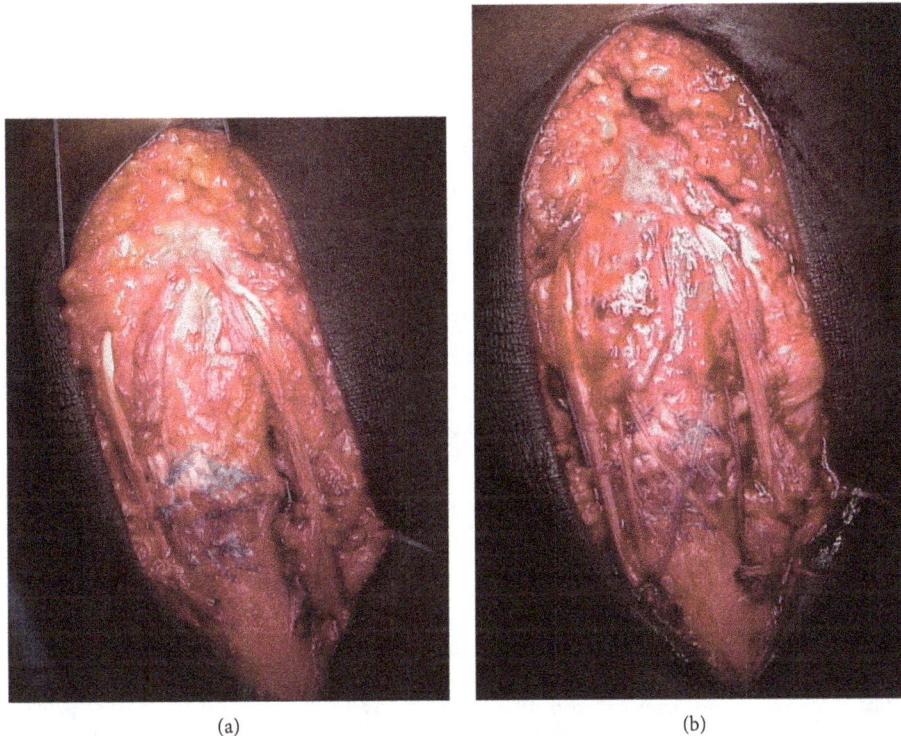

(a)   (b)

FIGURE 3: (a) The semitendinosus autograft is passed through the bone tunnel from medial to lateral and courses along the lateral aspect of the native patellar tendon. Small rents are created in the medial and lateral retinacula at the level of the superior pole of the patella, and the graft is woven transversely through the distal quadriceps tendon from lateral to medial. The graft is then brought down along the medial border of the native patellar tendon and passed through the bone tunnel from lateral to medial. The free ends cross in opposite directions within the tibial bone tunnel and are secured within the tibial tunnel using two interference screws (Tenodesis Screw, BioComposite, 6.25 × 15 mm; Arthrex, Naples, FL)—one from medial to lateral and one from lateral to medial. (b) An InternalBrace (Arthrex, Naples, FL) is used to augment and protect the reconstruction. Two 4.75 × 15 mm SwiveLock BioComposite suture anchors (Arthrex, Naples, FL) are placed into the distal pole of the patella securing the midpoint of one 2 mm FiberTape suture tape (Arthrex, Naples, FL) each. The free limbs of the FiberTape (Arthrex, Naples, FL) cross the repair site—one limb straight inferior and the other in an "X" fashion—and are then secured to the tibial tubercle using two 4.75 × 15 mm SwiveLock BioComposite suture anchors (Arthrex, Naples, FL).

4. Discussion

This report details our technique for treatment of neglected patellar tendon ruptures with patellar tendon reconstruction using a semitendinosus tendon autograft and suture tape augmentation. While the vast majority of patellar tendon ruptures are diagnosed and treated in a relatively timely manner, some go undiagnosed and lead to chronic injuries with significant retraction and scarring of the tendon. Although the prevalence and incidence of these undiagnosed injuries are unknown, their surgical management is challenging due to delay of diagnosis. Nonoperative management has limited indications and does not restore the function of the effected extremity. Late repair of chronic patellar tendon ruptures was first described in 1927, and several techniques have been described [25]. We advocate for autograft reconstruction as a method of tendon augmentation including the passage and incorporation through bone tunnels. Allograft reconstruction has an increased risk of infection and weakness secondary to radiation of the tendon graft. In addition, animal models have demonstrated that allograft extensor mechanism reconstruction shows a reduction in vascularity and cellularity when histologically compared to autograft reconstruction [26]. We also elected to use nonabsorbable sutures because we believe they add strength and longevity to the repair, which have been seen in a literature review of acute patellar tendon repair and an Achilles tendon repair model [27, 28].

The best method of treatment for neglected patellar tendon ruptures is controversial; however, we believe the technique above results in a robust construct that allows for the return of strength and function of the knee through early rehabilitation. Given the rare occurrence of neglected patellar tendon ruptures, there is a paucity of comparative literature to guide management. Future long-term studies are necessary to assess long-term outcomes with this injury and surgical technique.

5. Conclusion

Chronic patellar tendon rupture is a rare injury, and consensus for a gold standard approach to surgical management has yet to be reached. Previous cases of ipsilateral semitendinosus autograft reconstruction have shown positive outcomes and relatively rapid return to physical activity with rehabilitation. Our modified surgical technique involving suture tape augmentation provides a potentially stronger construct in addition to providing excellent range of motion and return to sporting activity at a six-month follow-up.

Conflicts of Interest

The authors declare that they have no conflicts of interest.

References

[1] C. W. Siwek and J. P. Rao, "Ruptures of the extensor mechanism of the knee joint," *The Journal of Bone & Joint Surgery*, vol. 63, no. 6, pp. 932–937, 1981.

[2] R. F. Zernicke, J. Garhammer, and F. W. Jobe, "Human patellar-tendon rupture," *The Journal of Bone & Joint Surgery*, vol. 59, no. 2, pp. 179–183, 1977.

[3] D. W. Kelly, V. S. Carter, F. W. Jobe, and R. K. Kerlan, "Patellar and quadriceps tendon ruptures—jumper's knee," *The American Journal of Sports Medicine*, vol. 12, no. 5, pp. 375–380, 1984.

[4] K. Y. Hsu, K. C. Wang, W. P. Ho, and R. W. Hsu, "Traumatic patellar tendon ruptures: a follow-up study of primary repair and a neutralization wire," *The Journal of Trauma: Injury, Infection, and Critical Care*, vol. 36, no. 5, pp. 658–660, 1994.

[5] A. Lamberti, G. Balato, P. P. Summa, A. Rajgopal, A. Vasdev, and A. Baldini, "Surgical options for chronic patellar tendon rupture in total knee arthroplasty," *Knee Surgery, Sports Traumatology, Arthroscopy*, vol. 26, no. 5, pp. 1429–1435, 2018.

[6] K. Belhaj, H. el Hyaoui, A. Tahir et al., "Long-term functional outcomes after primary surgical repair of acute and chronic patellar tendon rupture: series of 25 patients," *Annals of Physical and Rehabilitation Medicine*, vol. 60, no. 4, pp. 244–248, 2017.

[7] R. Papalia, S. Vasta, S. D'Adamio, E. Albo, N. Maffulli, and V. Denaro, "Complications involving the extensor mechanism after total knee arthroplasty," *Knee Surgery, Sports Traumatology, Arthroscopy*, vol. 23, no. 12, pp. 3501–3515, 2015.

[8] J. G. Enad, "Patellar tendon ruptures," *Southern Medical Journal*, vol. 92, no. 6, pp. 563–566, 1999.

[9] B. Chen, R. Li, and S. Zhang, "Reconstruction and restoration of neglected ruptured patellar tendon using semitendinosus and gracilis tendons with preserved distal insertions: two case reports," *The Knee*, vol. 19, no. 4, pp. 508–512, 2012.

[10] R. T. Burks and R. H. Edelson, "Allograft reconstruction of the patellar ligament. A case report," *The Journal of Bone and Joint Surgery-American Volume*, vol. 76, no. 7, pp. 1077–1079, 1994.

[11] B. Schliemann, N. Grüneweller, D. Yao et al., "Biomechanical evaluation of different surgical techniques for treating patellar tendon ruptures," *International Orthopaedics*, vol. 40, no. 8, pp. 1717–1723, 2016.

[12] A. Rothfeld, A. Pawlak, S. A. H. Liebler, M. Morris, and J. M. Paci, "Patellar tendon repair augmentation with a knotless suture anchor internal brace: a biomechanical cadaveric study," *The American Journal of Sports Medicine*, vol. 46, no. 5, pp. 1199–1204, 2018.

[13] A. Cadambi and G. A. Engh, "Use of a semitendinosus tendon autogenous graft for rupture of the patellar ligament after total knee arthroplasty. A report of seven cases," *The Journal of Bone & Joint Surgery*, vol. 74, no. 7, pp. 974–979, 1992.

[14] H. M. Chiou, M. C. Chang, and W. H. Lo, "One-stage reconstruction of skin defect and patellar tendon rupture after total knee arthroplasty. A new technique," *The Journal of Arthroplasty*, vol. 12, no. 5, pp. 575–579, 1997.

[15] L. S. Crossett, R. K. Sinha, V. F. Sechriest, and H. E. Rubash, "Reconstruction of a ruptured patellar tendon with Achilles tendon allograft following total knee arthroplasty," *The Journal of Bone and Joint Surgery-American Volume*, vol. 84, no. 8, pp. 1354–1361, 2002.

[16] M. Z. Milankov, N. Miljkovic, and M. Stankovic, "Reconstruction of chronic patellar tendon rupture with contralateral BTB autograft: a case report," *Knee Surgery, Sports Traumatology, Arthroscopy*, vol. 15, no. 12, pp. 1445–1448, 2007.

[17] C. Scuderi, "Ruptures of the quadriceps tendon; study of twenty tendon ruptures," *American Journal of Surgery*, vol. 95, no. 4, pp. 626–635, 1958.

[18] S. Fukuta, A. Kuge, and M. Nakamura, "Use of the Leeds-Keio prosthetic ligament for repair of patellar tendon rupture after total knee arthroplasty," *The Knee*, vol. 10, no. 2, pp. 127–130, 2003.

[19] P. B. Lewis, J. P. Rue, and B. Bach Jr, "Chronic patellar tendon rupture: surgical reconstruction technique using 2 Achilles tendon allografts," *The Journal of Knee Surgery*, vol. 21, no. 2, pp. 130–135, 2008.

[20] N. Maffulli, R. Papalia, G. Torre, and V. Denaro, "Surgical treatment for failure of repair of patellar and quadriceps tendon rupture with ipsilateral hamstring tendon graft," *Sports Medicine and Arthroscopy Review*, vol. 25, no. 1, pp. 51–55, 2017.

[21] N. Maffulli, A. del Buono, M. Loppini, and V. Denaro, "Ipsilateral hamstring tendon graft reconstruction for chronic patellar tendon ruptures: average 5.8-year follow-up," *The Journal of Bone & Joint Surgery*, vol. 95, no. 17, pp. e123-e1-e6, 2013.

[22] M. Spoliti, A. Giai Via, J. Padulo, F. Oliva, A. del Buono, and N. Maffulli, "Surgical repair of chronic patellar tendon rupture in total knee replacement with ipsilateral hamstring tendons," *Knee Surgery, Sports Traumatology, Arthroscopy*, vol. 24, no. 10, pp. 3183–3190, 2016.

[23] M. J. Matava, "Patellar tendon ruptures," *Journal of the American Academy of Orthopaedic Surgeons*, vol. 4, no. 6, pp. 287–296, 1996.

[24] M. A. Fazal, P. Moonot, and F. Haddad, "Radiographic features of acute patellar tendon rupture," *Orthopaedic Surgery*, vol. 7, no. 4, pp. 338–342, 2015.

[25] W. E. Gallie and A. B. Lemesurier, "The late repair of fractures of the patella and of rupture of the ligamentum patellae and quadriceps tendon," *The American Journal of Surgery*, vol. 2, no. 3, pp. 284–285, 1927.

[26] G. Chen, H. Zhang, Q. Ma et al., "Fresh-frozen complete extensor mechanism allograft versus autograft reconstruction in rabbits," *Scientific Reports*, vol. 6, no. 1, article 22106, 2016.

[27] M. R. Carmont, J. H. Kuiper, K. Grävare Silbernagel, J. Karlsson, and K. Nilsson-Helander, "Tendon end separation with loading in an Achilles tendon repair model: comparison of non-absorbable vs absorbable sutures," *Journal of Experimental Orthopaedics*, vol. 4, no. 1, p. 26, 2017.

[28] J. H. Gilmore, Z. J. Clayton-Smith, M. Aguilar, S. G. Pneumaticos, and P. V. Giannoudis, "Reconstruction techniques and clinical results of patellar tendon ruptures: evidence today," *The Knee*, vol. 22, no. 3, pp. 148–155, 2015.

8

Upper Extremity Compartment Syndrome in a Patient with Acute Gout Attack but without Trauma or Other Typical Causes

John G. Skedros ⓘ,[1] James S. Smith,[1] Marshall K. Henrie,[1] Ethan D. Finlinson,[1] and Joel D. Trachtenberg[2]

[1]*Department of Orthopaedic Surgery and Utah Orthopaedic Specialists, The University of Utah, 5323 South Woodrow Street, Salt Lake City, UT 84107, USA*
[2]*St. Marks Hospital, Salt Lake City, UT, USA*

Correspondence should be addressed to John G. Skedros; jskedrosmd@uosmd.com

Academic Editor: Zbigniew Gugala

We report the case of a 30-year-old Polynesian male with a severe gout flare of multiple joints and simultaneous acute compartment syndrome (ACS) of his right forearm and hand without trauma or other typical causes. He had a long history of gout flares, but none were known to be associated with compartment syndrome. He also had concurrent infections in his right elbow joint and olecranon bursa. A few days prior to this episode of ACS, high pain and swelling occurred in his right upper extremity after a minimal workout with light weights. A similar episode occurred seven months prior and was attributed to a gout flare. Unlike past flares that resolved with colchicine and/or anti-inflammatory medications, his current upper extremity pain/swelling worsened and became severe. Hand and forearm fasciotomies were performed. Workup included general medicine, rheumatology and infectious disease consultations, myriad blood tests, and imaging studies including Doppler ultrasound and CT angiography. Additional clinical history suggested that he had previously unrecognized recurrent exertional compartment syndrome that led to the episode of ACS reported here. Chronic exertional compartment syndrome (CECS) presents a difficult diagnosis when presented with multiple symptoms concurrently. This case provides an example of one such diagnosis.

1. Introduction

We report a case where a severe gout attack and acute compartment syndrome (ACS) of the upper extremity occurred simultaneously in a 30-year-old male. The compartment syndrome was not associated with trauma or other typical causes. The patient also had ipsilateral forearm cellulitis and culture-proven infections of the elbow joint and olecranon bursa. The temporal association of a gout flare with ACS and the concurrent infections confused all clinicians that cared for the patient in the hospital setting and in clinics several months thereafter. Because of this, the patient's workup was complex, reflecting a broad differential diagnosis. He eventually provided sufficient descriptions of prior episodes of bilateral upper extremity swelling and pain that allowed them to be clearly differentiated from his gout attacks. These episodes were more consistent with CECS, with the worst case being the episode of ACS that we report here.

CECS is a less common cause of compartment syndrome in the upper extremity, and to our knowledge, its coexistence with a severe gout attack has not been reported. It is important to note in this case report that it was mistakenly concluded that the patient had an initial one-time episode of ACS. Consequently, we describe the episode as ACS because this reflected the understanding that we had during the patient's September to November 2016 hospitalizations. Months later, it was understood that the episode of ACS was most likely the worst of a series of CECS episodes.

2. Case Report

The patient is a 30-year-old right-hand-dominant Polynesian (Tongan) male (height 182.9 cm, weight 141.9 kg, and BMI 42.6) with a long history of crystal-proven gout attacks. He had a chronic history of recurrent pain in his back, bilateral shoulders, elbows, hands/wrists, hips, knees, and

TABLE 1: Results of synovial fluid analysis.

	Normal range	Right wrist joint	Right elbow joint
WBC	0–200 mm^3	No cell count*	91,560 [H]
Crystals	None	CP	MU
RBC	None	No cell count*	21,000
Neutrophils	0–25%	79 [H]	85 [H]
Lymphocytes	0–78%	10	2
Monocytes	0–71%	8	13
Eosinophils	0–2%	3 [H]	None
Appearance	Clear	Bloody	Turbid
Color	Colorless	Red	Yellow

*Sample was clotted. CP = calcium pyrophosphate; MU = monosodium urate; RBC = red blood cell count; WBC = white blood cell count; [H] = high level.

ankles/feet. The patient had been prescribed febuxostat for chronic gout and hyperuricemia. Additional medical problems included a history of noninsulin dependent diabetes, but he was noncompliant with the medication prescribed for this. He is a two pack-a-day cigarette smoker and consumes alcohol only occasionally, but he denied consumption of alcohol for over one month. He also denied recent or past illicit drug use and had no prior history of local or systemic infections.

For four years, he was employed as a construction worker, which required heavy lifting, hammering nails, pulling cables, and other various repetitive activities. In August 2016, because of upper extremity swelling and joint pains caused by these work-related activities, he changed his manual work occupation to one that required less strenuous physical activity.

In mid-September 2016, he had been exercising with light weights for two consecutive days. He then noticed progressive swelling and pain in his right forearm, hand, and shoulder. The pain and moderate swelling persisted despite treatment with oral anti-inflammatory medications which had usually been sufficient to abate the majority of prior episodes of pain and swelling. The pain and swelling became tolerable when he reduced his activity level. Four days later, he was driving his car on a long trip, and after four hours had passed, he noted increased right shoulder pain with increased swelling of the right hand and forearm. He was treated in an emergency department (ED) with intravenous (i.v.) ketorolac tromethamine, oral prednisone and tramadol.

The following morning, he was seen in the ED of our hospital with worsening symptoms. He was admitted for a severe acute gout flare and emerging ACS of the right forearm and hand. He was afebrile but had what appeared to be right forearm/hand cellulitis. His blood pressure was 140/73, and heart rate was 89 beats/min. Results of lab tests performed during his hospitalization are summarized in Tables 1–3. Initial laboratory values included uric acid level of 7.7 (normal is <7.2), leukocytosis (13,800/μl), and a normal blood glucose level of 84. However, his blood glucose values were elevated several times during the remaining seven-day hospitalization (99–162). His CKMB (creatine kinase-MB) was normal at 2.5 ng/ml (normal range 0.5–3.6), and CK was mildly elevated at 245 U/liter (normal range

TABLE 2: Thyroid panel.

	Normal range	Result
T3 uptake	23–40%	37
T4	4.6–12 μg/dl	11.8
Free thyroxine index	1.4–4.5 ng/dl	4.366
TSH	0.34–4.82 U/ml	3.81

T3 = serum triiodothyronine; T4 = serum tetraiodothyronine; TSH = thyroid-stimulating hormone.

TABLE 3: General metabolic panels.

	Normal range	Result
Na	136–145 mmol/L	138
K	3.5–5.1 mmol/L	3.9
Cl	98–107 mmol/L	102
CO$_2$	23–32 mmol/L	26
Anion gap	4–12 mmol/L	19 [H]
Glucose	70–110 mg/dL	84
BUN	7–18 mg/dL	14
Creatinine	0.6–1.3 mg/dL	0.8
eGFR	>60	>60
PROT	6.4–8.2 g/dL	7.5
Albumin	3.4–5.0 g/dL	2.9 [L]
Calcium	8.5–10.1 mg/dL	8.6
BILI-TOT	0.1–1.2 mg/dL	0.3
AST	5–41 U/L	26
ALT	10–56 U/L	24
ALKPHOS	50–136 U/L	88

ALKPHOS = alkaline phosphatase; ALT = alanine aminotransferase; AST = aspartate aminotransferase; BILI-TOT = bilirubin total; BUN = blood urea nitrogen; Cl = chlorine; CO$_2$ = carbon dioxide; eGFR = estimated glomerular filtration rate; K = potassium; Na = sodium; PROT = protein; [H] = high level; [L] = low level.

35–224). He also tested negative for rheumatoid factor, thyroid abnormality, systemic lupus erythematous, and HIV-1 and HIV-2 antibodies. A blood toxicology screen was negative for narcotics, alcohol, and other elicit substances.

He was placed on colchicine, i.v. ketorolac tromethamine, and i.v. vancomycin (2,000 mg every 12 hours), and i.v. piperacillin/tazobactam (3.375 grams every six hours). A

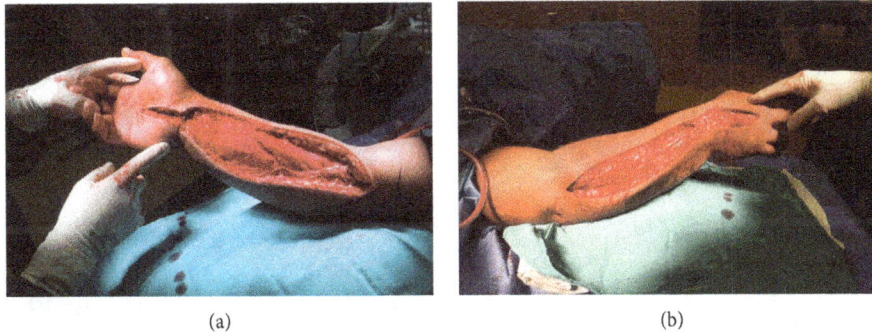

(a)   (b)

FIGURE 1: Intraoperative images of our patient's volar (a) and dorsal (b) fasciotomies of the right forearm and hand.

CT scan of his hand, forearm, and elbow revealed fluid accumulation in the right olecranon bursa and elbow joint. An MRI of his right shoulder did not reveal abnormalities. Needle aspirations of his right elbow joint, olecranon bursa, wrist, and shoulder were done. Aspiration of the right elbow joint revealed sodium urate crystals and had a white blood cell count of 91,650/mm^3. Aspirations of the right wrist revealed calcium pyrophosphate (pseudogout), but no organisms grew from the wrist culture. The white blood cell count could not be determined from the wrist aspiration because the sample had clotted. CT angiogram and Doppler ultrasound tests of his right upper extremity were negative for vein or artery pathology.

The patient was taken urgently to surgery for compartment fasciotomies because of clinically obvious compartment syndrome, including tense volar compartments, reduced sensation in all fingers, reduced capillary refill, and severe pain with passive finger stretch [1, 2]. His blood pressure was 160/98 mmHg at the time of compartment pressure measurements, which were made immediately prior to the induction of general anesthesia. Using a Stryker® Intra-Compartmental Pressure Monitor Set (Kalamazoo, Michigan, USA), his compartment pressures were measured twice in each of three locations. The volar compartments were measured between the mid and distal forearm, and the values were 20 and 24 mmHg. The carpal tunnel region and the mid palm ulnar to the median nerve each measured 45–48 mmHg. The dorsal forearm measured 12 and 14 mmHg. The dorsal forearm was not more than mild/moderately swollen. In view of the clinical findings and volar pressures exceeding 30 mmHg [3, 4], surgical releases were done for only the volar compartments, including the carpal tunnel and all volar hand compartments [4].

The volar forearm had bulging muscles that contracted with electrocautery stimulation, and there was no evidence of necrosis, pus, or odor (Figure 1(a)). Gouty tophi were not grossly observed in the fascia or muscle, but small tophi (~0.25–0.5 mm) were seen sporadically in the synovial sheaths of the flexor tendons, which can occur after many years in patients with poorly controlled gout [5]. The wounds were covered with sterile sponges attached to a conventional wound vacuum (V.A.C.Ulta™ Negative Pressure Wound Therapy System, KCI Medical, USA).

Because the swelling worsened over the 12 hours, especially in the dorsal hand and forearm, he was taken back to

surgery, and new dorsal fasciotomies were made (Figure 1(b)). The upper dorsal incision extended up to near the olecranon bursa, which allowed the superficial tissues to be elevated to access the olecranon bursa and elbow joint where infections were suspected in view of worsening white blood cell count and results of the elbow aspiration. The elbow joint was irrigated through a small arthrotomy and a bulb suction drain was placed.

Cultures from the tophitic/phlegmonous tissue obtained from the right olecranon bursa grew *Candida albicans*, which was treated with oral fluconazole. The fluid from the elbow aspiration grew *Staphylococcus haemolyticus*.

After a seven-day hospital stay, he was discharged to his home with four weeks of i.v. vancomycin and oral fluconazole and with outpatient wound vacuum sponge changes 2-3 times per week. Two weeks later, he was evaluated at a tertiary care hospital (University of Utah Medical Center) for a rheumatologic evaluation, which was not available at our hospital. In addition to having poorly controlled gout, he received the additional diagnosis of polyarthritis and oral prednisone and analgesics were recommended on an as-needed basis. At that time, all consulting physicians remained puzzled by the association of the patient's gout and joint pains with what was still considered a first-time episode of ACS.

Split-thickness skin grafts were successfully performed (Figure 2). He was seen again in the ED of our hospital on two additional occasions for crystal-proven gout flares of his shoulders and knees without significant limb compartment swelling. His CK levels were not elevated, and the symptoms improved with colchicine and anti-inflammatory medications.

When he returned to our clinic three months later, we obtained more details of his prior "gout attacks," including the duration, quality of pain and locations of swelling, and activities before their onset. It then became clear that what he believed, and had been told by all prior healthcare providers, were approximately 10 severe "gout attacks" over the past four years, which were more consistent with episodes of chronic exertional compartment syndrome (CECS) [1, 6, 7]. These episodes started several months after he began working in construction. Upon learning of the underlying diagnosis of CECS, the patient then stated that he was able to differentiate episodes of this condition from his gout flares because of what he considered to be distinct differences in pain and swelling intensity (gout-related pain and swelling was focused at the

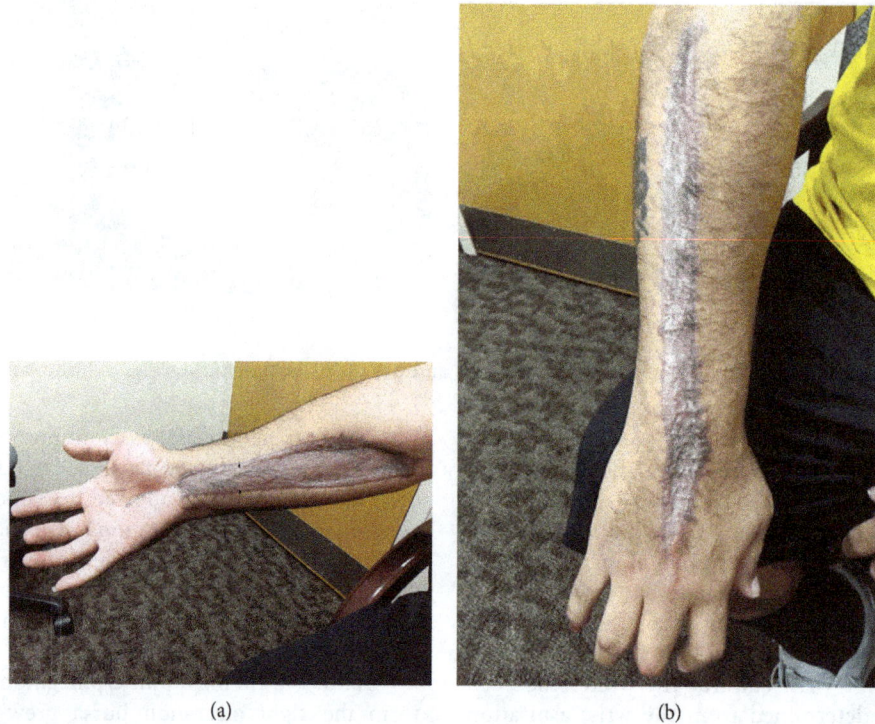

(a)   (b)

FIGURE 2: Three-month postoperative images showing healed skin grafts on the volar (a) and dorsal (b) aspects of our patient's right forearm and hand.

joint versus in CECS, the pain and swelling were of greater intensity and more diffuse in the limb).

At 12 months after the right upper extremity fasciotomies, the patient reported moderate weakness in grip strength and mild reduced motion of his finger joints. He did not return to manual labor and had no additional episodes of significant compartment swelling.

3. Discussion

This case is highly unusual because of the clinical presentation and diagnostic challenge. The rare concurrent diagnoses included (1) forearm/hand compartment syndrome, (2) calcium pyrophosphate crystals (pseudogout) in the wrist, (3) monosodium urate crystals, gouty tophi, and *S. haemolyticus* in the elbow, (4) *C. albicans* infection and gouty tophi in the olecranon bursa, and (5) elbow/forearm cellulitis. We initially incorrectly concluded that this was a first-time episode of ACS. Because of this, we focused on the possibility that the crystalline-induced arthritides and concurrent infections had somehow precipitated an atypical episode of ACS.

It is well known that gout attacks typically cause joint pain and swelling. There are only a few cases reported where gout or pseudogout crystal deposition cause high swelling of limb compartments [8]. In these rare cases, the limb compartment swelling usually subsides with rest and anti-inflammatory and/or antiuricemic medications [9–11]. Hence, these patients do not need surgical fasciotomies that are done for compartment syndrome. Our literature review (PubMed/Google Scholar) also revealed no evidence that

gout or pseudogout is causally related to ACS or CECS. However, prior to our recognition that our patient had CECS, case reports of carpal tunnel syndrome caused by gouty tophi [12–15] led us to consider the possibility that he had accumulated nonsynovial tophi (e.g., within the fascia) that precipitated ACS by reducing compliance of the fascia. But this hypothesis proved untenable in view of studies showing that tophi do not accumulate significantly in the fascia [5] and the fascia is not rendered thicker or stiffer by gout [16]. Nevertheless, possible additive effects of reduced fascial compliance and impaired venous return have been hypothesized as being causative factors for CECS for some patients [17]. Although gout can be associated with peripheral vascular disease [18], there was also no evidence that our patient had vascular disease.

We also considered the possibility that he had unrecognized metabolic deficiencies. For example, we considered acute rhabdomyolysis as a possible cause of his current episode of compartment syndrome [19, 20], which also led us to consider McArdle disease (glycogen storage disease type V) [21]. However, these conditions were excluded by CK levels that were only mildly elevated at each of the two hospital admissions and several ED visits made by our patient over a four month period. Fabry's disease was also considered as a possible underlying diagnosis because these patients exhibit, similar to our patient, increased levels of uric acid with associated pain and swelling in the distal extremities. Although some of these patients are diagnosed in the third or fourth decade of life, also resembling the age of our patient, his normal levels of α-galactosidase A eliminated this possibility [22–24].

Our patient also did not have unrecognized type I diabetes, which has been reported to be causally linked to spontaneous ACS (i.e., no trauma or other cause identified) [25, 26]. We also considered the possibility of a singular episode of ACS caused by Saturday night palsy resulting from prolonged limb ischemia after passing out during surreptitious binge use of alcohol and/or illicit drugs [27]. This possibility was ruled out by our patient's negative blood toxicology screen. Some additional more obscure causes of compartment syndrome include systemic disorders such as nephrotic syndrome, hypothyroidism, viral or drug-induced myositis, systemic capillary leak syndrome, and other rare metabolic disorders [21, 28–30]. These and additional rare causes listed elsewhere [26, 30] were also ruled-out as possible causes.

The concurrent infections seen in our patient suggest an immunocompromised state. Gout is not known to cause an immunocompromised state [31], but it can be misdiagnosed as cellulitis [32]. Our patient's cellulitis was relatively mild when compared to the more severe infections that can precipitate compartment syndrome [33–36]. Type 2 diabetes appears to be the most significant factor contributing to his immunocompromised state [37].

Our realization that our patient had prior episodes of exertional compartment syndrome was serendipitous, occurring after finding reports describing CECS after minimal exertion [1, 38, 39]. Pritchard et al. [38] found that the cause of CECS in 42 patients in the upper extremity (forearm) was rapid or strenuous repetitive tasks, such as keyboard and light assembly work or packing and heavy industrial assembly work (e.g., factory assembly workers). Brown et al. [1] described 12 patients with CECS of the forearm, all of which were treated with fasciotomies. One of their patients who had only partial resolution of symptoms were, like our patient, one with relatively low strenuous activities (46-year-old crane operator and golf player).

With this new information, it became clear that our patient's previous episodes of pain and swelling, which were diagnosed as "gout attacks" by various clinicians in different EDs, were actually multiple episodes of exertional compartment syndrome that occurred during his four-year employment as a construction worker. The episode of compartment syndrome described in this report was his worst even though it was precipitated by less strenuous activities.

Because CECS is rare, the diagnosis is often unclear or delayed [1, 17, 40]. In addition to pain, symptoms can include a feeling of tightness, hardness, or a "pumped up" sensation in the forearm, cramping, swelling, paraesthesiae of the fingers, weakness, and a feeling of loss of control of the hand [1]. The symptoms are often bilateral and are brought on by exertion and relieved by rest, recurring when the precipitating activity is resumed [1]. When a patient with an episode of CECS presents with these and other wide ranging symptoms, they can be—as in our patient—a red herring that distracts healthcare providers from determining the diagnosis in a timely fashion [6, 41]. Adding to the conclusion, the patients are also often asymptomatic at rest, showing minimal findings upon examination. Clinicians

need to consider CECS as a cause of activity-induced pain and swelling, and thus diagnostic compartment pressure measurements can be made before, during, and after exertion tests that reproduce the symptoms [6].

4. Conclusion

This report describes the rare association of an acute gout attack in a patient that presented to us with what was initially considered to be an isolated episode of ACS. Subsequent workup and more careful consideration of the patient's prior descriptions of some of his "gout attacks" ultimately revealed that he likely had been experiencing CECS. The worst episode of his recurrent CECS of the forearms and hands was the case we describe here. When patients present with ACS without typical causes, occupational/athletic history should be considered to determine if CECS is the cause of symptoms. Clinicians could improve their diagnostic acumen in similar cases by being more specific about the patient's prior episodes of joint pain and swelling versus limb pain and swelling.

Consent

The patient was informed and consented that data concerning the case would be submitted for publication.

Conflicts of Interest

The authors declare that there are no conflicts of interest regarding the publication of this article.

References

[1] J. S. Brown, P. C. Wheeler, K. T. Boyd, M. R. Barnes, and M. J. Allen, "Chronic exertional compartment syndrome of the forearm: a case series of 12 patients treated with fasciotomy," *Journal of Hand Surgery (European Volume)*, vol. 36, no. 5, pp. 413–419, 2011.

[2] T. E. Whitesides and M. M. Heckman, "Acute compartment syndrome: update on diagnosis and treatment," *Journal of the American Academy of Orthopaedic Surgeons*, vol. 4, no. 4, pp. 209–218, 1996.

[3] S. J. Mubarak, A. R. Hargens, C. A. Owen, L. P. Garetto, and W. H. Akeson, "The wick catheter technique for measurement of intramuscular pressure. A new research and clinical tool," *Journal of Bone and Joint Surgery, American Volume*, vol. 58, no. 7, pp. 1016–1020, 1976.

[4] A. H. Schmidt, "Acute compartment syndrome," *Orthopedic Clinics of North America*, vol. 47, no. 3, pp. 517–525, 2016.

[5] L. Qiu, Y. Chen, Z. Huang, L. Cai, and L. Zhang, "Widespread gouty tophi on 18F-FDG PET/CT imaging," *Clinical Nuclear Medicine*, vol. 39, no. 6, pp. 579–581, 2014.

[6] R. S. Paik, D. A. Pepple, and M. R. Hutchinson, "Chronic exertional compartment syndrome," *BMJ*, vol. 346, p. f33, 2013.

[7] M. J. Fraipont and G. J. Adamson, "Chronic exertional compartment syndrome," *Journal of the American Academy of Orthopaedic Surgeons*, vol. 11, no. 4, pp. 268–276, 2003.

[8] L. J. Forbess and T. R. Fields, "The broad spectrum of urate crystal deposition: unusual presentations of gouty tophi,"

Seminars in Arthritis and Rheumatism, vol. 42, no. 2, pp. 146–154, 2012.

[9] T. Neogi, T. L. Jansen, N. Dalbeth et al., "2015 Gout classification criteria: an American College of Rheumatology/European League Against Rheumatism collaborative initiative," *Annals of the Rheumatic Diseases*, vol. 74, no. 10, pp. 1789–1798, 2015.

[10] D. Khanna, J. D. Fitzgerald, P. P. Khanna et al., "2012 American College of Rheumatology guidelines for management of gout. Part 1: systematic nonpharmacologic and pharmacologic therapeutic approaches to hyperuricemia," *Arthritis Care and Research*, vol. 64, no. 10, pp. 1431–1446, 2012.

[11] S. Schlee, L. C. Bollheimer, T. Bertsch, C. C. Sieber, and P. Harle, "Crystal arthritides - gout and calcium pyrophosphate arthritis: Part 1: epidemiology and pathophysiology," *Zeitschrift für Gerontologie und Geriatrie*, 2017.

[12] A. Therimadasamy, Y. P. Peng, T. C. Putti, and E. P. Wilder-Smith, "Carpal tunnel syndrome caused by gouty tophus of the flexor tendons of the fingers: sonographic features," *Journal of Clinical Ultrasound*, vol. 39, no. 8, pp. 463–465, 2011.

[13] C. K. H. Chen, C. B. Chung, L. Yeh et al., "Carpal tunnel syndrome caused by tophaceous gout: CT and MR imaging features in 20 patients," *American Journal of Roentgenology*, vol. 175, no. 3, pp. 655–659, 2000.

[14] J. T. Rich, D. C. Bush, C. J. Lincoski, and T. M. Harrington, "Carpal tunnel syndrome due to tophaceous gout," *Orthopedics*, vol. 27, no. 8, 862–863, 2004.

[15] B. A. Silverstein, L. J. Fine, and T. J. Armstrong, "Occupational factors and carpal tunnel syndrome," *American Journal of Industrial Medicine*, vol. 11, no. 3, pp. 343–358, 1987.

[16] M. Dahl, P. Hansen, P. Stal, D. Edmundsson, and S. P. Magnusson, "Stiffness and thickness of fascia do not explain chronic exertional compartment syndrome," *Clinical Orthopaedics and Related Research*, vol. 469, no. 12, pp. 3495–3500, 2011.

[17] M. R. Bong, D. B. Polatsch, L. M. Jazrawi, and A. S. Rokito, "Chronic exertional compartment syndrome: diagnosis and management," *Bulletin Hospital for Joint Diseases*, vol. 62, no. 3-4, pp. 77–84, 2005.

[18] L. E. Clarson, S. L. Hider, J. Belcher, C. Heneghan, E. Roddy, and C. D. Mallen, "Increased risk of vascular disease associated with gout: a retrospective, matched cohort study in the UK clinical practice research datalink," *Annals of the Rheumatic Diseases*, vol. 74, no. 4, pp. 642–647, 2015.

[19] A. J. Ramme, S. Vira, M. J. Alaia, J. Van De Leuv, and R. C. Rothberg, "Exertional rhabdomyolysis after spinning: case series and review of the literature," *Journal of Sports Medicine and Physical Fitness*, vol. 56, no. 6, pp. 789–793, 2016.

[20] J. J. Wise and P. T. Fortin, "Bilateral, exercise-induced thigh compartment syndrome diagnosed as exertional rhabdomyolysis. A case report and review of the literature," *American Journal of Sports Medicine*, vol. 25, no. 1, pp. 126–129, 1997.

[21] A. B. Mull, J. I. Wagner, T. M. Myckatyn, and A. F. Kells, "Recurrent compartment syndrome leading to the diagnosis of McArdle disease: case report," *Journal of Hand Surgery (American Volume)*, vol. 40, no. 12, pp. 2377–2379, 2015.

[22] J. A. Kint, "Fabry's disease: alpha-galactosidase deficiency," *Science*, vol. 167, no. 3922, 1268–1269, 1970.

[23] D. Rob, J. Marek, G. Dostalova, L. Golan, and A. Linhart, "Uric acid as a marker of mortality and morbidity in Fabry disease," *PLoS One*, vol. 11, no. 11, Article ID e0166290, 2016.

[24] I. Pagnini, W. Borsini, F. Cecchi et al., "Distal extremity pain as a presenting feature of Fabry's disease," *Arthritis Care and Research*, vol. 63, no. 3, pp. 390–395, 2011.

[25] D. Edmundsson and G. Toolanen, "Chronic exertional compartment syndrome in diabetes mellitus," *Diabetic Medicine*, vol. 28, no. 1, pp. 81–85, 2011.

[26] R. M. Jose, N. Viswanathan, E. Aldlyami, Y. Wilson, N. Moiemen, and R. Thomas, "A spontaneous compartment syndrome in a patient with diabetes," *Journal of Bone and Joint Surgery*, vol. 86, pp. 1068–1070, 2004.

[27] D. A. Kimbrough, K. Mehta, and R. D. Wissman, "Case of the season: saturday night palsy," *Seminars in Roentgenology*, vol. 48, no. 2, pp. 108–110, 2013.

[28] K. Kyeremanteng, G. D'Egidio, C. Wan, A. Baxter, and H. Rosenberg, "Compartment syndrome as a result of systemic capillary leak syndrome," *Case Reports in Critical Care*, vol. 2016, Article ID 4206397, 4 pages, 2016.

[29] R. H. Brown, C. Downey, and S. Izaddoost, "Compartment syndrome in all four extremities: a rare case associated with systemic capillary leak syndrome," *Hand*, vol. 6, no. 1, pp. 110–114, 2011.

[30] S. E. Willick, A. J. Deluigi, M. Taskaynatan, D. J. Petron, and D. Coleman, "Bilateral chronic exertional compartment syndrome of the forearm: a case report and review of the literature," *Current Sports Medicine Reports*, vol. 12, no. 3, pp. 170–174, 2013.

[31] K. H. Yu, S. F. Luo, L. B. Liou et al., "Concomitant septic and gouty arthritis–an analysis of 30 cases," *Rheumatology*, vol. 42, no. 9, pp. 1062–1066, 2003.

[32] J. Y. Pyo, Y. J. Ha, J. J. Song, Y. B. Park, S. K. Lee, and S. W. Lee, "Delta neutrophil index contributes to the differential diagnosis between acute gout attack and cellulitis within 24 hours after hospitalization," *Rheumatology*, vol. 56, no. 5, pp. 795–801, 2017.

[33] K. J. Paley, W. T. Jackson, and R. J. Bielski, "Septicemia causing compartment syndrome," *Orthopedics*, vol. 19, no. 2, pp. 163–166, 1996.

[34] K. Wong, D. J. Nicholson, and R. Gray, "Lower limb compartment syndrome arising from fulminant Streptococcal sepsis," *ANZ Journal of Surgery*, vol. 75, no. 8, 728–729, 2005.

[35] J. Taylor and A. Wojcik, "Upper limb compartment syndrome secondary to streptococcus pyogenes (Group A streptococcus) infection," *Journal of Surgical Case Reports*, vol. 2011, no. 3, pp. 1–4, 2011.

[36] C. E. Paletta, R. Lynch, and A. P. Knutsen, "Rhabdomyolysis and lower extremity compartment syndrome due to influenza B virus," *Annals of Plastic Surgery*, vol. 30, no. 3, 272–273, 1993.

[37] J. J. Dubost, I. Fis, P. Denis et al., "Polyarticular septic arthritis," *Medicine*, vol. 72, no. 5, pp. 296–310, 1993.

[38] M. H. Pritchard, R. L. Williams, and J. P. Heath, "Chronic compartment syndrome, an important cause of work-related upper limb disorder," *Rheumatology*, vol. 44, no. 11, pp. 1442–1446, 2005.

[39] R. A. Pedowitz and F. M. Toutounghi, "Chronic exertional compartment syndrome of the forearm flexor muscles," *Journal of Hand Surgery (American Volume)*, vol. 13, no. 5, pp. 694–696, 1988.

[40] N. Shaikh and M. Barry, "Presentation of compartment syndrome without an obvious cause can delay treatment. A case report," *Acta Orthopaedica Belgica*, vol. 69, no. 6, pp. 566–567, 2003.

[41] R. Chatterjee, "Diagnosis of chronic exertional compartment syndrome in primary care," *British Journal of General Practice*, vol. 65, no. 637, pp. e560–e562, 2015.

9

Bilateral Multiligamentous Knee Injuries

Malynda S. Messer ⓘ **, Brendan Southam** ⓘ **, and Brian M. Grawe**

Department of Orthopaedic Surgery, University of Cincinnati Medical Center, 231 Albert Sabin Way, P.O. Box 670212, Cincinnati, OH 45267-0212, USA

Correspondence should be addressed to Brendan Southam; brendan.southam@uc.edu

Academic Editor: Johannes Mayr

Bilateral knee dislocations are rare musculoskeletal injuries. We report a case of a patient who sustained traumatic bilateral knee dislocations resulting in multiligamentous injuries to both knees. The patient subsequently underwent acute ligamentous reconstructions of both knees performed at 2 weeks and 3 weeks after the initial injury. One year after these procedures, the patient has achieved excellent functional outcomes and has returned to recreational sports.

1. Introduction

Multiligamentous knee injuries (MLI) occur as a result of both high- and low-energy traumas to the knee, most commonly due to motor vehicle accidents and sport-related injuries, respectively [1]. Ultra-low-velocity mechanisms have also been observed in obese patients that experience ground-level falls [2–4]. Knee dislocation, which is the primary cause of MLI, is an uncommon orthopaedic injury, only accounting for 0.02% of musculoskeletal trauma [5–7]. However, when such injuries are present, both vascular compromise and neurologic compromise can occur and may potentially threaten limb integrity. A MLI is typically defined as a disruption of at least two of the four major stabilizing ligaments of the knee [7].

Much of the existing literature on MLI has focused on the evaluation and treatment of isolated, unilateral knee injuries. Bilateral MLI are very rare, with most of the literature limited to case reports [8–11]. A recent retrospective case-control study comparing unilateral and bilateral MLI demonstrated a higher rate of concomitant injuries, as well as postoperative complications, in patients with bilateral knee injuries [11]. Furthermore, these patients represent a unique challenge to the surgeon who must evaluate and address numerous ligamentous, meniscal, and bony injuries at the time of reconstruction to effectively restore stability and improve functional outcomes.

This article details a patient who sustained bilateral knee dislocations resulting in MLI. The acute management, surgical reconstruction, and postoperative rehabilitation of this patient are described. Given the uncommon nature of these injuries and the relative paucity of literature regarding their management, increased emphasis has been given to considerations regarding the surgical reconstruction and perioperative management of the patient in this case. The authors obtained the patient's informed written consent for print and electronic publication of this case report.

2. Case Report

This case describes a 23-year-old male who was struck by a motor vehicle. Upon arrival at our hospital, the patient had a GCS of 8. FAST exam, chest radiograph, and computed topography (CT) of the head and cervical spine were obtained and were negative.

Exam of the lower extremities revealed abrasions over the left knee and tenderness over the lateral joint line with an effusion. The right knee was diffusely tender to palpation without effusion. The patient had palpable pulses in both feet with well-perfused extremities. Ankle brachial indices were

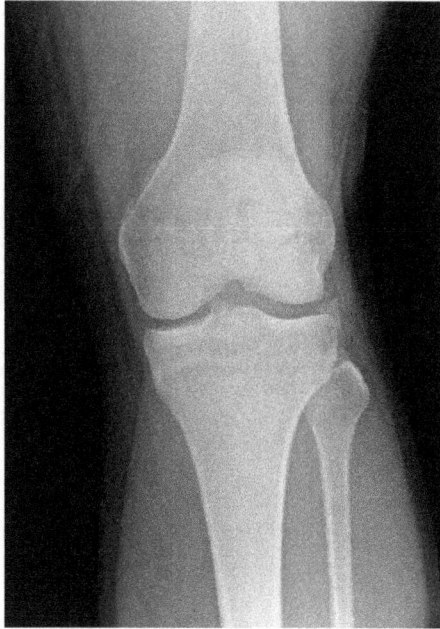

FIGURE 1: An anteroposterior radiograph of the patient's left knee demonstrating a Segond fracture.

performed and found to be >0.9. He demonstrated guarding and pain with the attempted Lachman maneuver of the left knee and slight opening of the left knee joint with varus stress. Radiographs were obtained and revealed a left knee Segond fracture (Figure 1).

Magnetic resonance imaging (MRI) of both knees was performed to evaluate for ligamentous injury. Left knee imaging demonstrated the Segond fracture along with a grade III lateral collateral ligament (LCL) tear with retraction (Figure 2), a grade II tear of the popliteus tendon and anterior cruciate ligament (ACL) (Figure 3), and a grade I medial collateral ligament (MCL) injury (Figure 4), as well as partial thickness tears of the biceps femoris and vastus medialis. Right knee imaging revealed a grade III tear of the ACL and MCL (Figure 5), grade II tears of the posterior cruciate ligament (PCL) (Figure 6), LCL, and popliteus tendon, and a medial meniscus tear. The patient was placed in bilateral hinged braces with the left knee unlocked and the right knee in locked extension to aid with transfers from a bed to a wheelchair. The patient was also given a left foot drop boot for a foot drop discovered during a secondary exam. On hospital day three, the patient was discharged home.

Nine days after the accident, the patient presented to the clinic. He noted that the left-sided foot drop was improving. On that side, he had 5/5 strength of his extensor hallucis longus and tibialis anterior (TA), without any sensory deficits in the peroneal nerve distributions. On the physical exam of the left knee, the Lachman maneuver was grade 2B (ACL injury with 5–10 mm translation without an endpoint), the varus stress test grade 3 (complete LCL tear with >10 mm opening of the lateral joint), and the valgus stress test grade 2 (MCL injury with 6–10 mm opening of the medial joint). The right lower extremity was also neurovascularly intact,

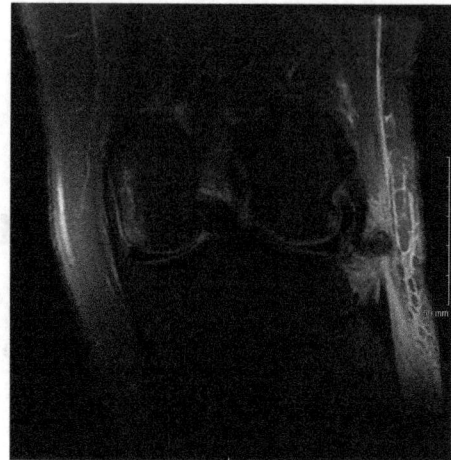

FIGURE 2: A T2 coronal MRI of the patient's left knee demonstrating a grade III lateral collateral ligament tear with retraction.

and the right knee exam revealed a grade 2A Lachman maneuver (ACL injury with 5–10 mm translation and a firm endpoint), a grade 3 posterior drawer test (complete tear of PCL with >10 mm posterior tibial translation), and a grade 3 valgus stress test (MCL injury with 11–15 mm opening of the medial joint), with a presumptive positive dial maneuver on the right side at 30 and 90 degrees (consistent with PCL and posterolateral corner (PLC) injury). However, given that the patient had bilateral PLC injuries, this physical exam finding was somewhat subjective without a reference point on the contralateral side. Subtle gapping with varus stress was also documented.

Multiligamentous reconstructions of both knees were recommended (Table 1). The left knee was addressed first in order to explore and decompress the common peroneal nerve. In regard to the right knee, preoperative physical therapy was performed to restore range of motion (ROM) before undergoing surgery.

Intraoperative findings of the left knee included a positive lateral gutter drive-through sign indicative of a PLC injury. The LCL was avulsed off the fibula, and the anterior lateral ligament (ALL) was also avulsed off the tibia. A greater than 50% disruption of the ACL was observed. Exam under anesthesia demonstrated a grade 2A Lachman maneuver, a grade 2 pivot shift, grade 3 varus instability, and instability on external rotation. The procedure included ACL reconstruction with a hamstring autograft augmented with an allograft, PLC reconstruction utilizing a TA allograft, and repair of the native avulsed LCL and ALL with suture anchors (Figure 7). First, the hamstrings were harvested and augmented with an allograft, and the tunnels for the ACL reconstruction were drilled. The PLC was then reconstructed using the anatomic technique described by Malanga et al. [12]. The native LCL was repaired using suture anchors with the overlying allograft reconstruction used to supplement it. The posterolateral capsule was then reefed into the LCL allograft reconstruction. Finally, the ACL graft was passed and fixed. Postoperatively, the patient was placed in a hinged brace locked in extension and was made toe-touch weight bearing.

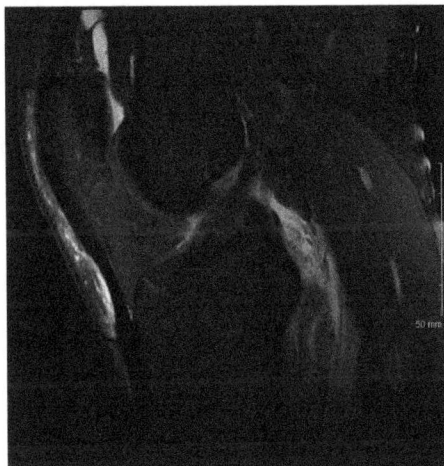

FIGURE 3: A T2 sagittal MRI of the patient's left knee demonstrating a grade II partial thickness tear of the anterior cruciate ligament.

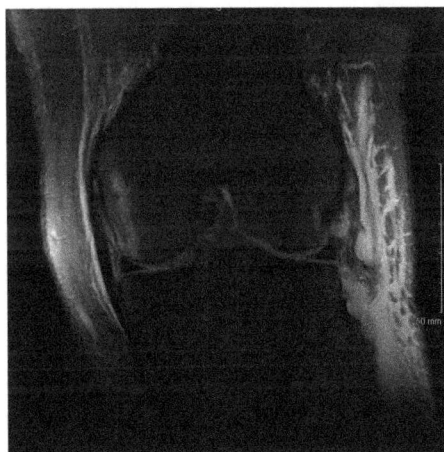

FIGURE 5: A T2 coronal MRI of the patient's right knee demonstrating a grade III MCL tear with partial extrusion of the medial meniscus.

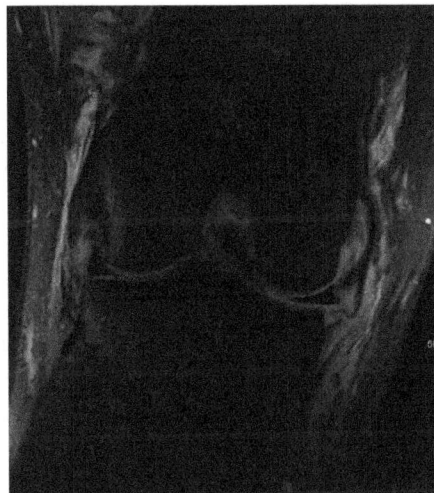

FIGURE 4: A T2 coronal MRI of the patient's left knee showing a grade I MCL injury with associated subchondral edema in the medial condyle.

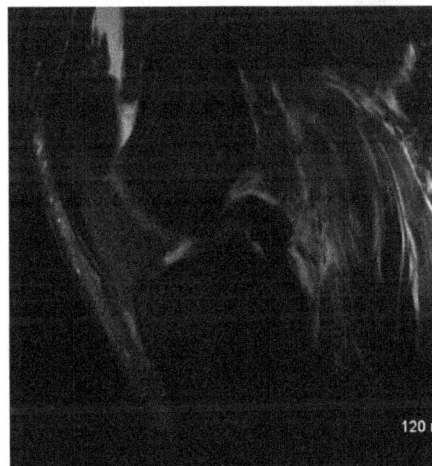

FIGURE 6: A T2 sagittal MRI of the patient's right knee demonstrating a grade II PCL tear.

The decision was made to proceed with the right knee reconstruction one week later. Exam under anesthesia revealed a grade 2A Lachman maneuver, grade 3 posterior drawer test, a grade 3 varus stress test, and a grade 2 valgus stress test. Surgery included ACL reconstruction with a bone-tendon-bone (BTB) autograft, PCL reconstruction with an Achilles allograft, MCL primary repair with additional Achilles allograft reconstruction, PLC reconstruction with TA allograft, and repair of the posterior horn of the medial meniscus (Figure 8). The lateral exposure for the PLC reconstruction was performed first, and the blind-ended sockets and fibular tunnel were drilled. An open approach to the MCL was then performed, and the injured MCL was found and tagged for later repair. The BTB autograft was then harvested for the ACL reconstruction. At this point, the posterior horn of the medial meniscus was confirmed to be torn from its root so this was repaired using sutures passed through a tibial tunnel. Guide pins were then passed for the ACL and PCL tunnels to ensure there was no convergence. Both tunnels were then reamed and the grafts passed. The

PCL was fixed first while the leg was flexed, and the ACL was then fixed with the leg in extension. The MCL repair and reconstruction with an allograft were completed using the surgical technique described by Sekiya et al. [13], followed by the PLC reconstruction which was carried out utilizing the same method noted previously. Postoperative immobilization and weight bearing status were the same as those in the contralateral side.

Range of motion and physical therapy rehabilitation began at 1 week postoperatively. Early exercises included isometric activities to strengthen the quadriceps and patella mobilization exercises. Both knees were kept in a brace locked in extension with minimal weight bearing the first six weeks following surgery. Six weeks after the initial reconstruction, the patient was instructed to begin weight bearing with crutch assistance, starting in extension and then unlocking the straight leg brace to 90° of flexion. At eight weeks post-op, the patient was transitioned out of knee braces and then given clearance to return to work ten weeks after surgery.

TABLE 1: Summary of knee injuries and surgical treatment.

	Left knee	Right knee
Injuries sustained		
ACL	Grade 2B	Grade 2A
PCL	Grade 2	Grade 3
MCL	Grade 2	Grade 3
LCL	Grade 3	Grade 2
Nerve injury	Common peroneal nerve	—
Time until surgery	2 weeks	3 weeks
Considerations	Decompression of the common peroneal nerve	Pre-op PT to improve ROM
Surgical treatment		
ACL	Hamstring autograft with allograft augmentation	Bone-tendon-bone autograft
PCL	N/A	Achilles allograft
MCL	N/A	Repair with Achilles allograft reconstruction
LCL	Repair with suture anchors	N/A
PLC	Reconstruction with a tibialis anterior allograft	Reconstruction with a tibialis anterior allograft
ALL	Repair with suture anchors	N/A
Medial meniscus	N/A	Posterior horn repair

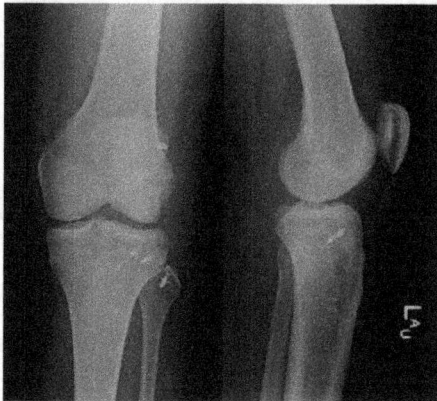

FIGURE 7: A postoperative anteroposterior and lateral radiograph of the patient's left knee following ACL reconstruction with a hamstring autograft augmented with an allograft, posterolateral corner reconstruction with an allograft, and repair of the native avulsed LCL and ALL with suture anchors.

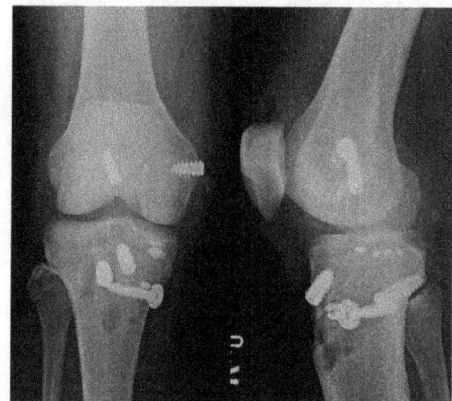

FIGURE 8: A postoperative anteroposterior and lateral radiograph of the patient's right knee following ACL reconstruction with a bone-tendon-bone autograft, PCL reconstruction with an allograft, MCL repair with additional allograft reconstruction, posterolateral corner reconstruction with an allograft, and repair of the posterior horn of the medial meniscus.

At six months post-op, the patient completed physical therapy. On the physical exam, the patient's knees demonstrated full ROM bilaterally with a grade 1A Lachman maneuver in both knees. The right knee also had a grade 2A posterior drawer test without sag. At that time, clearance was given to begin straight running. At one year post-op, the patient had returned to jogging and playing basketball recreationally and was able to participate in strenuous work (Table 2, Figure 9).

3. Discussion

Bilateral MLI occur as a result of high-energy mechanisms, with most reported cases resulting from motor vehicle accidents or motorcycle accidents [8–11]. Bilateral injuries

TABLE 2: Patient-reported functional outcomes of the left and right knee preoperatively compared to 12 months postoperatively using International Knee Documentation Committee (IKDC) and Knee Injury and Osteoarthritis Outcome Score (KOOS) patient-reported outcome measures.

	Pre-op	12-month follow-up
IKDC		
L knee	36.8	87.4
R knee	19.5	81.6
KOOS		
L knee	42.3	98.8
R knee	55.4	89.9

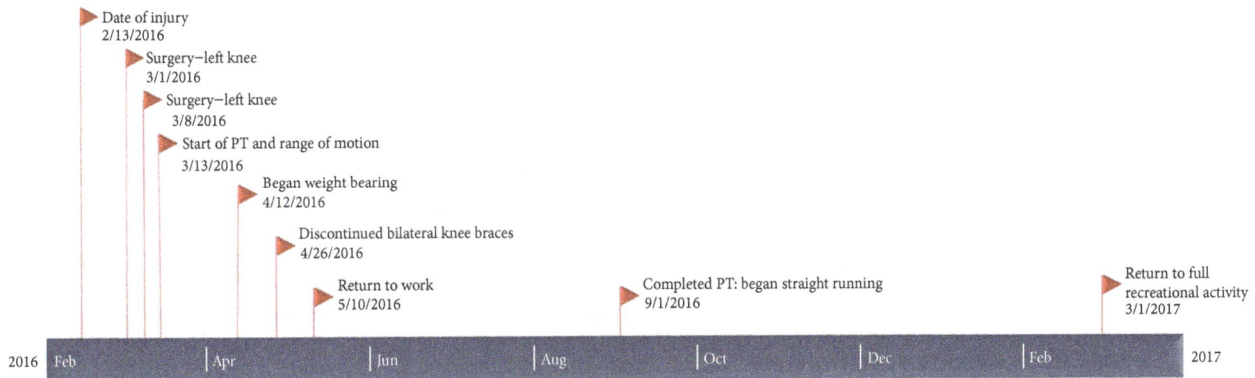

FIGURE 9: Timeline of the patient's surgical procedures and rehabilitation course.

are rare occurring in only 4-5% of all patients who sustain MLI. Compared to patients sustaining unilateral MLI, patients with bilateral injuries have significantly higher Injury Severity Scores, as well as more frequent chest, abdominal, and single-level spine injuries [11]. Given the higher incidence of concomitant injuries with these patients, careful evaluation in conjunction with a trauma team is crucial on presentation to assess for life- and limb-threatening injuries [5].

A thorough history and physical exam are necessary following knee dislocation to assess for MLI. In the acute setting, the examination can be severely limited due to patients' apprehension, guarding, and swelling [6]. Additionally, in the setting of bilateral MLI, the examiner has no contralateral reference point to compare the injured knee to when assessing for instability. Despite these challenges, a physical exam is imperative to assess the extent of ligamentous injuries following knee dislocation. Additionally, radiographs and advanced imaging should also be obtained to evaluate for the presence of periarticular fractures, tibial plateau fractures, and tendinous avulsion fractures [14]. MRI has been found to be highly sensitive to diagnosing meniscal, cruciate, and collateral ligament injuries of the knee [15].

The anterior drawer test and Lachman maneuver can both be used to detect and evaluate the extent of ACL tears, with the Lachman maneuver demonstrating higher sensitivity and specificity over the anterior drawer test [12]. In patients with MLI and concurrent PCL tears, posterior subluxation of the tibia can obscure findings from these exams [6]. Additionally, the pivot shift test used to assess for anterior knee instability loses some utility with MLI of the knee because of the inability to control for hip and leg position.

The posterior drawer test and posterior sag test are used to assess for PCL tears. In the case of a grade 3 posterior drawer test (>10 mm of posterior translation), a concomitant PCL and PLC injury should be suspected [13]. PLC stability is evaluated using the dial test. The knee is positioned at 30° and then 90° of flexion with external rotation applied to the foot. The evaluator then measures the amount of external rotation of the knee with ≥10° difference deemed significant. An isolated PLC injury is suspected with increased external rotation at 30° alone while a concomitant PCL and PLC injury is suspected with increased external rotation at both

30° and 90°. An isolated PCL injury is present with increased external rotation at 90° only [16]. This maneuver relies on contralateral comparison to determine significant differences, which, in the case of our patient with suspected bilateral PLC injuries, limited its utility. Furthermore, the dial test can also be positive in cases of isolated or combined medial-sided injuries. Therefore, it is important to concurrently examine a patient for the degree of anteromedial or posterolateral tibial rotation to distinguish PLC versus posteromedial injury of the knee [17].

Valgus and varus stress tests are used to evaluate the MCL and LCL, respectively. Increased medial joint opening with valgus stress while the knee is in full extension suggests concomitant cruciate and/or posteromedial capsular injury. Excessive lateral joint opening with varus stress suggests concomitant PLC and/or cruciate ligament injury [18]. Furthermore, varus and valgus stress radiographs provide useful adjuncts to the physical examination as they can be used to further evaluate the extent of these injuries preoperatively.

Careful assessment for a vascular injury is critical as failure to recognize such an injury may result in loss of the limb if not addressed emergently. A recent systematic review of 862 patients who experienced knee dislocations in the literature demonstrated a weighted frequency of 18% who sustained vascular injuries [19]. Conversely, a larger study of 8050 limbs with knee dislocations identified from a large private-payer database demonstrated 267 concomitant vascular injuries for an overall frequency of 3.3% [20]. While routine arteriography was previously the standard of care [19], more recent recommendations suggest selective arteriograms for cases in which an ankle-brachial index < 0.8 is observed with a well-perfused foot, with any changes in color and temperature, or with diminished pulsations in the ipsilateral foot, or for the case of an expanding hematoma. If the ABI is normal (≥0.9), no further testing is necessary, but serial exams should be performed to closely monitor the vascular status of the affected extremity.

Early identification of nerve injuries will help guide management of these injuries and potentially prevent permanent damage. In a retrospective study performed investigating MLI patterns at a level I trauma center, the incidence of peroneal nerve injury was 25% and highly associated with PLC injuries [5]. The mechanism of injury typically involves traction on the peroneal nerve resulting from a substantial varus force applied to the knee [21]. In the case of incomplete nerve palsy, the majority of patients will make a complete recovery of nerve function. Surgical intervention is indicated for all patients with complete palsies [21].

3.1. Surgical Management.

3.1. Surgical Management. Previous literature has demonstrated superior outcomes in surgically treated patients compared to those managed nonoperatively [7, 22–24]. In a recent review, operatively managed knee dislocations had superior functional outcomes with lower rates of contracture and instability and increased return to preinjury levels of activity [23]. In patients with significant comorbidities and severe concomitant injuries or those with limited functional status, nonoperative treatment may be considered. Due to this patient's young age and preinjury activity level, he was felt to be an ideal surgical candidate.

Timing of multiligamentous reconstruction has been an area of ongoing debate. Acute reconstructions refer to those that occur within 2-3 weeks of injury, while delayed reconstructions are those performed after that time [7, 11, 22]. There has been an increasing consensus that acute interventions produce superior subjective and objective functional outcomes as well as improved ligamentous stability [22, 25–29]. A systematic review by Mook et al. demonstrated that acute reconstructions are associated with significantly higher odds of residual anterior knee instability, flexion deficits, and the need for additional surgeries for manipulation or arthrolysis [30]. Arguments for delayed reconstruction include the opportunity to increase ROM of the injured knee prior to surgery as well as to allow other injuries in extra-articular structures and soft tissue to have increased time to heal, potentially avoiding further operative interventions [22, 31].

3.2. Operative Technique and Literature Review with a Focus on Controversies. Reconstructive techniques have shown improved results and decreased failure rates compared to primary repairs of injuries to the MCL, posteromedial corner, and PLC [32, 33]. Often, reconstruction of cruciate ligaments of the knee is augmented with allografts or autografts due to decreased failure rates and residual laxity compared to earlier reconstructive/repair techniques [32–35].

3.2.1. ACL. Due to lack of studies comparing different ACL reconstruction techniques in the setting of the MLI, surgical techniques are typically dictated by a surgeon's preference [36]. The current patient underwent ACL reconstruction with a hamstring autograft of the left knee, augmented with an allograft. The hamstring autograft was favored because it has shown to have less donor site morbidity and pain when compared to the bone-tendon-bone autograft [37–39]. Augmentation of the hamstring autograft was performed because the native autograft has a diameter of <8 mm, which has been shown to portend failure [40–42]. The right knee underwent ACL reconstruction with a bone-tendon-bone autograft. A hamstring autograft was not preferred on the right knee given concomitant MCL injury and the role of hamstring tendons in dynamic stabilization of the medial knee.

3.2.2. PCL. No graft or surgical technique as the gold standard for PCL reconstructions in MLI exists. The leading technique options include tibial inlay and transtibial reconstructions [36, 43]. Many grafts have been utilized including the Achilles allograft or hamstring and patellar tendon autograft [36, 43]. Right knee PCL reconstruction utilizing an Achilles allograft was the preferred method in our patient.

3.2.3. MCL and PMC. Depending on the severity of injury to medial-sided structures of the knee, both repair and reconstruction may be considered. Avulsion of the MCL can often be repaired using suture anchors for reattachment, while midsubstance damage will typically require reconstruction with or without graft augmentation [32]. Irrespective of the technique used, anatomic and isometric arrangement is crucial and should be tested arthroscopically during range of motion manipulation [43, 44]. Newer techniques promote the use of an Achilles allograft or a modified Bosworth technique using a semitendinosus graft [44, 45]. Our patient's right knee underwent primary repair of the MCL with an Achilles allograft as well as medial meniscus repair.

3.2.4. LCL and PLC. Techniques to address PLC injuries include both primary repair and reconstruction. Repair should be considered with osseous injuries such as an arcuate complex avulsion [36, 43]. The preferred reconstructive technique is an anatomic approach to restore native anatomy [43, 46–48]. Isolation of the peroneal nerve for protection is imperative, regardless of the technique utilized. Autograft tissues including those of semitendinosus tendon, biceps tendon, and split biceps tendon are used. Allograft tissues including those of TA, Achilles tendon, and bone-patellar tendon bone can also be used [36]. In our patient, the left knee underwent PLC reconstruction utilizing a semitendinosus allograft with repair of the native LCL and repair of the ALL with suture anchors, while the right knee underwent PLC repair with a TA allograft.

3.3. Complications and Comorbidities. Postsurgical complications occur at a much higher incidence in MLI as compared to single-cruciate-ligament injuries [49–52]. Some studies have suggested a direct correlation between the increased number of injured ligaments and obesity with the overall rate of complications [2, 49, 53]. Common complications that studies have addressed include high postoperative infection rates, arthrofibrosis, residual laxity, failure rates, and posttraumatic osteoarthritis. Infection rates can range anywhere from 0% to 17.4% in MLI [2, 49]. Arthrofibrosis is more common after severe injuries, acute reconstruction, and medial-sided injury repair [7, 22, 30, 36, 44, 45, 49]. Posttraumatic osteoarthritis can emerge in up to 53% of knees, due to cartilage injury and residual instability postoperatively [36, 43].

4. Conclusion

Bilateral knee dislocations are rare, and literature detailing the treatment of these types of injuries is largely limited to unilateral knee injuries. We detailed the perioperative management and operative techniques used to treat a patient with bilateral MLI who went on to regain excellent function one year postoperatively. This case highlights that each MLI represents a unique challenge to the treating surgeon regarding timing, sequence of reconstruction, and postoperative rehabilitation protocol.

Conflicts of Interest

The authors declare that there is no conflict of interest regarding the publication of this article.

References

[1] R. Rossi, F. Dettoni, M. Bruzzone, U. Cottino, D. G. D'Elicio, and D. E. Bonasia, "Clinical examination of the knee: know your tools for diagnosis of knee injuries," *Sports Medicine, Arthroscopy, Rehabilitation, Therapy & Technology*, vol. 3, no. 1, 2011.

[2] B. C. Werner, F. W. Gwathmey Jr., S. T. Higgins, J. M. Hart, and M. D. Miller, "Ultra-low velocity knee dislocations: patient characteristics, complications, and outcomes," *The American Journal of Sports Medicine*, vol. 42, no. 2, pp. 358–363, 2014.

[3] F. M. Azar, J. C. Brandt, R. H. Miller III, and B. B. Phillips, "Ultra-low-velocity knee dislocations," *The American Journal of Sports Medicine*, vol. 39, no. 10, pp. 2170–2174, 2011.

[4] A. G. Georgiadis, S. T. Guthrie, and A. D. Shepard, "Beware of ultra-low-velocity knee dislocation," *Orthopedics*, vol. 37, no. 10, pp. 656–658, 2014.

[5] E. H. Becker, J. D. Watson, and J. C. Dreese, "Investigation of multiligamentous knee injury patterns with associated injuries presenting at a level I trauma center," *Journal of Orthopaedic Trauma*, vol. 27, no. 4, pp. 226–231, 2013.

[6] J. G. Skendzel, J. K. Sekiya, and E. M. Wojtys, "Diagnosis and management of the multiligament-injured knee," *The Journal of Orthopaedic and Sports Physical Therapy*, vol. 42, no. 3, pp. 234–242, 2012.

[7] N. R. Howells, L. R. Brunton, J. Robinson, A. J. Porteus, J. D. Eldridge, and J. R. Murray, "Acute knee dislocation: an evidence based approach to the management of the multiligament injured knee," *Injury*, vol. 42, no. 11, pp. 1198–1204, 2011.

[8] J. E. Voos, B. E. Heyworth, D. P. Piasecki, R. F. Henn III, and J. D. MacGillivray, "Traumatic bilateral knee dislocations, unilateral hip dislocation, and contralateral humeral amputation: a case report," *HSS Journal*, vol. 5, no. 1, pp. 40–44, 2009.

[9] A. Foad and R. F. LaPrade, "Bilateral luxatio erecta humeri and bilateral knee dislocations in the same patient," *American Journal of Orthopedics-Belle Mead*, vol. 36, no. 11, pp. 611–613, 2007.

[10] S. Colen, M. P. J. van den Bekerom, and J. Truijen, "High-energy bilateral knee dislocations in a young man: a case report," *Journal of Orthopaedic Surgery*, vol. 21, no. 3, pp. 396–400, 2013.

[11] M. T. Burrus, B. C. Werner, J. M. Cancienne, and M. D. Miller, "Simultaneous bilateral multiligamentous knee injuries are associated with more severe multisystem trauma compared to unilateral injuries," *Knee Surgery, Sports Traumatology, Arthroscopy*, vol. 23, no. 10, pp. 3038–3043, 2015.

[12] G. A. Malanga, S. Andrus, S. F. Nadler, and J. McLean, "Physical examination of the knee: a review of the original test description and scientific validity of common orthopedic tests," *Archives of Physical Medicine and Rehabilitation*, vol. 84, no. 4, pp. 592–603, 2003.

[13] J. K. Sekiya, D. R. Whiddon, C. T. Zehms, and M. D. Miller, "A clinically relevant assessment of posterior cruciate ligament and posterolateral corner injuries: evaluation of isolated and combined deficiency," *The Journal of Bone and Joint Surgery-American Volume*, vol. 90, no. 8, pp. 1621–1627, 2008.

[14] T. M. Moore, "Fracture–dislocation of the knee," *Clinical Orthopaedics and Related Research*, vol. 156, pp. 128–140, 1981.

[15] J. Halinen, M. Koivikko, J. Lindahl, and E. Hirvensalo, "The efficacy of magnetic resonance imaging in acute multiligament injuries," *International Orthopaedics*, vol. 33, no. 6, pp. 1733–1738, 2009.

[16] R. F. LaPrade, T. V. Ly, F. A. Wentorf, and L. Engebretsen, "The posterolateral attachments of the knee: a qualitative and quantitative morphologic analysis of the fibular collateral ligament, popliteus tendon, popliteofibular ligament, and lateral gastrocnemius tendon," *The American Journal of Sports Medicine*, vol. 31, no. 6, pp. 854–860, 2003.

[17] J. Chahla, G. Moatshe, C. S. Dean, and R. F. LaPrade, "Posterolateral corner of the knee: current concepts," *Archives of Bone and Joint Surgery*, vol. 4, no. 2, pp. 97–103, 2016.

[18] A. L. Merritt and C. Wahl, "Initial assessment of the acute and chronic multiple-ligament injured (dislocated) knee," *Sports Medicine and Arthroscopy Review*, vol. 19, no. 2, pp. 93–103, 2011.

[19] O. Medina, G. A. Arom, M. G. Yeranosian, F. A. Petrigliano, and D. R. McAllister, "Vascular and nerve injury after knee dislocation: a systematic review," *Clinical Orthopaedics*, vol. 472, no. 9, pp. 2621–2629, 2014.

[20] K. M. Natsuhara, M. G. Yeranosian, J. R. Cohen, J. C. Wang, D. R. McAllister, and F. A. Petrigliano, "What is the frequency of vascular injury after knee dislocation?," *Clinical Orthopaedics and Related Research®*, vol. 472, no. 9, pp. 2615–2620, 2014.

[21] M. O'Malley, A. Pareek, P. Reardon, A. Krych, M. Stuart, and B. Levy, "Treatment of peroneal nerve injuries in the multiligament injured/dislocated knee," *The Journal of Knee Surgery*, vol. 29, no. 4, pp. 287–292, 2016.

[22] B. A. Levy, K. A. Dajani, D. B. Whelan et al., "Decision making in the multiligament-injured knee: an evidence-based systematic review," *Arthroscopy: The Journal of Arthroscopic & Related Surgery*, vol. 25, no. 4, pp. 430–438, 2009.

[23] C. J. Peskun and D. B. Whelan, "Outcomes of operative and nonoperative treatment of multiligament knee injuries: an evidence-based review," *Sports Medicine and Arthroscopy Review*, vol. 19, no. 2, pp. 167–173, 2011.

[24] B. T. Dedmond and L. C. Almekinders, "Operative versus nonoperative treatment of knee dislocations: a meta-analysis," *The American Journal of Knee Surgery*, vol. 14, no. 1, pp. 33–38, 2001.

[25] G. C. Fanelli, B. F. Giannotti, and C. J. Edson, "Arthroscopically assisted combined posterior cruciate ligament/posterior lateral complex reconstruction," *Arthroscopy: The Journal of Arthroscopic & Related Surgery*, vol. 12, no. 5, pp. 521–530, 1996.

[26] C. D. Harner, R. L. Waltrip, C. H. Bennett, K. A. Francis, B. Cole, and J. J. Irrgang, "Surgical management of knee dislocations," *The Journal of Bone and Joint Surgery. American Volume*, vol. 86-A, no. 2, pp. 262–273, 2004.

[27] R. Y. L. Liow, M. McNicholas, J. F. Keating, and R. W. Nutton, "Ligament repair and reconstruction in traumatic dislocation of the knee," *The Journal of Bone and Joint Surgery. British Volume*, vol. 85, no. 6, pp. 845–851, 2003.

[28] D. C. Wascher, J. R. Becker, J. G. Dexter, and F. T. Blevins, "Reconstruction of the anterior and posterior cruciate ligaments after knee dislocation: results using fresh-frozen nonirradiated allografts," *The American Journal of Sports Medicine*, vol. 27, no. 2, pp. 189–196, 1999.

[29] M. Tzurbakis, A. Diamantopoulos, T. Xenakis, and A. Georgoulis, "Surgical treatment of multiple knee ligament injuries in 44 patients: 2–8 years follow-up results," *Knee Surgery, Sports Traumatology, Arthroscopy*, vol. 14, no. 8, pp. 739–749, 2006.

[30] W. R. Mook, M. D. Miller, D. R. Diduch, J. Hertel, Y. Boachie-Adjei, and J. M. Hart, "Multiple-ligament knee injuries: a systematic review of the timing of operative intervention and postoperative rehabilitation," *The Journal of Bone and Joint Surgery. American Volume*, vol. 91, no. 12, pp. 2946–2957, 2009.

[31] B. A. Levy, G. C. Fanelli, D. B. Whelan et al., "Controversies in the treatment of knee dislocations and multiligament reconstruction," *The Journal of the American Academy of Orthopaedic Surgeons*, vol. 17, no. 4, pp. 197–206, 2009.

[32] J. P. Stannard, B. S. Black, C. Azbell, and D. A. Volgas, "Posteromedial corner injury in knee dislocations," *The Journal of Knee Surgery*, vol. 25, no. 5, pp. 429–434, 2012.

[33] B. A. Levy, K. A. Dajani, J. A. Morgan, J. P. Shah, D. L. Dahm, and M. J. Stuart, "Repair versus reconstruction of the fibular collateral ligament and posterolateral corner in the multiligament-injured knee," *The American Journal of Sports Medicine*, vol. 38, no. 4, pp. 804–809, 2010.

[34] B. S. Black and J. P. Stannard, "Repair versus reconstruction in acute posterolateral instability of the knee," *Sports Medicine and Arthroscopy Review*, vol. 23, no. 1, pp. 22–26, 2015.

[35] R. Kovachevich, J. P. Shah, A. M. Arens, M. J. Stuart, D. L. Dahm, and B. A. Levy, "Operative management of the medial collateral ligament in the multi-ligament injured knee: an evidence-based systematic review," *Knee Surgery, Sports Traumatology, Arthroscopy*, vol. 17, no. 7, pp. 823–829, 2009.

[36] G. C. Fanelli and C. J. Edson, "Surgical treatment of combined PCL-ACL medial and lateral side injuries (global laxity): surgical technique and 2- to 18-year results," *The Journal of Knee Surgery*, vol. 25, no. 4, pp. 307–316, 2012.

[37] A. Matsumoto, S. Yoshiya, H. Muratsu et al., "A comparison of bone-patellar tendon-bone and bone-hamstring tendon-bone autografts for anterior cruciate ligament reconstruction," *The American Journal of Sports Medicine*, vol. 34, no. 2, pp. 213–219, 2006.

[38] K. B. Freedman, M. J. D'Amato, D. D. Nedeff, A. Kaz, and B. R. Bach, "Arthroscopic anterior cruciate ligament reconstruction: a metaanalysis comparing patellar tendon and hamstring tendon autografts," *The American Journal of Sports Medicine*, vol. 31, no. 1, pp. 2–11, 2003.

[39] L. Ejerhed, J. Kartus, N. Sernert, K. Köhler, and J. Karlsson, "Patellar tendon or semitendinosus tendon autografts for anterior cruciate ligament reconstruction?," *The American Journal of Sports Medicine*, vol. 31, no. 1, pp. 19–25, 2003.

[40] B. M. Grawe, P. N. Williams, A. Burge et al., "Anterior cruciate ligament reconstruction with autologous hamstring: can preoperative magnetic resonance imaging accurately predict graft diameter?," *Orthopaedic Journal of Sports Medicine*, vol. 4, no. 5, 2016.

[41] E. J. Conte, A. E. Hyatt, C. J. Gatt Jr., and A. Dhawan, "Hamstring autograft size can be predicted and is a potential risk factor for anterior cruciate ligament reconstruction failure," *Arthroscopy: The Journal of Arthroscopic & Related Surgery*, vol. 30, no. 7, pp. 882–890, 2014.

[42] M. R. Boniello, P. M. Schwingler, J. M. Bonner, S. P. Robinson, A. Cotter, and K. F. Bonner, "Impact of hamstring graft diameter on tendon strength: a biomechanical study," *Arthroscopy: The Journal of Arthroscopic & Related Surgery*, vol. 31, no. 6, pp. 1084–1090, 2015.

[43] F. W. Gwathmey Jr., D. A. Shafique, and M. D. Miller, "Our approach to the management of the multiple-ligament knee injury," *Operative Techniques in Sports Medicine*, vol. 18, no. 4, pp. 235–244, 2010.

[44] R. G. Marx and I. Hetsroni, "Surgical technique: medial collateral ligament reconstruction using Achilles allograft for combined knee ligament injury," *Clinical Orthopaedics*, vol. 470, no. 3, pp. 798–805, 2012.

[45] E. Argintar, "Multiligamentous knee reconstruction," *Orthopedics*, vol. 36, no. 7, pp. 527–528, 2013.

[46] S. A. Kuzma, R. M. Chow, W. M. Engasser, M. J. Stuart, and B. A. Levy, "Reconstruction of the posterolateral corner of the knee with Achilles tendon allograft," *Arthroscopy Techniques*, vol. 3, no. 3, pp. e393–e398, 2014.

[47] P. Djian, "Posterolateral knee reconstruction," *Orthopaedics & Traumatology: Surgery & Research*, vol. 101, no. 1, pp. S159–S170, 2015.

[48] W. A. van der Wal, P. J. C. Heesterbeek, T. G. van Tienen, V. J. Busch, J. H. M. van Ochten, and A. B. Wymenga, "Anatomical reconstruction of posterolateral corner and combined injuries of the knee," *Knee Surgery, Sports Traumatology, Arthroscopy*, vol. 24, no. 1, pp. 221–228, 2016.

[49] S. Cook, T. J. Ridley, M. A. McCarthy et al., "Surgical treatment of multiligament knee injuries," *Knee Surgery, Sports Traumatology, Arthroscopy*, vol. 23, no. 10, pp. 2983–2991, 2015.

[50] J. Halinen, J. Lindahl, and E. Hirvensalo, "Range of motion and quadriceps muscle power after early surgical treatment of acute combined anterior cruciate and grade-III medial collateral ligament injuries: a prospective randomized study," *The Journal of Bone and Joint Surgery-American Volume*, vol. 91, no. 6, pp. 1305–1312, 2009.

[51] S.-I. Bin and T.-S. Nam, "Surgical outcome of 2-stage management of multiple knee ligament injuries after knee dislocation," *Arthroscopy: The Journal of Arthroscopic & Related Surgery*, vol. 23, no. 10, pp. 1066–1072, 2007.

[52] A. K. L. Tay and P. B. MacDonald, "Complications associated with treatment of multiple ligament injured (dislocated) knee," *Sports Medicine and Arthroscopy Review*, vol. 19, no. 2, pp. 153–161, 2011.

[53] L. Engebretsen, M. A. Risberg, B. Robertson, T. C. Ludvigsen, and S. Johansen, "Outcome after knee dislocations: a 2–9 years follow-up of 85 consecutive patients," *Knee Surgery, Sports Traumatology, Arthroscopy*, vol. 17, no. 9, pp. 1013–1026, 2009.

10

Talus Bipartitus: A Rare Anatomical Variant Presenting as an Entrapment Neuropathy of the Tibial Nerve within the Tarsal Tunnel

M. O. Abrego ⓘ,[1] **F. L. De Cicco,**[1] **N. E. Gimenez,**[1] **M. O. Marquesini,**[2] **P. Sotelano,**[1] **M. N. Carrasco,**[1] **and M. G. Santini Araujo**[1]

[1]*Trauma and Orthopaedics Institute "Carlos Ottolenghi", Italian Hospital of Buenos Aires, Peron 4190, C11000ABD CABA, Argentina*
[2]*Center for Diagnostic Imaging, Italian Hospital of Buenos Aires, Peron 4190, C11000ABD CABA, Argentina*

Correspondence should be addressed to M. O. Abrego; mariano.abrego@hospitalitaliano.org.ar

Academic Editor: Bayram Unver

Tarsal tunnel syndrome is an entrapment neuropathy of the tibial nerve within the tarsal tunnel that lies beneath the retinaculum on the medial side of the ankle. It is often underdiagnosed. Talus bipartitus is a rare anatomical variant; only a few cases have been described in medical literature. We report a case of a 36-year-old female with tarsal tunnel syndrome secondary to a talus bipartitus undergoing surgical treatment with good clinical outcome. To our knowledge, talus bipartitus presenting as tarsal tunnel syndrome has no previous reports. Image studies and physical examination are crucial to reach precise diagnosis.

1. Introduction

Tarsal tunnel syndrome (TTS) is an entrapment neuropathy of the tibial nerve or its branches within the tarsal tunnel that lies beneath the retinaculum on the medial side of the ankle. This condition is frequently underdiagnosed. Main symptoms are burning, cramping, and pain along the foot plantar region. The typical clinical profile includes worsening of symptoms as the day goes on and nocturnal awakening with tingling feet [1, 2].

Clinical tests include the dorsiflexion-eversion provocative manoeuvre in which the tibial nerve is compressed by positioning the ankle in passively maximally eversion and dorsiflexion while all of the metatarsophalangeal joints are maximally dorsiflexed and held in this position for five to ten seconds [3]. Tinel's sign is present in most of the cases, having a 92% sensibility and 100% specificity, with a predictive value of 85%. The use of electromyography may also be helpful [2, 4]. TTS aetiology varies from heel varus,

arthritis, tendinopathy, osteophytes, lipomas, perineural fibrosis, trauma, systemic diseases, and venous pathology to postsurgical injuries [4–6]. There is also a considerable number of idiopathic cases.

Talus bipartitus (TB) is a rare anatomical anomaly of the talus. It consists of two talar fragments separated by the presence of articular cartilage. There are less than 30 reported cases of TB in medical literature. There is no information about the prevalence of this infrequent condition.

We present a case of a 36-year-old female with tarsal tunnel syndrome due to a talus bipartitus with a medial prominence, undergoing surgical treatment with good clinical outcome.

2. Case Report

A 36-year-old female patient presented with a 4-year history of right ankle pain. She had significate loss of weight and started physical activity just before the symptoms appeared

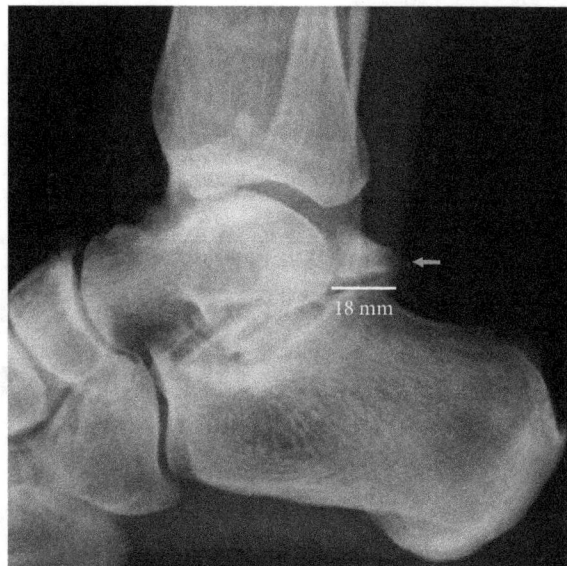

FIGURE 1: X-ray of the hind foot, lateral view, showing a 1.8 cm accessory posterior bone fragment (arrow).

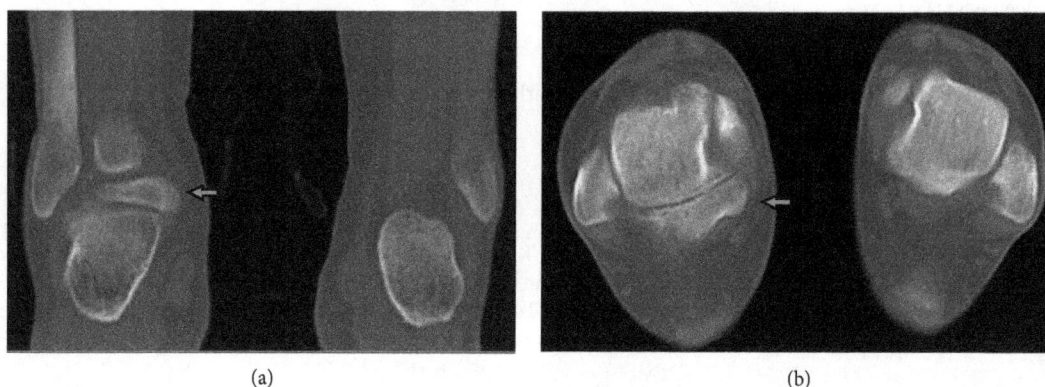

(a)   (b)

FIGURE 2: Comparative CT scan showing posterior bone process, displacing into the medial side (arrow) in both coronal (a) and axial (b) view.

four years ago. No history of trauma was reported. First diagnosis was synovitis, for which the patient underwent physical therapy with torpid outcome. She experienced paraesthesia along the posterior and medial aspect of the ankle and foot. Symptoms got worse at the end of the day, with cramping episodes in the foot. Physical examination revealed a positive dorsiflexion-eversion test provoking numbness of the foot. Tinel's sign was positive. Ankle range of motion was limited due to pain, scored 8 using the Visual Analog Score (VAS). The patient had a preoperative score of 40 points, according to the American Orthopaedic Foot and Ankle Society (AOFAS). Bilateral electromyography (EMG) was performed, disclosing abnormal adductor hallucis and adductor digiti quinti neurophysiologic parameters in comparison to the asymptomatic side.

Initial plain radiographs showed a considerable (1.8 cm) posterior bone fragment in relation with the talus (Figure 1). CT scan was then performed, which showed the presence of an articulated accessory bone. At this point, talus bipartitus (TB) diagnosis was suspected (Figure 2). MRI disclosed the presence of an inflammatory process, bone

fragment covered with cartilage, and what appears to be a degenerative synchondrosis as a consequence of posteromedial impingement (Figure 3).

In this scenario, a surgical procedure was indicated due to increasing symptoms and several conservative treatment trials with no response.

Preoperatory assessment included three-dimensional CT scan images to get full awareness of the bone fragment's specific anatomy. Anatomic relationship between the tibial nerve, posterior tibial artery, flexor hallucis longus, flexor digitorium longus, and tibialis posterior tendon and the bone fragment was assessed with the help of MRI. Though fixation of the accessory bone has been previously reported, in the index case, this was not an option because of its particular shape, with a medial protuberance invading the tarsal tunnel.

Excision of the bone fragment was performed. A medial approach was used. Both tibialis posterior tendon and neurovascular bundle were identified and carefully preserved. The bone fragment was removed and the tunnel was released (Figure 4). Postoperative care included cast immobilization and a 30-day weight-bearing restriction. Postoperative

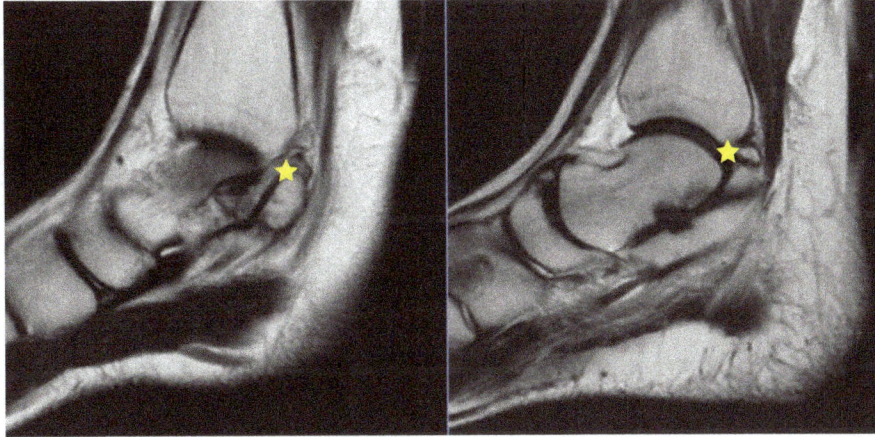

FIGURE 3: MRI, sagittal view of the ankle; the presence of cartilage between the talar body and the accessory bone can be appreciated (stars).

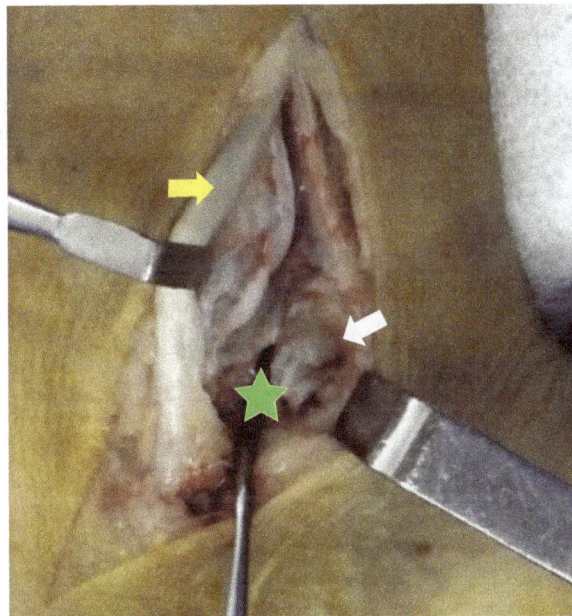

FIGURE 4: Medial approach with exposure of the pseudoarticular space (star), tibialis posterior retracted forward (yellow arrow), and the accessory bone fragment (white arrow).

radiographs showed the complete absence of residual bone fragment (Figure 5). Histological findings disclosed mature bone with articular cartilage surface. After 6 months of follow-up, the patient had a VAS score of 2 and an AOFAS score of 87. At a 2-year follow-up, VAS was 1 and AOFAS was 96. Patient had no residual pain and no recurrence of neurological symptoms.

3. Discussion

All image studies suggested that the cause of our patient's pain and neurological condition was attributable to the presence of the unusual bone fragment. Furthermore, the particular anatomical shape of this bone fragment with a clear prominence towards the medial aspect of the ankle reinforced the diagnosis.

However, image studies were not able to confirm as a gold standard method whether this bone prominence was indeed entrapping any nerve structure or even in contact with. Though it may have seemed that diagnosis in this index case was easy to achieve, the patient lingered for a while with no diagnosis.

MRI is a good method for identifying pathologic causes of TTS, specific space occupying lesions [7]. McSweeney and Cichero [8] demonstrated in their study that MRI could identify the cause of TTS in 88% of patients with symptoms. That being said, TTS diagnosis is not always easy to achieve and is regularly underdiagnosed [4, 7]. Physical examination is crucial. TTS specific cause can be identified in up to 80% of cases [9, 10]; provocative tests such as Tinel's sign are mandatory to reach neuropathy diagnosis [11, 12]. When clinical findings are not conclusive, axonal injury can be

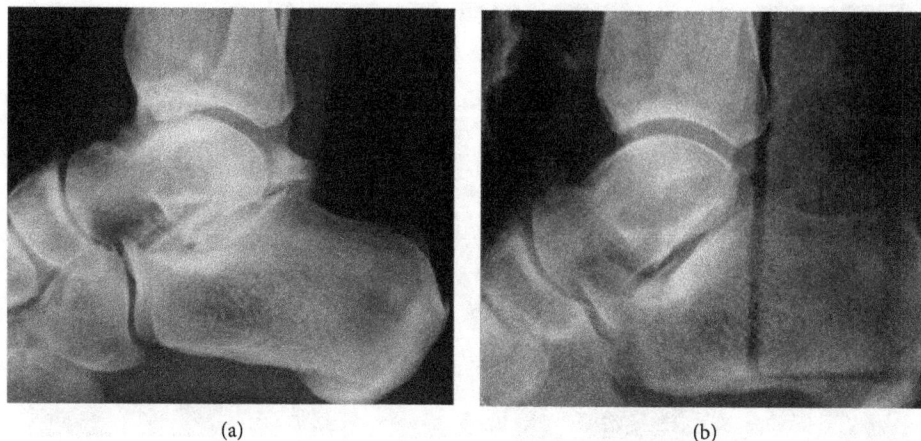

(a)   (b)

FIGURE 5: Comparative preoperative (a) and postoperative X-rays with no residual bone (b).

demonstrated with an EMG. In this particular case, both MRI and EMG worked together to achieve proper diagnosis. EMG by itself will never spur a suspicion of any bone anatomical variation. MRI is helpful to study the anatomy of the tarsal tunnel and to reinforce TB diagnosis (presence of cartilage). CT scan is even a better method to reach TB diagnosis and to study its particular anatomy.

Reichert et al [5]. reported a series of 31 patients with TTS undergoing surgical treatment. Only in 9 patients an internal cause was found (ganglion, neuroma, tendinopathy, and lipoma). They concluded that knowing the cause of TTS improves the effectiveness of treatment.

Surgical treatment of TTS is still challenging. Gondring et al. [13] showed in their study that only 51% of the patients with TTS had better quality of life after surgical decompression. Other series have been reported, with only 42% satisfactory outcome in patients with TTS postsurgery [14].

To our knowledge, only 1 case of TTS has been reported secondary to a skeletal anomaly (accessory ossicle) [15]. TB is a very rare skeletal variation. Tsuruta et al. [16] performed a radiological study with more than 3000 feet without finding TB. According to medical literature, its aetiology still remains uncertain. It usually constitutes about one-third of the posterior aspect of the talar body and is separated from that structure by a frontal split [17].

In the clinical practice, TB is vaguely seen and most physicians tend to attribute symptoms to more frequent conditions. Differential diagnosis of TB includes the presence of an os trigonum, which lacks of articular surface and has a higher incidence (13%). Zwiers et al. [18] identified only 23 reported cases of TB in their systematic review. None of them involved neuropathy entrapment. Main symptoms described were pain, swelling, and restricted range of motion. Surgical treatment included removal or fixation of the accessory bone.

In this index case, surgical technique was focused in removing the bone fragment, preserving structures and recognizing any nerve injury if present. We cannot provide any reliable information about surgical approach to TTS release by reporting one single case, which may vary according to aetiology.

We present what it seems to be the first reported case of tarsal tunnel syndrome secondary to talus bipartitus. TTS is relatively common but has many different causes. Clinical findings and proper imaging are crucial to reach precise diagnosis and to conduct preoperatory planning.

Disclosure

All authors certify that their institution has approved the reporting of this case.

Conflicts of Interest

All authors declare that there are no competing interests regarding the publication of this paper.

Acknowledgments

The study was performed at the Italian Hospital of Buenos Aires, Argentina.

References

[1] S. Nayagam, G. M. Slowvik, and L. Klenerman, "The tarsal tunnel syndrome: a study of pressures within the tunnel and review of the anatomy," *The Foot*, vol. 1, no. 2, pp. 93–96, 1991.

[2] A. L. Dellon, "The four medial ankle tunnels: a critical review of perceptions of tarsal tunnel syndrome and neuropathy," *Neurosurgery Clinics of North America*, vol. 19, no. 4, pp. 629–648, 2008.

[3] M. Kinoshita, R. Okuda, J. Morikawa, T. Jotoku, and M. Abe, "The dorsiflexion-eversion test for diagnosis of tarsal tunnel syndrome," *The Journal of Bone and Joint Surgery. American Volume*, vol. 83-A, no. 12, pp. 1835–1839, 2001.

[4] M. Ahmad, K. Tsang, P. J. Mackenney, and A. O. Adedapo, "Tarsal tunnel syndrome: a literature review," *Foot and Ankle Surgery*, vol. 18, no. 3, pp. 149–152, 2012.

[5] P. Reichert, K. Zimmer, W. Wnukiewicz, S. Kuliński, P. Mazurek, and J. Gosk, "Results of surgical treatment of tarsal tunnel syndrome," *Foot and Ankle Surgery*, vol. 21, no. 1, pp. 26–29, 2015.

[6] G. J. Sammarco and L. Chang, "Outcome of surgical treatment of tarsal tunnel syndrome," *Foot & Ankle International*, vol. 24, no. 2, pp. 125–131, 2003.

[7] P. E. Doneddu, D. Coraci, C. Loreti, G. Piccinini, and L. Padua, "Tarsal tunnel syndrome: still more opinions than evidence. Status of the art," *Neurological Sciences*, vol. 38, no. 10, pp. 1735–1739, 2017.

[8] S. C. McSweeney and M. Cichero, "Tarsal tunnel syndrome - a narrative literature review," *The Foot*, vol. 25, no. 4, pp. 244–250, 2015.

[9] D. S. Bailie and A. S. Kelikian, "Tarsal tunnel syndrome: diagnosis, surgical technique, and functional outcome," *Foot & Ankle International*, vol. 19, no. 2, pp. 65–72, 1998.

[10] W. R. Cimino, "Tarsal tunnel syndrome: review of the literature," *Foot & Ankle*, vol. 11, no. 1, pp. 47–52, 1990.

[11] M. Mondelli, S. Passero, and F. Giannini, "Provocative tests in different stages of carpal tunnel syndrome," *Clinical Neurology and Neurosurgery*, vol. 103, no. 3, pp. 178–183, 2001.

[12] A. T. Patel, K. Gaines, R. Malamut et al., "Usefulness of electrodiagnostic techniques in the evaluation of suspected tarsal tunnel syndrome: an evidence-based review," *Muscle & Nerve*, vol. 32, no. 2, pp. 236–240, 2005.

[13] W. H. Gondring, B. Shields, and S. Wenger, "An outcomes analysis of surgical treatment of tarsal tunnel syndrome," *Foot & Ankle International*, vol. 24, no. 7, pp. 545–550, 2003.

[14] P. J. Ward and M. L. Porter, "Tarsal tunnel syndrome: a study of the clinical and neurophysiological results of decompression," *Journal of the Royal College of Surgeons of Edinburgh*, vol. 43, no. 1, pp. 35-36, 1998.

[15] T. A. Sweed, S. A. Ali, and S. Choudhary, "Tarsal tunnel syndrome secondary to an unreported ossicle of the talus: a case report," *The Journal of Foot and Ankle Surgery*, vol. 55, no. 1, pp. 173–175, 2016.

[16] T. Tsuruta, Y. Shiokawa, A. Kato et al., "Radiological study of the accessory skeletal elements in the foot and ankle (author's transl)," *Nippon Seikeigeka Gakkai Zasshi*, vol. 55, no. 4, pp. 357–370, 1981.

[17] S. Rammelt, H. Zwipp, and A. Prescher, "Talus bipartitus: a rare skeletal variation," *The Journal of Bone and Joint Surgery. American Volume*, vol. 93, no. 6, pp. e21(1)–e21(9), 2011.

[18] R. Zwiers, P. A. J. de Leeuw, G. M. M. J. Kerkhoffs, and C. N. van Dijk, "Talus bipartitus: a systematic review and report of two cases with arthroscopic treatment," *Knee Surgery, Sports Traumatology, Arthroscopy*, vol. 26, no. 7, pp. 2131-2141, 2018.

11

Surgical Treatment of Intrapelvic Pseudotumour after Hip Resurfacing Arthroplasty

Cristian Barrientos,[1,2] Julian Brañes,[3] José-Luis Llanos,[4] Alvaro Martinez,[3] and Maximiliano Barahona ⓘ[1,2]

[1]Orthopaedic Department at Hospital Clinico Universidad de Chile, Santos Dumontt 999, Santiago, Chile
[2]Hospital Clinico Universidad de Chile, 999 Santos Dumont av., Independencia, Santiago 8380456, Chile
[3]Orthopaedic Department at Hospital San José, 1196 San Jose av. Independencia, Santiago 8380419, Chile
[4]Coloproctology Surgery at Hospital Clinico Universidad de Chile, Santos Dumontt 999, Santiago, Chile

Correspondence should be addressed to Maximiliano Barahona; maxbarahonavasquez@gmail.com

Academic Editor: Koichi Sairyo

Hip replacement is the surgery of the last century due to its impact on the quality of life. A pseudotumour is a rare complication of hip arthroplasty, and it is related to a metal-bearing surface. Pseudotumour is a challenging scenario for hip surgeons due to poor clinical outcomes. The patient consulted for hip pain and paresthesia in the left lower extremity, and analyses showed that the cause was a sizeable intrapelvic pseudotumour. A multidisciplinary team surgery was planned. At first, an infraumbilical approach was made to resect the intrapelvic-retroperitoneum portion of the pseudotumour. Then, a posterolateral hip approach was performed, to resect the remaining portion of the pseudotumour and revision arthroplasty. At five years of follow-up, there are no clinical or imaging signs of recurrence of the pseudotumour. Treatment evidence is limited to a series of cases and expert opinions; we encourage complete resection and revision arthroplasty.

1. Introduction

Hip replacement is the surgery of the last century due to its impact on the life of quality [1]. Different types of prosthesis design exist. In traditional total hip replacement (THR), the head of the femur is removed, and a stem is placed inside the femoral metaphysis. In the early 1990s, hip resurfacing arthroplasty (HRA) was introduced; there was no significant difference in the acetabulum component, but in the femoral side, only the femur head is replaced and a short stem is used; therefore, the metaphysis of the femur remains intact. So, compared to THR, HRA preserves more bone, has lower stress shielding, and has lower surgery morbidity (i.e., less bleeding). A few case series have shown good results in the short and medium terms [2, 3].

Two major concerns for HRA are described: a higher incidence of neck fracture because, for design, more stress is placed in the neck of the femur and the other concern is metal ion risk [4]. All prosthesis models have a bearing surface: one in the acetabulum and other in the femoral head. Different materials have been used as a bearing surface, such as polyethylene, ceramic, and metal. The amount and size of the debris depend on the material used as a bearing surface and are associated with the aseptic loosening of the prosthesis [5]. HRA uses metal on metal-bearing surface only, and this bearing surface is related to a particular complication known as a pseudotumour.

The most specific histological finding of a pseudotumor is a lymphocytic immune response described as an aseptic lymphocytic injury-associated vasculitis (ALVAL) [6]. Its formation has been associated with high serum levels of cobalt and chromium; however, the physiopathology remains unclear given that the most frequent findings consist of an infiltrate of monocytes, reparative tissue, giant cells, and areas of necrosis [7, 8].

The surgical treatment of pseudotumour is a theme of discussion, and only a few clinical series have been published [9]. Treatment should include pseudotumour resection and revision hip arthroplasty (RHA). The extension of the pseudotumour resection is on a debate and, sometimes due to its extension, is not completely resected. RHA consists of removing all the prosthetic components, including the bearing surface and replacing them with a new prosthesis [10].

Our purpose is to report the case of a patient in which a complete resection of an intrapelvic pseudotumor that compromised the retroperitoneum, following an HRA, was performed, showing no signs of recurrence after five years of follow-up.

2. Case Report

A 46-year-old female patient underwent a left hip resurfacing arthroplasty (Birmingham®, UK) for severe hip osteoarthritis, secondary to developmental hip dysplasia, in 2005. She had a good initial outcome with no complications. The surgery was performed in another centre.

She consulted with us for the first time six years later (2011) complaining about hip pain and paresthesia in the anterior left thigh, which progressively compromised her function. She denied fever or other signs of infection. Physical exams revealed a mild claudication gait and limited active and passive hip flexion. No palpable masses or skin lesions were observed. Laboratory analyses showed a WBC, ESR, and CRP within normal limits. No signs of osteolysis were found in the hip anteroposterior radiography; nevertheless, a vertical cup was noted (Figure 1). It was compared with the immediate postsurgery radiography, and no change was noted.

Computed tomography and an MRI demonstrated a biloculate hypodense mass of approximately 34×19 cm that extended from the retroperitoneum, compromising the left iliopsoas muscle and an intimate contact with the femoral vessels, to the left hip and the left femoral-cutaneous nerve (Figures 2 and 3). A routine hip arthrocentesis was performed to rule out infection. The cytochemical and Gram analyses were negative for infection. Cultures were negative after 14 days.

Thus, a pseudotumour was the diagnosis, and surgery led by an orthopaedic surgeon and a coloproctology surgeon was planned. The aim was to remove the pseudotumor entirely and to perform an RHA. As the CT shows (Figure 2(d)), the intrapelvic mass was significant, so it was decided to start with a laparotomy by the coloproctology surgeon.

First, the patient was positioned supine, and an infraumbilical laparotomy was performed; the left paracolic gutter was dissected to address the retroperitoneum. The iliac vessels and the left ureter were protected, and an irregular cystic mass was observed in direct contact with the psoas muscle and femoral bundle. It was punctured, and an abundant grey milky-like fluid was obtained. The membrane of the cyst was carefully removed, protecting the vessels and the femoral nerve. The lesion was completely resected, and samples were sent for biopsy and cultures (Figure 4).

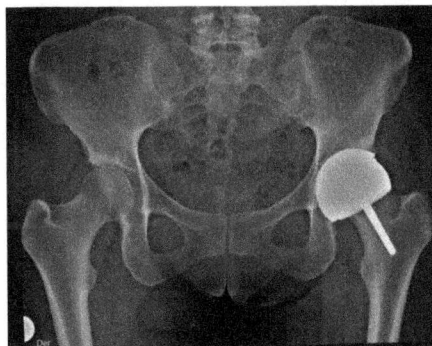

FIGURE 1: Postoperative AP radiograph showing the left hip's resurfacing arthroplasty. Femoral head was 46 mm. Acetabular cup was 52 mm and was placed too vertical; malposition of the components is a risk factor for pseudotumour [8].

Then, the patient was repositioned in lateral decubitus, and a posterolateral hip approach was performed. The capsule was looking distend; it was punctured and then, a 30 cc fluid was obtained, similar to the liquid found in the retroperitoneum. After capsulotomy and femoral neck osteotomy, all arthroplasty components were removed, noticing an anterosuperior wall defect in the acetabulum. After complete pseudotumour resection, RHA was performed (Figure 5). The acetabular cup component was a cementless 56 mm Dynasty® (Wright Medical, Memphis, USA), and the femoral component was a high offset femoral cementless stem (Stellaris®, Mathys, Bettlach, Switzerland, no. 17). The bearing surface used was polyethylene-ceramic, being Dynasty® polyethylene liner, on the acetabulum and a 40 mm ceramic on the femoral head (BIOLOX®, Mathys, Bettlach, Switzerland). Post surgery, an anteroposterior pelvic radiograph was taken (Figure 6). After fourteen days, tissue cultures obtained at surgery were negative for infection.

Histopathological findings confirm the pseudotumour. The analyses reported an extensive aseptic inflammatory infiltrate of macrophages with detritus inside near a necrotic tissue area (Figure 7(a)). A PAS histochemical stain confirmed these findings. No signs of ALVAL were observed. Also, reparative tissue was found with black particulate material corresponding to the prosthetic material near the neoformation of blood vessels and fibroblast (Figure 7(b)).

No early- or late-surgery complication is reported. Since post surgery, the patient progressively recovers the hip's range of motion and normal gait. In the last follow-up, 60 months postoperatively, the patient is in excellent condition with no functional limitations and a full hip range of motion. Radiological exams, which included an annual MRI, showed no pseudotumour formation and no arthroplasty loosening. The MRI at five years of follow-up is shown in Figure 8.

3. Discussion

Pseudotumour is a rare complication of hip arthroplasty, and it is related to a metal-bearing surface [11]. The treatment planned in this case, which included complete resection of

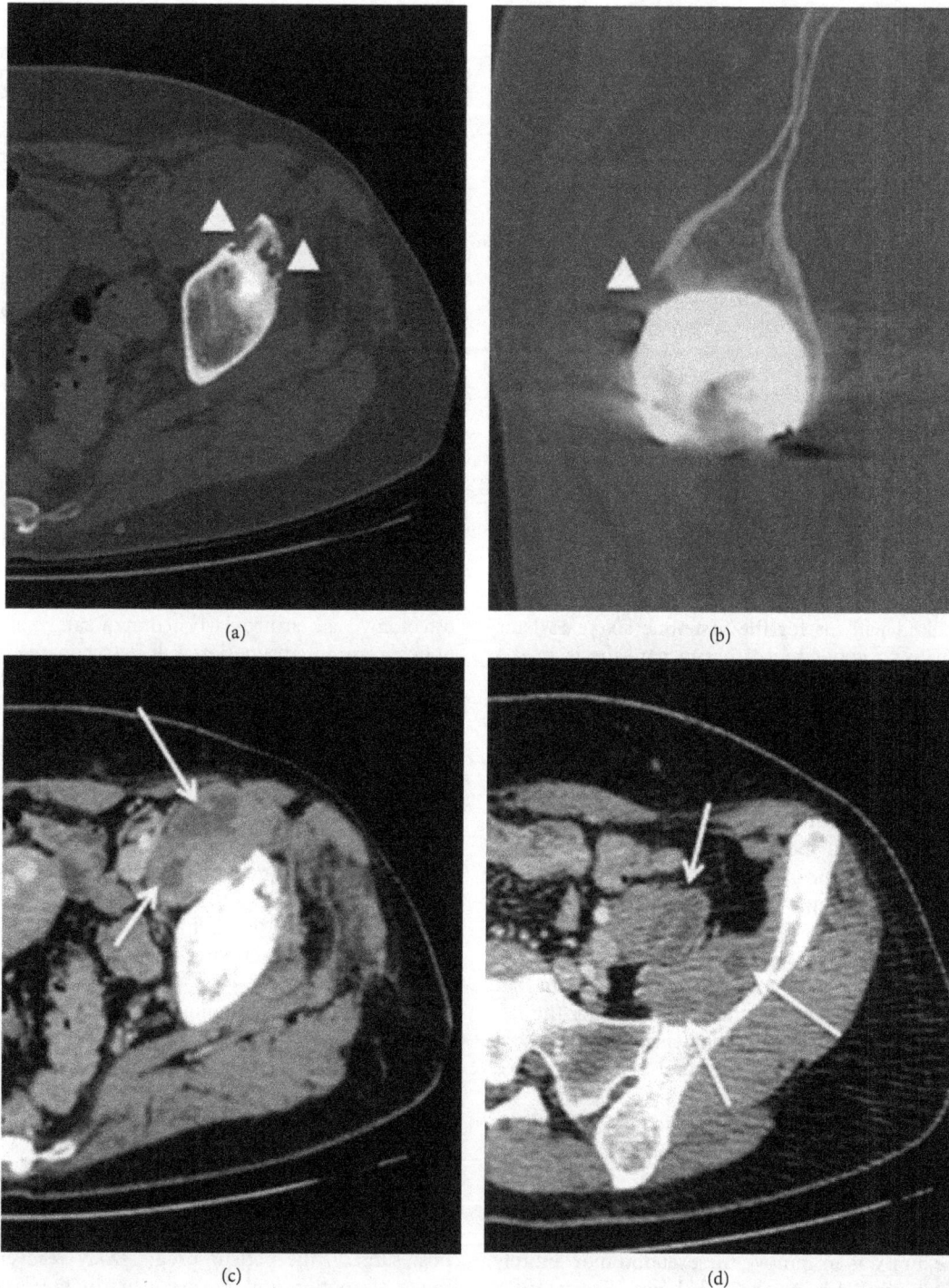

FIGURE 2: Computed tomography of the left hip: axial (a) and sagittal (b) views show periprosthetic osteolytic lesions (arrow head) in the anterior acetabular roof. Axial views (c, d) show a polylobate cystic lesion in the retroperitoneum compromising the left iliopsoas muscle with white arrows.

the pseudotumour and RHA, achieves excellent clinical outcomes, as the patient had no signs of pseudotumour after five years of follow-up.

It is well known that pseudotumour goes underdiagnosed; recent studies show that the prevalence of pseudotumour could be higher than previously reported [12]. In a cohort of 125 patients (143 hips, Birmingham® HRA), 28% had pseudotumour in the CT study. Most patients (72.5%) were asymptomatic. The most common symptoms described were a hip pain, a palpable mass, or paresthesia [13]. Another study showed a substantially higher incidence of pseudotumour formation in metal-on-metal THA, reaching 42 patients (39%) diagnosed with a pseudotumour, while 13 (12%) of these were symptomatic and were revised [9].

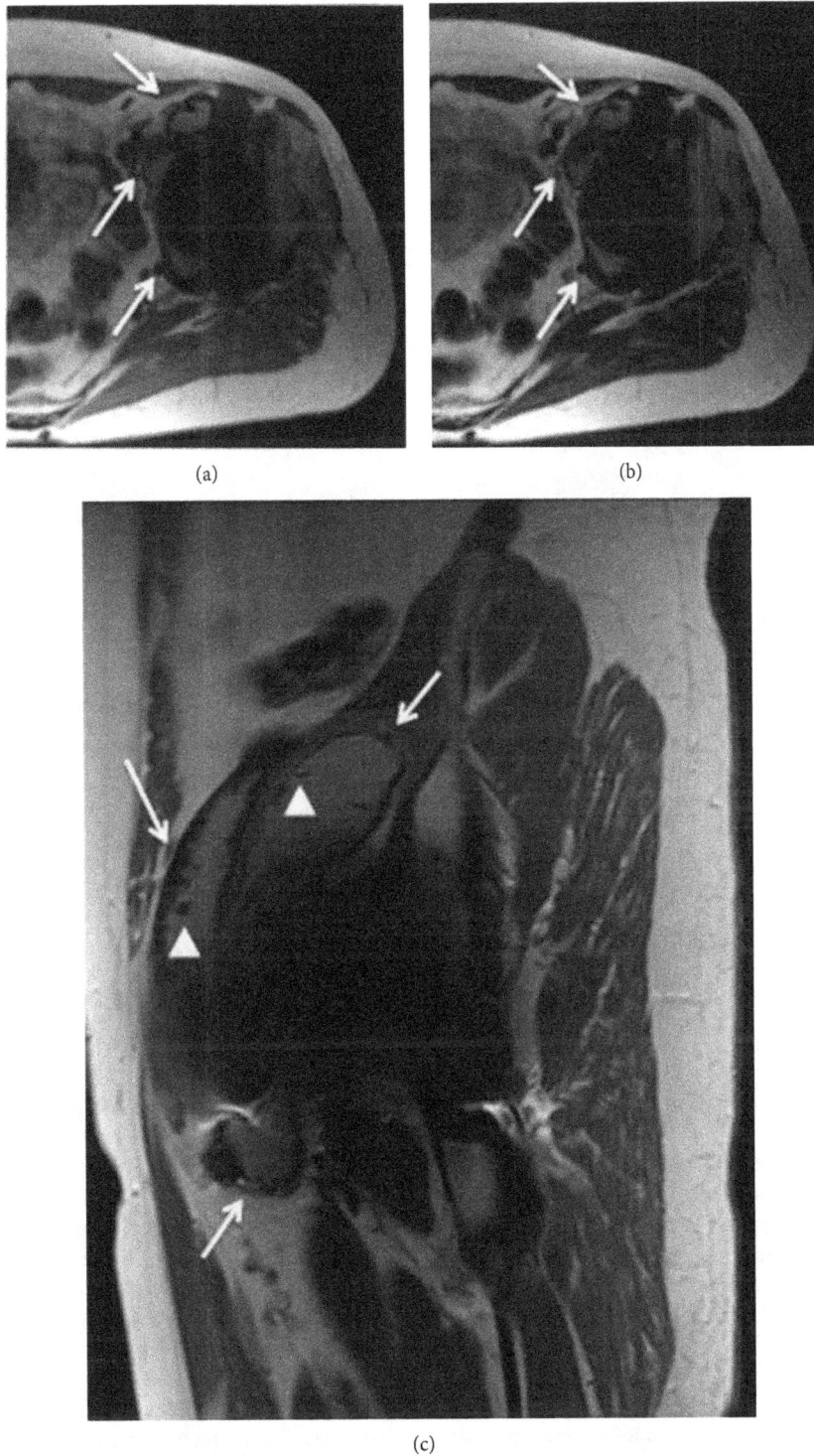

FIGURE 3: In the metal artefact reduction sequence magnetic resonance imaging (MARS MRI), axial T1 (a), axial T2 (b), and sagittal T1 (c) show the presence of two lesions of thick walls located anterior to the psoas and iliacus (arrows) muscle. Within the lesion, a small focus of artefact is seen (arrow heads). This finding is critical to determining that the aetiology of the pseudotumour is "metallosis."

Moreover, delayed diagnosis drives to increase the size of the pseudotumour with more bone and soft tissue damage; therefore, there are more complications and poor clinical revision outcomes [14–16]. It is critical to remark that the longer the follow-up is, the higher the incidence of pseudotumour and its symptoms is.

Pseudotumour diagnosis is not easy as patients remain asymptomatic for a long time. As it is a well-known complication, screening with images must be performed on all prosthesis with a metal-bearing surface [17]. Moreover, we believe that the imaging study should include an MRI, which features high sensitivity and specificity for diagnosis, and a

(a)

(b)

(c)

(d)

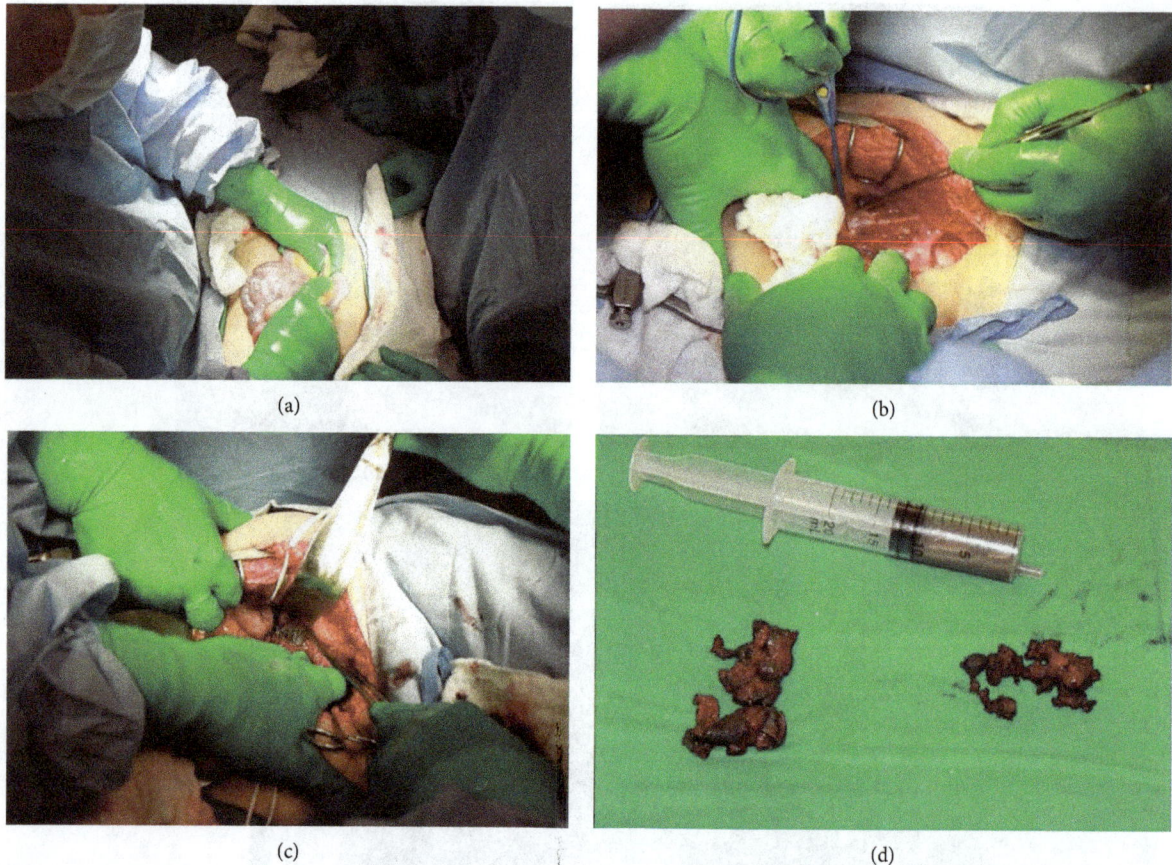

FIGURE 4: Four images from the first step of the surgery are shown. After a midline longitudinal infraumbilical approach, the left paracolic gutter was addressed (a) to obtain access to the retroperitoneum (b); a cystic tumour was observed in intimate contact with the iliopsoas muscle and the femoral nerve and vessels (c). The pseudotumour was punctured, and a grey milky-like fluid was obtained; then, the tumour was completely resected (d).

better definition of pseudotumour for diagnosis and operative planning [14, 18], especially in places where the measurement of metal ions in the blood is not available as it is in our case [19, 20].

Another issue that cannot be missed is that infection must be ruled out, as it is also a complication of THA and it transcends all prosthesis design [21]. For this, joint arthrocentesis and a synovial fluid analysis must be performed routinely. The liquid obtained must be sent to a traditional study and prolonged microbiological cultures for two weeks, according to international publications [22].

Regarding the aetiology of pseudotumours, current evidence attributes it to an adverse reaction to metal debris. Some studies indicate that this is due to a local inflammatory response to wear of the metal surface, which develops a granulomatous-like reaction proportional to the amount of the wear debris, and it correlates with the amount of metal ions in plasma [23, 24]. Beside the bearing surface, it has been reported as risk factor of hip dysplasia, malposition of prosthesis components, and larger size of the femoral head of the prosthesis hip dysplasia—all of them associated to excessive wear [8]. On the other hand, Willert et al. describe that pseudotumour is an aseptic lymphocyte-dominated vasculitis- (ALVAL-) associated lesion which is a delayed hypersensitivity reaction type and seems to be mildly related

to the amount of wear debris. The most characteristic histological features of ALVAL were diffuse and perivascular infiltrates of lymphocytes and plasma cell infiltrates of eosinophilic granulocytes and necrosis. Only a few metal particles were detected [6, 25–27]. According to the recently published histopathological classification of joint implant-related pathology, this case corresponds to a "type 1: particle type," in which the hallmark is the infiltrate of macrophages often with foamy feature and multinuclear giant cell, in which prosthesis wear can be detected [22].

Pseudotumour, as it has been established in previous paragraphs, is not an exclusive complication of RHA, but of those that use metal on metal-bearing surface. Even more, few cases have been reported supporting that pseudotumour could also be triggered by metal ion release from the head-neck taper junction in cases were no metal on metal-bearing surface was used [28]. The highest incidence of this complication in resurfacing prosthesis happens because they use only metal on metal-bearing surface [29]. A series with extended follow-ups of Birmingham® HRA had shown a significant rate of early failure, being the most frequent cause of a metal ion adverse reaction confirmed by histological analysis [2, 30]. Ollivere et al. report a series of 463 Birmingham® hip resurfacing [31], in which 9 of them had macroscopic and histological evidence of adverse

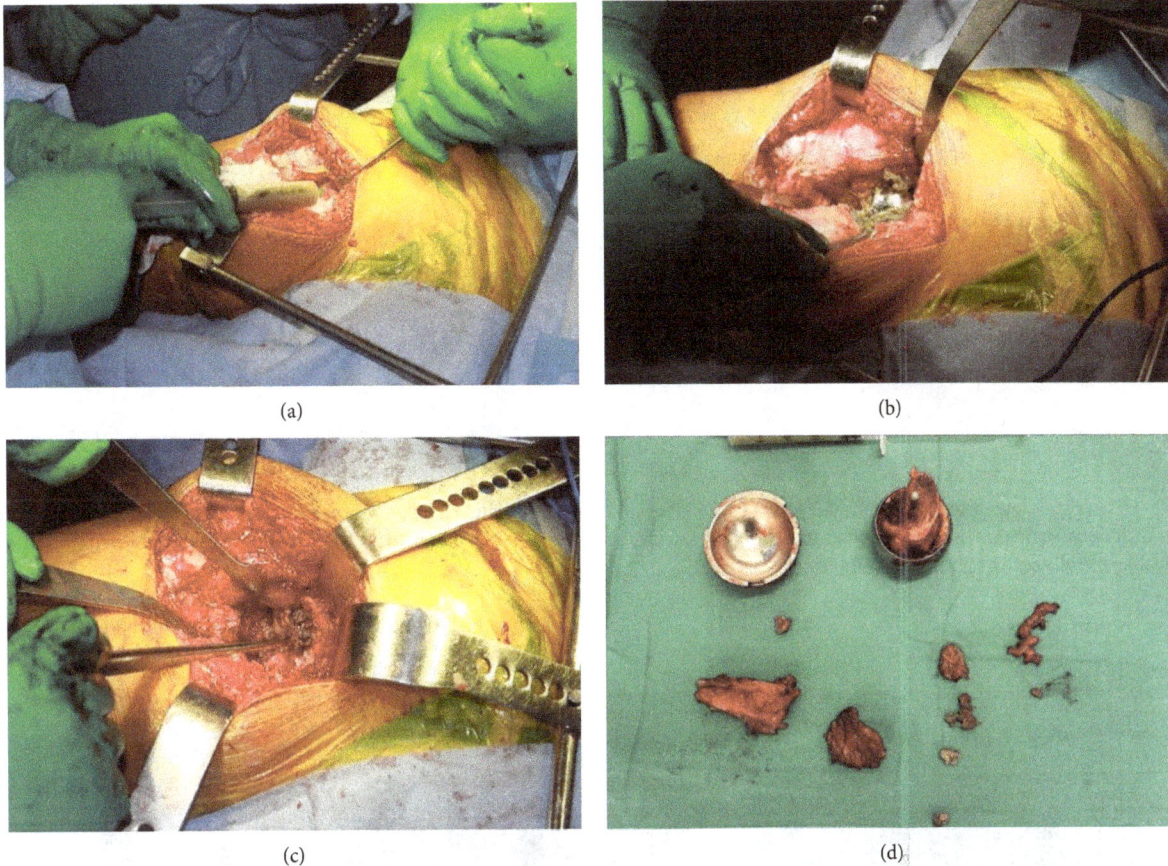

FIGURE 5: Four images from the second step of the surgery are shown. Through a posterolateral hip approach, an RHA was performed. The capsule was looking distend, so it was punctured (a), after capsulotomy the pseudotumour was evident (b), all components were removed, and an anterosuperior acetabulum wall defect was observed (c). Tumour sample, liquid and the hip prosthesis removed are shown in (d).

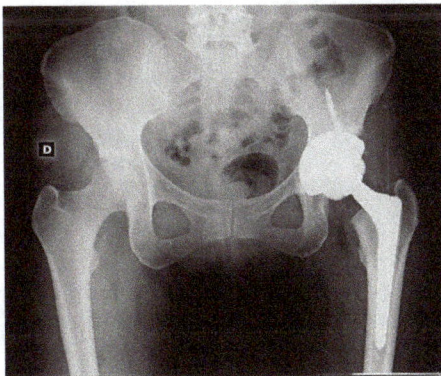

FIGURE 6: In an immediate post-RHA pelvis anteroposterior X-ray, an adequate position of the components is seen.

reaction to metal debris. The main risk factors in this study were female gender, a small femoral component, a high abduction angle, and obesity. They do not recommend the use of Birmingham® HRA in these patients [31]. A more extensive series of 4226 hips with three types of HRA found 58 failures associated with adverse reaction to metal debris. The median ion concentrations in the failed group were significantly higher than those in the control group. Increased wear from the metal-on-metal-bearing surface

was associated with an increased rate of failure secondary to an adverse reaction. Moreover, revision surgery seems to be useful to decrease the blood concentration of metal ions [32].

There are only case report evidences of the surgical treatment of this pathology [33–35]. Consensus exists to perform pseudotumour resection and RHA, mainly changing the metal-bearing surface; however, the amount of pseudotumour resection is not precise, and some authors prefer to resect what is around the hip, leaving the pseudotumor in more difficult areas to address such as the retroperitoneum [9, 36]. In our case, an aggressive tumour resection by a double approach was decided after considering the pseudotumour extension and neurological compromise. We believe that the complete resection of the pseudotumour is related to successful outcomes, and it is supported by some authors [32]. Until our last follow-up almost five years later, the patient had no clinical signs of pseudotumour, and annual MR imaging examinations had been negative. Tumour size and location matter, so it was technically challenging to remove it, as it was in close relation to the iliac and the femoral vessels. Retroperitoneum compromise is not often; Bosker et al. [9] described two cases where the pseudotumour extends into the abdominal space along the iliopsoas muscle. We believe that it is essential to perform surgery by a

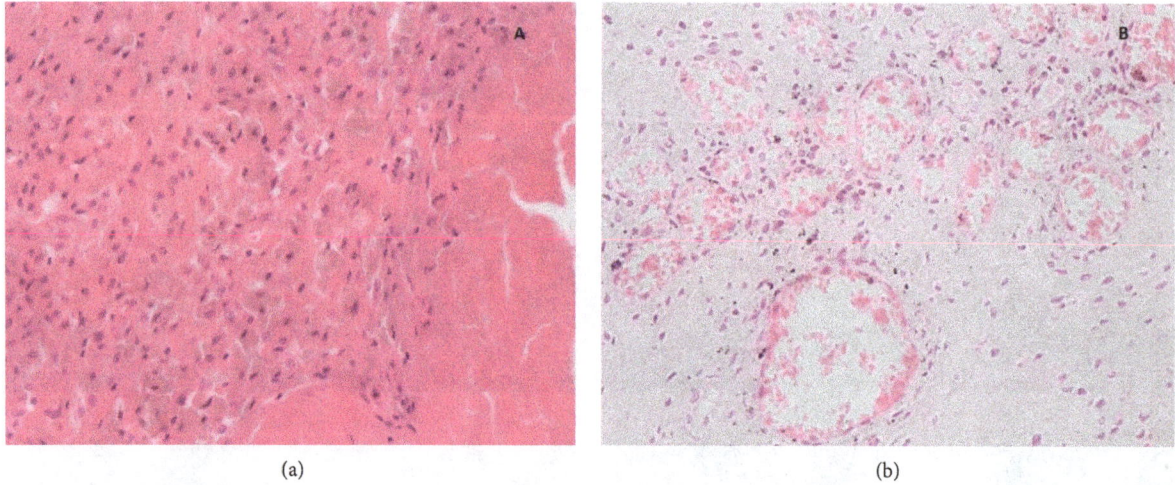

(a) (b)

FIGURE 7: Histologic view of the soft tissue mass. (a) (40x) Hematoxylin and eosin (HE) shows an infiltrate of the macrophages with brown contents and detritus inside, near a necrotic area. (b) (100x) HE shows black particulates from the prosthetic material in a reparative tissue with fibroblast and neoformation of blood vessels.

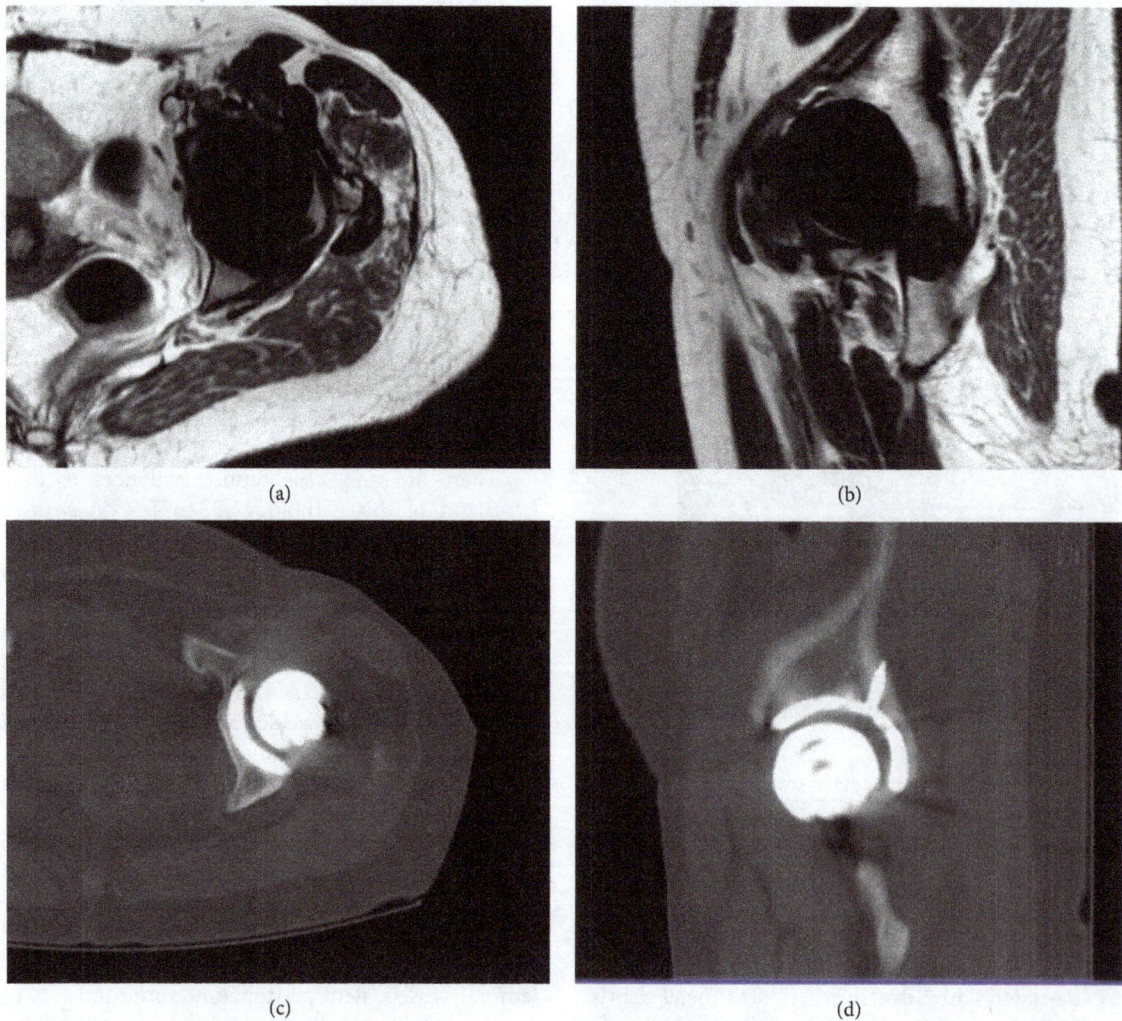

(a) (b)

(c) (d)

FIGURE 8: MRI (a) and (b) and CT (c) and (d) images taken five years post-RHA. There were no signs of pseudotumour after an extended follow-up.

multidisciplinary team and complete resection of the pseudotumour [37]. A vascular surgeon was prepared if needed in our case, and the first step was performed by a surgeon, which was more familiar with the retroperitoneum approach.

Regarding RHA, a bone defect caused by the pseudotumour is an issue. In this case, fortunately, it was resolved by standard components, and it was not necessary to use complex revision arthroplasty components that add morbidity to the surgery. However, we consider that performing a RHA is not easy or risk exempt. In a study that compares the result of 53 revisions of different implants of Birmingham® hip resurfacing, the author concluded that the incidence of major complications after RHAs for pseudotumour (50%) was significantly higher than that of after RHAs for other causes (14%). The authors concluded that the outcome of revision for pseudotumour (16 cases) is poor, so consideration should be given to an early RHA before the tumour grows and a significant bone defect is present [10].

4. Conclusions

This case represents a rare but devastating complication related to metal-bearing surface arthroplasty, particularly to HRA. Currently, the evidence shows that the incidence of pseudotumours and the rate of revision for pseudotumours are higher than initially reported. So, the indication of a metal-bearing surface is questionable given the higher rate of early RHA compared to other bearing surfaces such as polyethylene or ceramic. The most remarkable of this case is that after complete pseudotumour resection and RHA, at five years of follow up, the patient achieved a complete range of motion, no pain, no limp, and no sign of recurrence in MRI. We encourage that for such cases, MRI for diagnosis should be performed, arthrocentesis to rule out infection, and complete resection of the pseudotumour and hip revision for treatment led by a multidisciplinary team. Also, we are in favour of not using the metal-bearing surface as the first option [38].

Conflicts of Interest

The authors declare no conflict of interest.

Acknowledgments

We thank the invaluable collaboration of Facundo Las Heras, MD, for his histopathological analysis of this and other related cases. He is a pathologist at our centre dedicated to musculoskeletal pathology and a professor at the University of Chile. Also, we would like to thank Jorge Diaz, MD, for his collaboration in the interpretation of CT and MRI images. Dr. Diaz is the chief of the musculoskeletal unit in the radiology department at the Hospital Clinico Universidad de Chile.

References

[1] I. D. Learmonth, C. Young, and C. Rorabeck, "The operation of the century: total hip replacement," *The Lancet*, vol. 370, no. 9597, pp. 1508–1519, 2007.

[2] J. Daniel, P. Pynsent, and D. McMinn, "Metal-on-metal resurfacing of the hip in patients under the age of 55 years with osteoarthritis," *The Journal of Bone and Joint Surgery. British volume*, vol. 86-B, no. 2, pp. 177–184, 2004.

[3] A. Shimmin, P. E. Beaule, and P. Campbell, "Metal-on-metal hip resurfacing arthroplasty," *The Journal of Bone and Joint Surgery. American Volume*, vol. 90, no. 3, pp. 637–654, 2008.

[4] C. Delaunay, I. Petit, I. D. Learmonth, P. Oger, and P. A. Vendittoli, "Metal-on-metal bearings total hip arthroplasty: the cobalt and chromium ions release concern," *Orthopaedics & Traumatology, Surgery & Research*, vol. 96, no. 8, pp. 894–904, 2010.

[5] P. F. Lachiewicz, L. T. Kleeman, and T. Seyler, "Bearing surfaces for total hip arthroplasty," *The Journal of the American Academy of Orthopaedic Surgeons*, vol. 26, no. 2, pp. 45–57, 2018.

[6] H. G. Willert, G. H. Buchhorn, A. Fayyazi et al., "Metal-on-metal bearings and hypersensitivity in patients with artificial hip joints: A clinical and histomorphological study," *The Journal of Bone & Joint Surgery*, vol. 87, no. 1, pp. 28–36, 2005.

[7] P. Campbell, E. Ebramzadeh, S. Nelson, K. Takamura, K. De Smet, and H. C. Amstutz, "Histological features of pseudotumor-like tissues from metal-on-metal hips," *Clinical Orthopaedics and Related Research*, vol. 468, no. 9, pp. 2321–2327, 2010.

[8] H. Pandit, S. Glyn-Jones, P. McLardy-Smith et al., "Pseudotumours associated with metal-on-metal hip resurfacings," *The Journal of Bone and Joint Surgery. British volume*, vol. 90-B, no. 7, pp. 847–851, 2008.

[9] B. H. Bosker, H. B. Ettema, M. van Rossum et al., "Pseudotumor formation and serum ions after large head metal-on-metal stemmed total hip replacement. Risk factors, time course and revisions in 706 hips," *Archives of Orthopaedic and Trauma Surgery*, vol. 135, no. 3, pp. 417–425, 2015.

[10] G. Grammatopolous, H. Pandit, Y.-M. Kwon et al., "Hip resurfacings revised for inflammatory pseudotumour have a poor outcome," *The Journal of Bone and Joint Surgery. British volume*, vol. 91-B, no. 8, pp. 1019–1024, 2009.

[11] D. Fu, W. Sun, J. Shen, X. Ma, Z. Cai, and Y. Hua, "Inflammatory pseudotumor around metal-on-polyethylene total hip arthroplasty in patients with ankylosing spondylitis: description of two cases and review of literature," *World Journal of Surgical Oncology*, vol. 13, no. 1, p. 57, 2015.

[12] B. Bosker, H. Ettema, M. Boomsma, B. Kollen, M. Maas, and C. Verheyen, "High incidence of pseudotumour formation after large-diameter metal-on-metal total hip replacement," *The Journal of Bone and Joint Surgery. British Volume*, vol. 94-B, no. 6, pp. 755–761, 2012.

[13] R. Bisschop, M. F. Boomsma, J. J. Van Raay, A. T. Tiebosch, M. Maas, and C. L. Gerritsma, "High prevalence of pseudotumors in patients with a Birmingham hip resurfacing prosthesis: a prospective cohort study of one hundred and twenty-nine patients," *The Journal of Bone & Joint Surgery*, vol. 95, no. 17, pp. 1554–1560, 2013.

[14] G. Grammatopoulos, H. Pandit, A. Kamali et al., "The correlation of wear with histological features after failed hip resurfacing arthroplasty," *The Journal of Bone & Joint Surgery*, vol. 95, no. 12, article e81, 2013.

[15] R. A. Brand and J. L. Marsh, "Particulate debris osteolysis simulating malignant tumor," *The Iowa Orthopaedic Journal*, vol. 24, p. 111, 2004.

[16] C. Jeanrot, M. Ouaknine, P. Anract, M. Forest, and B. Tomeno, "Massive pelvic and femoral pseudotumoral osteolysis secondary to an uncemented total hip arthroplasty," *International Orthopaedics*, vol. 23, no. 1, pp. 37–40, 1999.

[17] H. Wynn-Jones, R. Macnair, J. Wimhurst et al., "Silent soft tissue pathology is common with a modern metal-on-metal hip arthroplasty," *Acta Orthopaedica*, vol. 82, no. 3, pp. 301–307, 2011.

[18] O. Lainiala, P. Elo, A. Reito, J. Pajamaki, T. Puolakka, and A. Eskelinen, "Comparison of extracapsular pseudotumors seen in magnetic resonance imaging and in revision surgery of 167 failed metal-on-metal hip replacements," *Acta Orthopaedica*, vol. 85, no. 5, pp. 474–479, 2014.

[19] F. Hannemann, A. Hartmann, J. Schmitt et al., "European multidisciplinary consensus statement on the use and monitoring of metal-on-metal bearings for total hip replacement and hip resurfacing," *Orthopaedics & Traumatology: Surgery & Research.*, vol. 99, no. 3, pp. 263–271, 2013.

[20] E. Robinson, J. Henckel, S. Sabah, K. Satchithananda, J. Skinner, and A. Hart, "Cross-sectional imaging of metal-on-metal hip arthroplasties: can we substitute MARS MRI with CT?," *Acta orthopaedica.*, vol. 85, no. 6, pp. 577–584, 2014.

[21] M. M. Mikhael, A. D. Hanssen, and R. J. Sierra, "Failure of metal-on-metal total hip arthroplasty mimicking hip infection: a report of two cases," *The Journal of Bone & Joint Surgery*, vol. 91, no. 2, pp. 443–446, 2009.

[22] V. Krenn, L. Morawietz, G. Perino et al., "Revised histopathological consensus classification of joint implant related pathology," *Pathology, Research and Practice*, vol. 210, no. 12, pp. 779–786, 2014.

[23] D. Langton, T. Joyce, S. Jameson et al., "Adverse reaction to metal debris following hip resurfacing," *The Journal of Bone and Joint Surgery. British volume*, vol. 93, no. 2, pp. 164–171, 2011.

[24] R. Sidaginamale, T. Joyce, J. Lord et al., "Blood metal ion testing is an effective screening tool to identify poorly performing metal-on-metal bearing surfaces," *Bone & Joint Research*, vol. 2, no. 5, pp. 84–95, 2013.

[25] J. R. Berstock, R. P. Baker, G. C. Bannister, and C. P. Case, "Histology of failed metal-on-metal hip arthroplasty; three distinct sub-types," *Hip International*, vol. 24, no. 3, pp. 243–248, 2014.

[26] A. K. Matthies, J. A. Skinner, H. Osmani, J. Henckel, and A. J. Hart, "Pseudotumors are common in well-positioned low-wearing metal-on-metal hips," *Clinical Orthopaedics and Related Research*, vol. 470, no. 7, pp. 1895–1906, 2012.

[27] T. S. Watters, D. M. Cardona, K. S. Menon, E. N. Vinson, M. P. Bolognesi, and L. G. Dodd, "Aseptic lymphocyte-dominated vasculitis-associated lesion: a clinicopathologic review of an underrecognized cause of prosthetic failure," *American Journal of Clinical Pathology*, vol. 134, no. 6, pp. 886–893, 2010.

[28] P. Bisseling, T. Tan, Z. Lu, P. A. Campbell, and J. L. Susante, "The absence of a metal-on-metal bearing does not preclude the formation of a destructive pseudotumor in the hip—a case report," *Acta Orthopaedica*, vol. 84, no. 4, pp. 437–441, 2013.

[29] A. J. Hart, A. Matthies, J. Henckel, K. Ilo, J. Skinner, and P. C. Noble, "Understanding why metal-on-metal hip arthroplasties fail: a comparison between patients with well-functioning and revised Birmingham hip resurfacing arthroplasties. AAOS exhibit selection," *The Journal of Bone and Joint Surgery. American Volume*, vol. 94, no. 4, article e22, 2012.

[30] J. W. Griffin, M. D'Apuzzo, and J. A. Browne, "Management of failed metal-on-metal total hip arthroplasty," *World Journal of Orthopedics*, vol. 3, no. 6, pp. 70–74, 2012.

[31] B. Ollivere, S. Duckett, A. August, and M. Porteous, "The Birmingham hip resurfacing: 5-year clinical and radiographic results from a district general hospital," *International Orthopaedics*, vol. 34, no. 5, pp. 631–634, 2010.

[32] O. Lainiala, A. Reito, P. Elo, J. Pajamaki, T. Puolakka, and A. Eskelinen, "Revision of metal-on-metal hip prostheses results in marked reduction of blood cobalt and chromium ion concentrations," *Clinical Orthopaedics and Related Research*, vol. 473, no. 7, pp. 2305–2313, 2015.

[33] R. A. Clayton, I. Beggs, D. M. Salter, M. H. Grant, J. T. Patton, and D. E. Porter, "Inflammatory pseudotumor associated with femoral nerve palsy following metal-on-metal resurfacing of the hip," *The Journal of Bone and Joint Surgery-American Volume*, vol. 90, no. 9, pp. 1988–1993, 2008.

[34] T. von Schewelov and L. Sanzen, "Catastrophic failure due to aggressive metallosis 4 years after hip resurfacing in a woman in her forties–a case report," *Acta Orthopaedica*, vol. 81, no. 3, pp. 402–404, 2010.

[35] D. Boardman, F. Middleton, and T. Kavanagh, "A benign psoas mass following metal-on-metal resurfacing of the hip," *The Journal of Bone and Joint Surgery. British volume*, vol. 88-B, no. 3, pp. 402–404, 2006.

[36] A. Rajpura, M. L. Porter, A. K. Gambhir, A. J. Freemont, and T. N. Board, "Clinical experience of revision of metal on metal hip arthroplasty for aseptic lymphocyte dominated vasculitis associated lesions (ALVAL)," *Hip International*, vol. 21, no. 1, pp. 43–51, 2011.

[37] R. Berber, Y. Pappas, M. Khoo et al., "A new approach to managing patients with problematic metal hip implants: the use of an internet-enhanced multidisciplinary team meeting," *The Journal of Bone and Joint Surgery*, vol. 97, no. 4, article e20, 2015.

[38] C. A. Engh Jr., H. Ho, and C. A. Engh, "Metal-on-metal hip arthroplasty: does early clinical outcome justify the chance of an adverse local tissue reaction?," *Clinical Orthopaedics and Related Research*, vol. 468, no. 2, pp. 406–412, 2010.

12

Extensive Bone Lengthening for a Patient with Linear Morphea

Kenichi Mishima ⓘ, Hiroshi Kitoh ⓘ, Masaki Matsushita, Tadashi Nagata, Yasunari Kamiya, and Naoki Ishiguro

Department of Orthopaedic Surgery, Nagoya University Graduate School of Medicine, 65 Tsurumai, Showa-ku, Nagoya, Aichi 466-8550, Japan

Correspondence should be addressed to Hiroshi Kitoh; hkitoh@med.nagoya-u.ac.jp

Academic Editor: Hitesh N. Modi

Localized scleroderma, also known as morphea, is a rare condition characterized by progressive sclerosis of the skin and associated atrophy of the underlying tissues. The linear type of localized scleroderma is the most frequent form in childhood, usually affecting unilateral extremities. Fibrosclerosis of the fasciae and muscles can spread across joints and impair the range of motion of the joint. Dysplastic and/or atrophic bones of the affected lower extremity can lead to clinically significant leg length discrepancy (LLD). Limb reconstruction surgery has rarely been indicated for LLD in patients with linear morphea. We report on a case of extensive bone lengthening for appreciable LLD in a pediatric patient with linear morphea. A Japanese girl with linear morphea underwent staged simultaneous lengthening of the femur and tibia twice at seven and eleven years of age using a unilateral external fixator. A healing index exceeded 100 days/cm except for the first femoral lengthening that was complicated by regenerate fracture. At the final follow-up, LLD of 38 mm remained, but she could walk independently without a brace or a crutch. Due to soft tissue tightness and poor regenerative ability in the affected limb, cautions should be taken to prevent regenerate fracture and/or malalignment of the limb.

1. Introduction

Localized scleroderma (LS), also known as morphea, is a rare condition characterized by progressive sclerosis of the skin and associated atrophy of the underlying tissues [1]. LS is classified into five types, including plaque type, generalized type, bullous type, linear type, and deep type [2]. The linear type is the most frequent form of LS in childhood, usually affecting unilateral extremities [3]. Fibrosclerosis of the fasciae and muscles can spread across joints and impair the range of motion of the joint. Dysplastic and/or atrophic bones of the affected lower extremity can lead to clinically significant leg length discrepancy (LLD) [4]. Severe joint contracture and LLD inevitably cause significant physical disability in patients with the linear type of LS, linear morphea (LM), for whom bone shortening or amputation has been indicated, whereas extensive bone lengthening has rarely performed. To our knowledge, there is only one case report describing limb reconstruction surgery in a patient with LM [5]. We report on a juvenile LM case who underwent extensive bone lengthening to correct substantial LLD.

2. Case Presentation

A four-year-old Japanese girl with no remarkable medical history was referred to our orthopedic clinic for treatment of 2 cm of LLD. She had a two-year history of progressive LM in a wide range of the posteromedial aspect of the right thigh and the medial aspect of the right lower leg. At the first presentation, skin lesions exhibited hyperpigmentation, induration, and xerosis. The range of motion of the right knee was full extension to 80° of flexion. Radiographs of the right lower extremity revealed dysplastic/atrophic femur and tibia. LLD increased with time and reached nearly 10 cm at seven years of age (Figure 1(a)). As she and her parents refused to undergo epiphysiodesis of the unaffected side of the lower extremity, we performed simultaneous lengthening of the right femur and tibia using a unilateral external

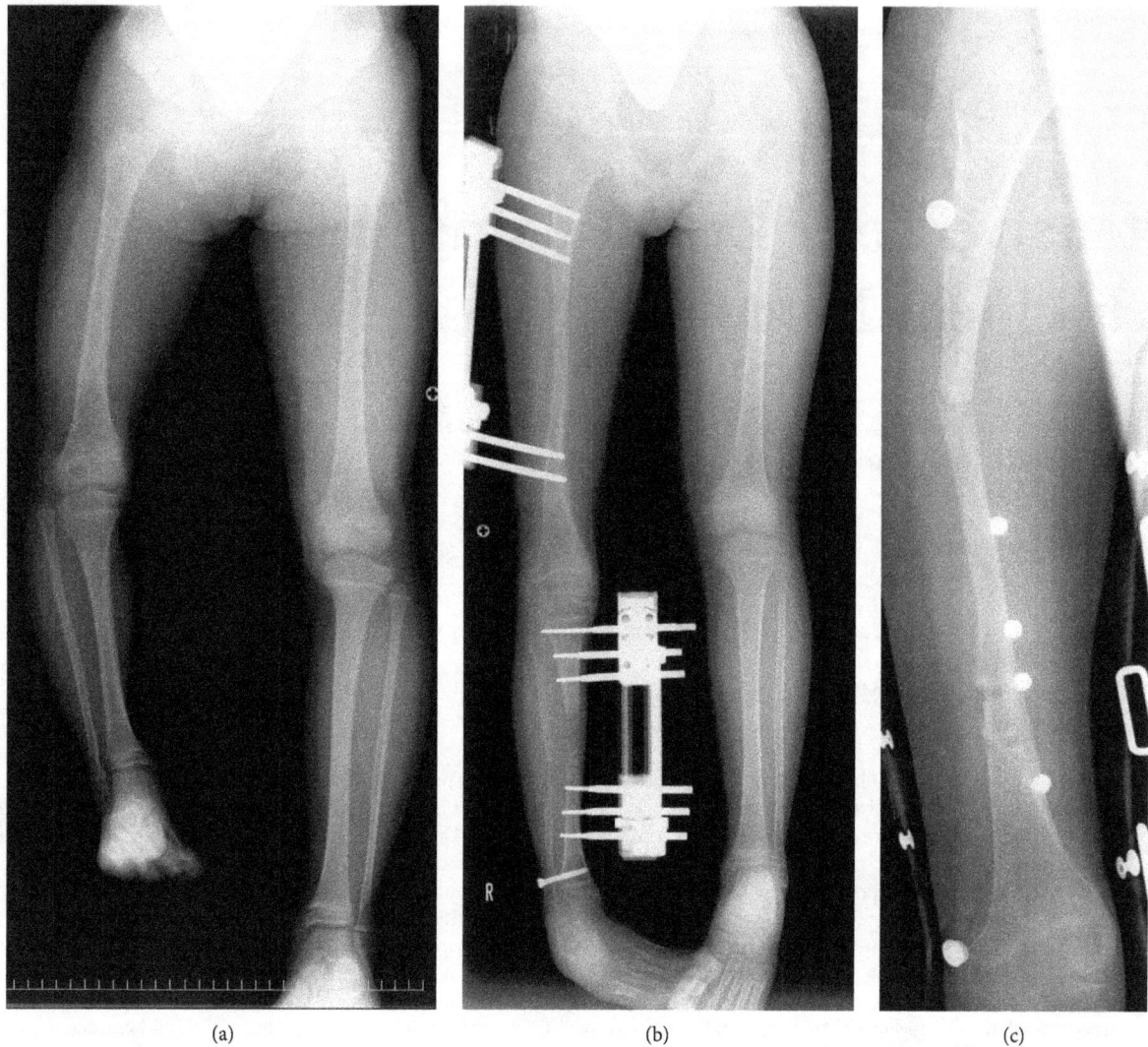

FIGURE 1: Radiographs of the lower extremities at the time of the first lengthening. (a) An anteroposterior standing radiograph of the lower extremities at seven years of age showing LLD of nearly 10 cm with the right foot placed on a block. (b) An anteroposterior supine radiograph of the lower extremities at the end of the lengthening period of the first lengthening demonstrating 83 mm and 37 mm of lengthening in the femur and tibia, respectively. (c) An anteroposterior radiograph of the right femur showing regenerate fracture at the site of the lengthened callus.

fixator (EBI/Zimmer Biomet Carbon Rail Deformity System; Warsaw, Indiana, USA). She had taken low-dose prednisolone every day or every second day prior to the first lengthening procedure. The dosage regimen had been dependent on the disease activity based on clinical and thermographic assessment. Tibial osteotomy was performed with the Gigli saw, whereas femoral osteotomy was done with a multiple drilling technique. No postoperative immobilization was used, and full-weight bearing was encouraged from the second postoperative day. After 14 days of the waiting period, distraction of the femur and tibia was commenced at a rate of 1 mm and 0.5 mm per day, respectively. Femur was lengthened at the same rate throughout the distraction period, whereas the distraction speed of the tibia was gradually decreased after the lengthening callus showed thin and sparse on radiographs. Distraction of the tibia was occasionally interrupted until the callus width and continuity were reestablished. As a result, the lengthening period/amount of

lengthening of the femur and tibia were 90 days/83 mm and 163 days/37 mm, respectively, and an overall leg length was 7 mm longer in the affected limb at the end of the lengthening period (Figure 1(b)). During the neutralizing period, an accordion technique and daily low-intensity pulsed ultrasound (LIPUS) exposure were applied to the tibia to stimulate callus maturation. She received LIPUS treatment using a sonic accelerated fracture healing system (SAFHS; Teijin Pharma Ltd., Tokyo, Japan) once a day for 20 minutes without interruption. After 84 days and 194 days of the neutralizing period in the femur and tibia, respectively, the device was loosened to allow dynamization of the lengthened callus so that it could fully mature. The dynamization period reached 49 days in the femur and 58 days in the tibia to obtain matured callus exhibiting fusiform/cylindrical shape and similar density to that of the adjacent cortical bone on radiographs. Before pin removal, we dislodged the fixator frame with the fixation pins leaving in situ for a while to monitor

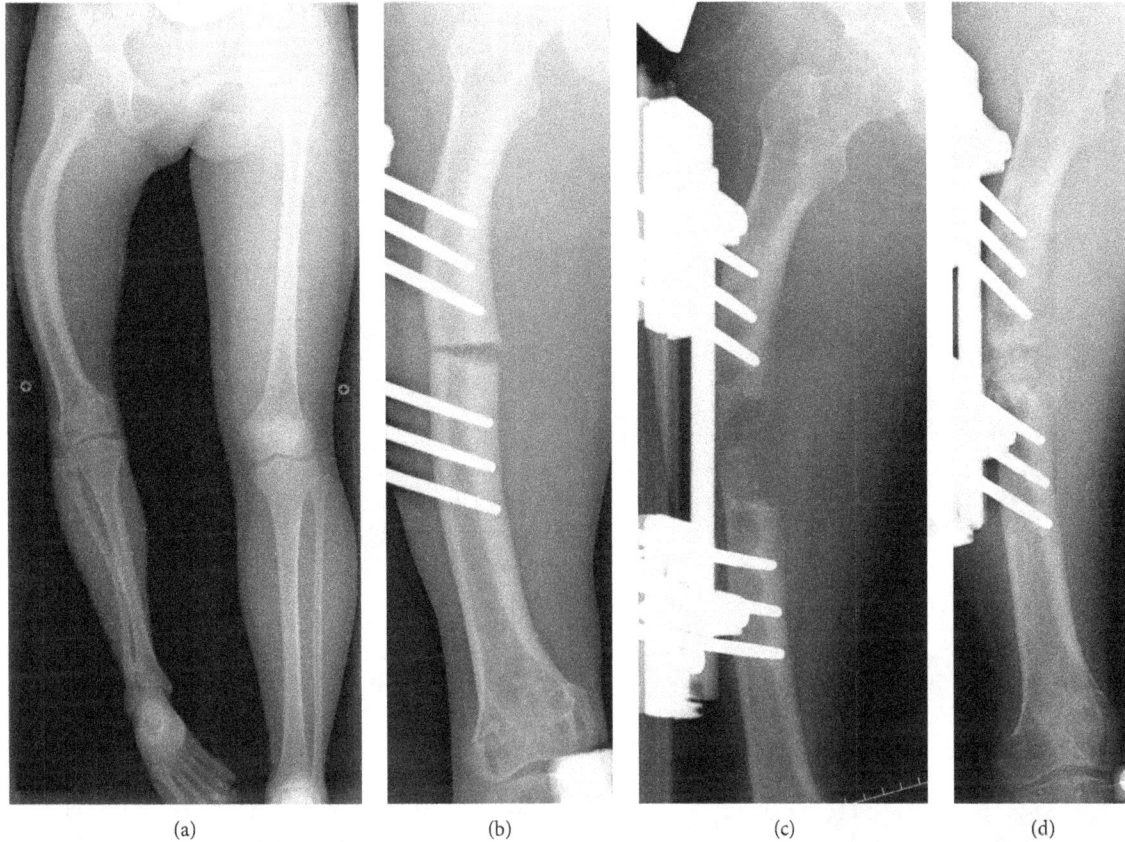

(a) (b) (c) (d)

FIGURE 2: Radiographs of the lower extremities at the time of the second lengthening. (a) An anteroposterior supine radiograph of the lower extremities at eleven years of age before the second lengthening revealing LLD of 11 cm. (b) A radiograph of the right femur just after the femoral osteotomy demonstrating acute correction of an anterolateral bowing deformity. (c, d) Radiographs of the right femur before (c) and after (d) the chipping surgery.

the development of regenerate bone fracture or bending. The monitoring period was 47 days for the tibia and only one day for the femur, because the femoral pins had already been loosened. A healing index (HI) was 29 days/cm and 129 days/cm in the femur and tibia, respectively. Regenerate fracture of the femur, however, occurred due to minor trauma three days after the pin removal (Figure 1(c)). Since parental consent for open reduction and internal fixation was not obtained, she was treated conservatively with skin traction, resulting in malunion associated with a marked anterolateral bowing.

After the first lengthening procedure, LLD gradually increased again and reached 11 cm at eleven years of age (Figure 2(a)), when the flexion angle of the right knee decreased to 30 degrees. The second simultaneous lengthening of the femur and tibia was performed through percutaneous osteotomy using a multiple drilling technique. In the femur, acute correction of the bowing was done at the osteotomy site with the use of a fixator. The angulation was corrected up to 25 degrees using a proximal rotational clamp, followed by mechanical realignment of the bone axis using a distal translational clamp. After correction of the angular deformity, the osteotomy site was compressed (Figure 2(b)). Distraction by 1 mm and 0.5 mm per day was initiated at 14

days postoperatively in the femur and tibia, respectively. During the lengthening period, the rate of distraction was adjusted appropriately in order not to deteriorate the continuity of the callus on radiographs. Since the callus was poorly consolidated in the femur (Figure 2(c)), a modified "chipping and lengthening technique" was performed to enhance bone regeneration at nine months postoperatively (Figure 2(d)) [6]. Briefly, both ends of the osteotomy site and the callus were drilled with a 3.0 mm Kirschner wire in advance and then broken into smaller pieces with an osteotome. Subsequently, the comminuted bones were compressed until a radiolucent area was no longer recognized. Hard callus that obliterated the medullary cavity at the ends of the osteotomy site was removed with a sharp spoon. Two weeks after the chipping surgery, the distraction was resumed at a rate of 0.5 mm per day. The lengthening period/amount of the femur and tibia were 435 days/55 mm and 209 days/29 mm, respectively, and an overall leg length was 31 mm shorter in the affected limb at the end of the lengthening period. Symptomatic pin tract infection occasionally occurred during the treatment period and was resolved with oral antibiotics without any sequelae. The HI of the femur and tibia was 182 days/cm and 222 days/cm, respectively. Currently, two or three years have passed since the final removal of the femoral or

(a)

(b)

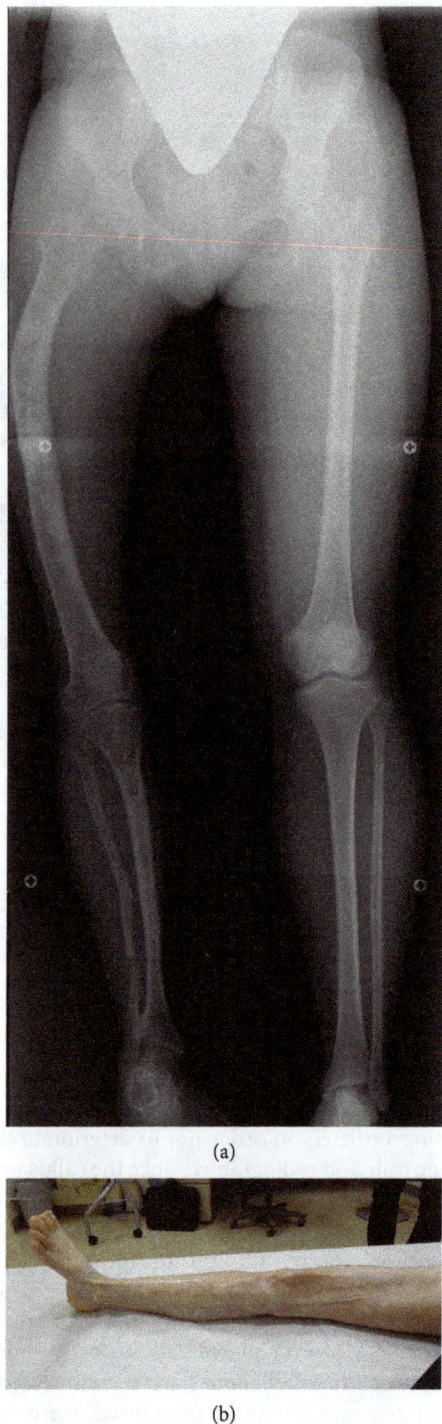

FIGURE 3: Current radiograph and view of the lower extremities. (a) An anteroposterior supine radiograph of the lower extremities at 17 years of age showing an anterolateral bowing of the right femur and a medial bowing of the right tibia. (b) A postoperative view of the right lower extremity showing atrophic skin surfaces on the posteromedial aspect of the thigh and the medial aspect of the lower leg, where brown pigmented cutaneous lesions were observed at the first presentation.

tibial pins, respectively, and 38 mm of LLD is left with acceptable lower limb alignment (Figure 3). The range of motion of the right knee is 20° of flexion and 0° of extension, but she

can walk independently without a brace or a crutch. She and her parents are satisfied with the outcome despite the long treatment period.

3. Discussion

Unlike the nonlinear type of LS, LM can cause significant LLD due to its unilateral involvement and early onset during childhood [3]. The bone lengthening procedure has not been indicated for LM cases, partly because it was thought to increase pathological sclerosis and contracture of the affected soft tissues [4]. Besides, the affected limb is thought to possess less bone-regenerating ability since the adipose tissue, a potent source of stem cells that can differentiate into bone-forming osteoblastic cells [7], has been shown to be replaced by poorly vasculated fibrous tissues in advanced LS [3]. Growth factors and nutrient supply necessary for osteoblastic differentiation obviously require abundant vascularization [8]. Therefore, LM-associated LLD has been managed primarily by epiphysiodesis and/or bone shortening, and, in some severe cases, by limb amputation [4]. In this case, however, the patient and her parents eagerly desired limb reconstruction surgery, although we expected that soft tissue tightness and poor regenerative ability in the affected limb would hamper successful extensive bone lengthening.

Juvenile LS patients have shown higher levels of IFN-γ and GM-CSF and lower levels of TNF-α [9]. These cytokines directly or indirectly regulate osteoclastogenesis, with IFN-γ and GM-CSF suppressing [10, 11] and TNF-α activating osteoclast differentiation [12]. Osteoclast-mediated resorption of calcified tissues is indispensable for proper bone remodeling [8]. The predominance of suppressed osteoclastogenesis may thus lead to the delay in callus maturation, which is presumably responsible for regenerate fracture as occurred in the first femoral lengthening. Tibial lengthening and the second femoral lengthening, on the other hand, necessitated an extremely long treatment period but were not associated with regenerate fractures. We thus consider that acceptable bone lengthening in LM patients may require a slow rate of distraction to preserve the integrity of the lengthened callus and quite a long neutralizing and dynamization period to ensure the consolidation and maturation of the callus.

The regenerate fracture malunited, and the extension contracture of the knee deteriorated after the first femoral lengthening. A review of MRI findings of LS has shown that fascial thickening and enhancement were notable in addition to subcutaneous septal thickening [13]. In our case, contractured fasciae at the posteromedial side of the thigh could distort the fractured femur as if a strained string had bent a bow. Open reduction and osteosynthesis should be done for regenerate fractures to prevent bowing deformity and keep bone length in this specific disease.

Limb reconstruction by extensive bone lengthening can be achieved even in severe LM patients, although it may need an extremely long period of an external fixation. We thus recommend the combination of bone lengthening of the affected side and epiphysiodesis of the healthy side to minimize LLD expansion and the amount of lengthening required.

In addition, we propose the conversion of external fixation to rigid internal fixation after the lengthening period not only to protect against regenerate fractures but also to shorten the period of external fixation. In severe LM cases, staged lengthening is indispensable to correct a large amount of LLD. To this end, conversion to plate fixation rather than intramedullary nailing may be preferable, because the endosteum, which is important for bone regeneration, should be preserved for a subsequent lengthening procedure [14].

We report on a rare case of extensive bone lengthening for LLD in a patient with linear morphea. Satisfactory correction of LLD can be attained even in severe cases of linear morphea by extensive bone lengthening alone despite an extremely long treatment period. Due to soft tissue tightness and poor regenerative ability in the affected limb, cautions should be taken to prevent regenerate fracture and/or malalignment of the limb.

Conflicts of Interest

The authors declare that they have no competing interests.

References

[1] F. Zulian, G. Cuffaro, and F. Sperotto, "Scleroderma in children: an update," *Current Opinion in Rheumatology*, vol. 25, no. 5, pp. 643–650, 2013.

[2] L. S. Peterson, A. M. Nelson, and W. P. D. Su, "Classification of morphea (localized scleroderma)," *Mayo Clinic Proceedings*, vol. 70, no. 11, pp. 1068–1076, 1995.

[3] M. F. Careta and R. Romiti, "Localized scleroderma: clinical spectrum and therapeutic update," *Anais Brasileiros de Dermatologia*, vol. 90, no. 1, pp. 62–73, 2015.

[4] S. L. Buckley, S. Skinner, P. James, and R. K. Ashley, "Focal scleroderma in children: an orthopaedic perspective," *Journal of Pediatric Orthopedics*, vol. 13, no. 6, pp. 784–790, 1993.

[5] M. Z. Handler, A. J. Wulkan, S. J. Stricker, and L. A. Schachner, "Linear morphea and leg length discrepancy: treatment with a leg-lengthening procedure," *Pediatric Dermatology*, vol. 30, no. 5, pp. 616–618, 2013.

[6] T. Matsushita and Y. Watanabe, "Chipping and lengthening technique for delayed unions and nonunions with shortening or bone loss," *Journal of Orthopaedic Trauma*, vol. 21, no. 6, pp. 404–406, 2007.

[7] P. A. Zuk, M. Zhu, P. Ashjian et al., "Human adipose tissue is a source of multipotent stem cells," *Molecular Biology of the Cell*, vol. 13, no. 12, pp. 4279–4295, 2002.

[8] S. Khosla, J. J. Westendorf, and M. J. Oursler, "Building bone to reverse osteoporosis and repair fractures," *The Journal of Clinical Investigation*, vol. 118, no. 2, pp. 421–428, 2008.

[9] K. S. Torok, K. Kurzinski, C. Kelsey et al., "Peripheral blood cytokine and chemokine profiles in juvenile localized scleroderma: T-helper cell-associated cytokine profiles," *Seminars in Arthritis and Rheumatism*, vol. 45, no. 3, pp. 284–293, 2015.

[10] R. Lari, A. J. Fleetwood, P. D. Kitchener et al., "Macrophage lineage phenotypes and osteoclastogenesis–complexity in the control by GM-CSF and TGF-beta," *Bone*, vol. 40, no. 2, pp. 323–336, 2007.

[11] H. Takayanagi, K. Ogasawara, S. Hida et al., "T-cell-mediated regulation of osteoclastogenesis by signalling cross-talk between RANKL and IFN-gamma," *Nature*, vol. 408, no. 6812, pp. 600–605, 2000.

[12] J. Lam, S. Takeshita, J. E. Barker, O. Kanagawa, F. P. Ross, and S. L. Teitelbaum, "TNF-alpha induces osteoclastogenesis by direct stimulation of macrophages exposed to permissive levels of RANK ligand," *The Journal of Clinical Investigation*, vol. 106, no. 12, pp. 1481–1488, 2000.

[13] S. Schanz, G. Fierlbeck, A. Ulmer et al., "Localized scleroderma: MR findings and clinical features," *Radiology*, vol. 260, no. 3, pp. 817–824, 2011.

[14] P. Merloz, "Bone regeneration and limb lengthening," *Osteoporosis International*, vol. 22, no. 6, pp. 2033–2036, 2011.

13

Tibia Adamantinoma Resection and Reconstruction with a Custom-Made Total Tibia Endoprosthesis

Gilber Kask⑩,[1] **Toni-Karri Pakarinen,**[1] **Jyrki Parkkinen,**[2] **Hannu Kuokkanen,**[3] **Jyrki Nieminen,**[4] **and Minna K. Laitinen**⑩[1]

[1]*Department of Orthopaedics and Traumatology, Unit of Musculoskeletal Surgery, Tampere University Hospital, Teiskontie 35, 33521 Tampere, Finland*
[2]*Fimlab Laboratories, Arvo Ylpön katu 4, 33520 Tampere, Finland*
[3]*Division of Plastic Surgery, Helsinki University Central Hospital, Topeliuksenkatu 5, 00260 Helsinki, Finland*
[4]*Coxa Hospital for Joint Replacement, Biokatu 6, 33520 Tampere, Finland*

Correspondence should be addressed to Gilber Kask; gilber.kask@gmail.com

Academic Editor: Wan Ismail Faisham

This case study describes a total tibia resection and reconstruction with a custom-made endoprosthetic replacement (EPR) and a long-term, 8-year follow-up. The patient underwent a total tibia adamantinoma resection in 2009. Reconstruction was performed with a custom-made total tibia EPR, where both the knee joint and ankle joint were reconstructed. Two muscle flaps, latissimus dorsi free flap and a pedicled medial gastrocnemius flap, were used for soft tissue reconstruction. The patient returned to normal life as a kindergarten teacher, without complications for eight years. This case demonstrated the importance of successful multidisciplinary teamwork in close collaboration with industry. In our best knowledge, no over 2 years of follow-up of total tibia replacement reports have been published.

1. Introduction

Adamantinoma is a rare malignant bone tumor, accounting for approximately 0.1–0.5% of all primary bone tumors [1]. There is a slight male predominance [1–3]. Tibia is involved in 85–90% of cases, but the other sites, including the fibula, ulna, femur, humerus, and radius, have been also reported [2, 4].

There have been no definitive guidelines for a treatment of adamantinoma. The preferred treatment is surgical management with wide margins, reconstruction if necessary and possible, or amputation [1]. Methods of limb salvage with reconstruction include distraction osteogenesis, allografts, vascularized fibular autografts, nonvascularized autogenous bone grafts, or endoprosthetic reconstructions (EPRs) [5]. Chemotherapy and radiotherapy in adamantinoma treatment have not been shown to be effective [2, 6, 7], and therefore

surgery remains the only curative option. After successful surgery with wide margins, the overall 10-year survival rates vary from 82% to 87% [1, 6]. In the literature, reported limb salvage rate for long bone adamantinoma patients is about 84% [3] and amputation compared with the limb preserving surgery has not been proved to improve survival rate [5].

Reconstruction after resection surgery for adamantinoma, in long bones, is dependent on the site and size of tumor. In the most common site, tibia, reconstruction is often EPR which is associated with a high rate of complications (48%) [3]. One of the most serious complication in EPR surgery is a periprosthetic joint infection (PJI). Deep infection in EPR around the knee is reported to be 4–45% [8]. Furthermore, limb reconstruction with extensive customized endoprosthesis is associated with an even higher incidence of serious complications. PJI is the main indication for a secondary amputation in EPR of the proximal tibia [9].

In cases where tumor affects the entire tibia, a wide excision with a clear margin is achievable with knee disarticulation, or higher amputation, or with a total tibia resection and reconstruction. In the current literature, only two cases of total tibia reconstruction have been published [10, 11]. One total EPR had a short follow-up of two years without early complications, and one case was reconstructed with a total tibia allograft, subsequently ending in a complication leading to amputation. To our best knowledge, no midterm or long-term results over 2 years of follow-up of total tibia replacement case reports have been published.

This study describes a case of complete tibia resection and total tibia custom-made EPR, with a long-term follow-up and functional outcome. This case study highlights the rarity of the reconstruction, multidisciplinary team work, and the good long-term functional result.

2. Case Presentation

A 48-year-old female with known breast carcinoma was screened for possible dissemination with whole-body computed tomography (CT) and a bone scintigraphy scan. The bone scan revealed a tumor in the entire right tibia. The patient reported no symptoms from the tibia tumor. A plain X-ray and magnetic resonance image (MRI) confirmed an intraosseal tumor that extended from 4 cm below the knee joint proximally to about 4 cm from the ankle joint distally (Figure 1). An open biopsy confirmed an adamantinoma histology. Different treatment options were thoroughly discussed with the patient, including a lower leg amputation with disarticulation of the knee, a total tibia resection and reconstruction with a tibia allograft, or a custom-made tibia EPR, which was eventually selected.

The tumor was resected with an extensive anteromedial approach, and the defect was reconstructed with a custom-made, silver-coated, modular endoprosthesis of the Modular Universal Tumor and Revision System (Implantcast®, Buxtehüde, Germany) (Figure 2). The knee joint was reconstructed with a metal-on-poly articulation with a (unique) metal-on-metal hinge mechanism (Figure 3). The ankle joint was reconstructed with a metal-on-poly hinge joint with a talar replacement, stabilized with a trans-talar and trans-calcanear hydroxyapatite-coated stem. A supplementary screw was used to add stability in the subtalar joint. The endoprosthesis was enveloped in a Trevira (Implantcast®) tube to facilitate the attachment of soft tissues and the patella tendon (Figure 4). A microvascular latissimus dorsi musculocutaneous flap was anastomosed to the tibia artery (end-to-side) and concomitant vein and wrapped around the prosthesis to avoid dead space and allow tension-free closure. In addition, a medial gastrocnemius muscle flap was transposed to cover the patellar tendon region; this was covered with a meshed split-thickness skin graft.

A histological analysis of the resected specimen showed an adamantinoma that had spread throughout the entire tibia and the margins were wide: an unaffected periosteum as an anatomic barrier and a minimum of clear soft tissue margin of 3 mm. Due to intracortical location of the tumor, no massive muscle excision was needed.

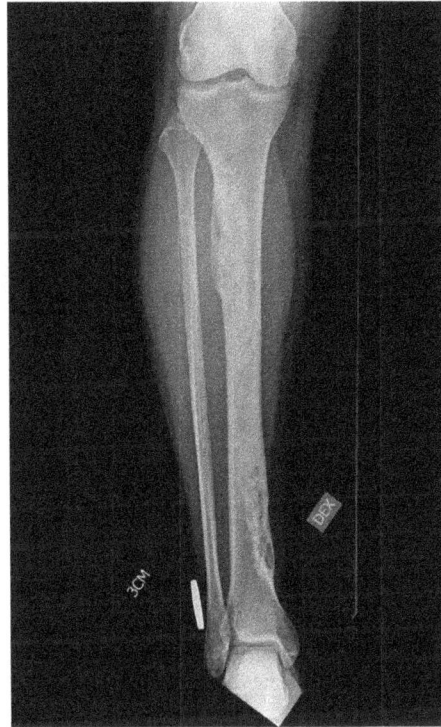

FIGURE 1: Preoperative X-ray from a right tibia. A plain X-ray from a right tibia with an intraosseal tumor that extended from 4 cm below the knee joint proximally to about 4 cm from the ankle joint distally.

The knee joint was immobilized in extension for 6 weeks to facilitate patella ligament attachment to the tube. Then, the joint was gradually mobilized. After 6 months, the patient's gait was almost normal, with mild limping. Local MRI and chest radiographs performed during the 8 years of follow-up showed no signs of local recurrence or distant metastasis. No loosening of the stem or other mechanical problem was reported. In a routine follow-up, in addition to radiographs, we used a local MRI with a metal artifact reduction sequence (MARS) technique [12], which enables to observe local recurrences of the tumor around the massive titanium endoprosthesis.

Eight years postoperatively, the patient had most of the time no pain and could mobilize freely. The patient resumed working full-time as a kindergarten teacher, and she has maintained her previous active lifestyle (except downhill skiing). On her latest follow-up visit (at 8 years), the knee range of motion was 0–105 degrees, ankle dorsiflexion was 5 degrees, and ankle flexion was 35 degrees. In the latest follow-up visit, we used 4 patient-related outcome (PRO) measures. The Musculoskeletal Society Tumor Score (MSTS) was 77%; the Oxford Knee score (OKS) was 35/48; the Toronto Extremity Salvage Score (TESS) was 80/100; and the 15D was 0.87/1.

The metal-on-metal prosthesis caused an increase in metal ion concentrations: cobalt was 6 ppb and chromium was 8 ppb. The silver coating created a mild, local skin argyria pigmentation, with cosmetic discomfort [13] (Figure 5).

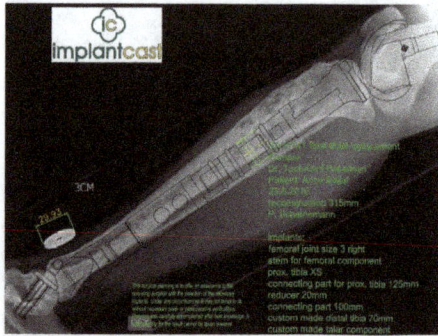

FIGURE 2: The preoperative planning of a custom-made total tibia endoprosthesis. The preoperative planning for total tibia resection and reconstruction with a custom-made, silver-coated, modular endoprosthesis of the Modular Universal Tumor and Revision System.

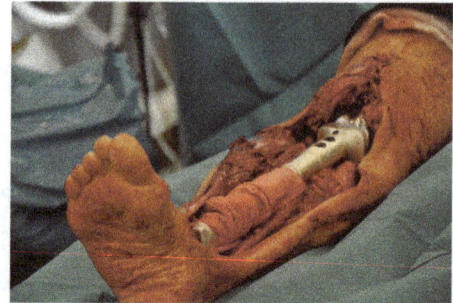

FIGURE 4: Perioperative image of the total tibia resection and reconstruction. The tibia tumor is totally resected, and the tibia is replaced with a custom-made endoprosthesis. The endoprosthesis was enveloped in a Trevira tube to facilitate the attachment of soft tissues and the patella tendon.

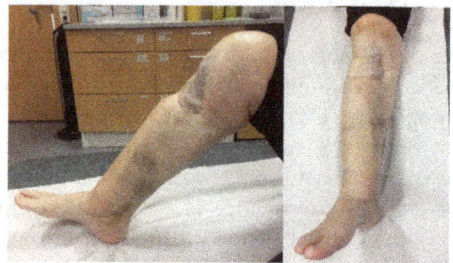

FIGURE 5: Patient's right lower extremity image in an 8-year follow-up visit. The silver coating created a mild, local skin argyria pigmentation, with cosmetic discomfort.

3. Discussion

Due to the subcutaneous location of the tibia and its close proximity to vital neurovascular and musculotendinous structures, limb salvage surgery can be difficult to achieve in tibia bone malignancies. Complication rates are higher in the proximal and distal tibia than at other locations, and they are highest with total tibia reconstructions [8]. PJIs, particularly in tibia locations, comprise the main indication for a secondary amputation. The 10-year implant survival rates are reported to be 40–74%, following tumor resection and reconstruction with different types of EPRs. However, those studies mostly investigated implant survival for fixed- or rotating-hinge knee prostheses, with some total femoral prostheses, but none investigated a total tibia replacement [9].

In our opinion, it is essential to use a well-vascularized flap after implant reconstruction. Muscle flaps have demonstrated good adherence to implants, and thus they resist seroma formation and lower the risk of infection. Technically, a free flap is relatively easy to use in the primary operation, because vascular structures are well exposed.

The soft tissue reconstruction is very important to prevent infection complications. In present case, a free latissimus dorsi flap was wrapped around the prosthesis to avoid dead space. Rotational medial gastrocnemius was used to cover the defects. In preankle area, it is very important to avoid dead space, cover the defects and get good vascularity, to prevent infection.

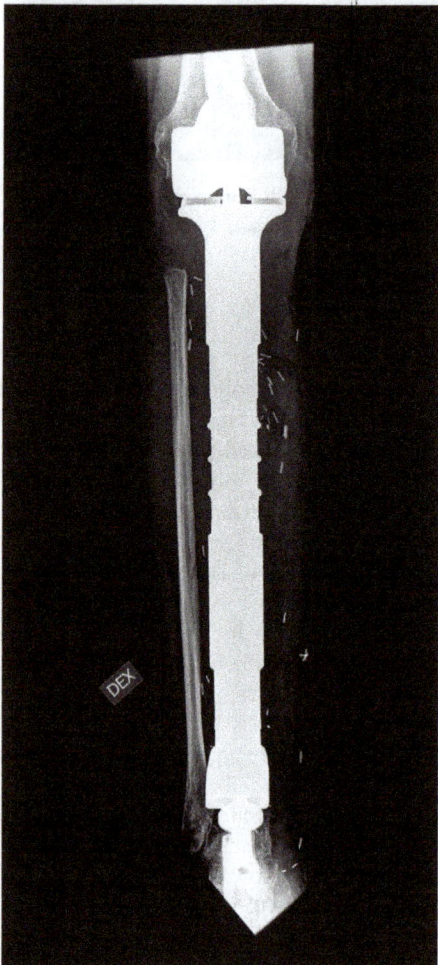

FIGURE 3: Postoperative X-ray from a right tibia. The knee joint was reconstructed with a metal-on-poly articulation with a (unique) metal-on-metal hinge mechanism, and the ankle joint was reconstructed with a metal-on-poly hinge joint with a talar replacement, stabilized with a trans-talar and trans-calcanear hydroxyapatite-coated stem. A supplementary screw was used to add stability in the subtalar joint.

The antimicrobial activity of silver has gained interest in the orthopaedic community, especially among orthopaedic surgeons using megaendoprostheses. The main advantage of using silver-coated EPR includes the reduction of the incidence of PJI with a low level of toxicity [14–16]. Several side effects in silver-coated implants have been reported, including argyria, as seen in our patient, kidney and liver damage, leukopenia, and toxicity in neural tissues. The systemic effects have been reported with blood concentrations exceeding 300 ppb. In large clinical series of silver-coated EPR, silver levels in blood samples did not exceed 56 ppb and were considered nontoxic [17, 18]. Local asymptomatic argyria has been described to occur even in 23% of patients with silver-coated EPR [19].

Eight years postoperatively, the patient resumed working full-time as a kindergarten teacher, and except downhill skiing, she has maintained her previous active lifestyle. On her latest follow-up visit, the motions of knee and ankle ranges were good. In addition, we used 4 PRO measures in the latest follow-up visit (MSTS, OKS, TESS, and 15D). Based on these measures, patient had some limitations in walking and participating in usual leisure activities. She had mild pain from the knee, limping problems, and impossibility to kneel. In addition, patient had moderate difficulties in putting shoes on, gardening, getting in and out of the bath, walking upstairs and downstairs, and getting out of a car. The 15D questionnaire showed that patient had mild sleeping problems and mild sadness. In our opinion, patient's overall functional outcome was good.

Local MRI with a MARS technique enables to observe local recurrences of the tumor around the massive titanium endoprosthesis. This technique reduces the artifacts caused by endoprosthesis, improves the quality of the images at the periprosthetic region, and leads to reliable diagnosis of endoprosthesis-related problems [12].

Due to the rarity of a total tibia EPR, we could identify only one previous case report with a relatively short follow-up. In the literature case report [11], a total tibia EPR was performed for a patient with Ewing sarcoma. They described a 2-year follow-up, with no early-stage complications. In addition, another study has presented a 17-year follow-up of tibia replacement [20]. However, in this osteosarcoma case report, it was not a total tibia replacement as no total ankle joint replacement was made, since part of the distal tibia was not removed. Anterior part of the ankle is a critical location for complications, because of the movement and subcutaneous position of the joint. Also, one reconstruction with a total tibia allograft has been published [10]. In this report, eight months after the surgery, the patient reappeared with rapidly increased pain and the allograft was fractured. About 1 year after the initial diagnosis, a knee disarticulation was performed and the patient was supplied with an exoprosthesis. In this case, authors have discussed that using a prosthesis system instead of the allograft might have saved the limb of their patient [10].

The present report demonstrated that a complex total tibia EPR is feasible with a functionally good outcome. It is important to use a well-vascularized flap after implant reconstruction. Technically, a free flap is relatively easy to use in the primary operation. Muscle flaps have demonstrated good adherence to implants: they resist seroma formation and decrease the risk of infection. However, we emphasize that long-term success required a multidisciplinary team working closely in collaboration with the endoprosthesis industry.

Consent

The patient has given informed consent for the case report to be published.

Conflicts of Interest

The authors declare that they have no conflicts of Interest.

Authors' Contributions

Gilber Kask and Minna K. Laitinen analyzed and interpreted the patient data regarding the oncological disease and the surgery. Surgery was performed by Minna K. Laitinen, Toni-Karri Pakarinen, Hannu Kuokkanen, and Jyrki Nieminen. Jyrki Parkkinen performed the histological examination of the tumor. Gilber Kask and Minna K. Laitinen were a major contributor in writing the manuscript. Minna K. Laitinen, Toni-Karri Pakarinen, and Jyrki Nieminen provided writing assistance. All authors read and approved the final manuscript.

References

[1] P. J. Papagelopoulos, A. F. Mavrogenis, E. C. Galanis, O. D. Savvidou, C. Y. Inwards, and F. H. Sim, "Clinicopathological features, diagnosis, and treatment of adamantinoma of the long bones," *Orthopedics*, vol. 30, pp. 211–215, 2007.

[2] M. Szendrői, I. Antal, and G. Arató, "Adamantinoma of long bones: a longterm follow-up study of 11 cases," *Pathology Oncology Research*, vol. 15, no. 2, pp. 209–216, 2009.

[3] A. A. Qureshi, S. Shott, B. A. Mallin, and S. Gitelis, "Current trends in the management of adamantinoma of long bones," *The Journal of Bone and Joint Surgery-American Volume*, vol. 82, no. 8, pp. 1122–1131, 2000.

[4] V. Y. Jo and C. D. M. Fletcher, "WHO classification of soft tissue tumours: an update based on the 2013 (4th) edition," *Pathology*, vol. 46, no. 2, pp. 95–104, 2014.

[5] D. Jain, V. K. Jain, R. K. Vasishta, P. Ranjan, and Y. Kumar, "Adamantinoma: a clinicopathological review and update," *Diagnostic Pathology*, vol. 3, no. 1, p. 8, 2008.

[6] G. L. Keeney, K. K. Unni, J. W. Beabout, and D. J. Pritchard, "Adamantinoma of long bones. A clinicopathologic study of 85 cases," *Cancer*, vol. 64, no. 3, pp. 730–737, 1989.

[7] C. Khémiri, D. Mrabet, H. Mizouni et al., "Adamantinoma of the tibia and fibula with pulmonary metastasis: an unusual presentation," *BML Case Reports*, vol. 2011, no. oct16 1, p. bcr0620114318, 2011.

[8] T. Morii, H. Morioka, T. Ueda et al., "Deep infection in tumor endoprosthesis around the knee: a multi-institutional study by the Japanese musculoskeletal oncology group," *BMC Musculoskeletal Disorders*, vol. 14, no. 1, p. 51, 2013.

[9] G. J. C. Myers, A. T. Abudu, S. R. Carter, R. M. Tillman, and R. J. Grimer, "The longterm results of endoprosthetic replacement of the proximal tibia for bone tumours," *The Journal of*

Bone and Joint Surgery. British volume, vol. 89-B, no. 12, pp. 1632–1637, 2007.

[10] S. P. Frey, J. Hardes, H. Ahrens, W. Winkelmann, and G. Gosheger, "Total tibia replacement using an allograft (in a patient with adamantinoma). Case report and review of literature," *Journal of Cancer Research and Clinical Oncology*, vol. 134, no. 4, pp. 427–431, 2008.

[11] G. Gosheger, J. Hardes, B. Leidinger et al., "Total tibial endoprosthesis including ankle joint and knee joint replacement in a patient with Ewing sarcoma," *Acta Orthopaedica*, vol. 76, no. 6, pp. 944–946, 2005.

[12] D. Yue, C. Fan Rong, C. Ning et al., "Reduction of metal artifacts from unilateral hip arthroplasty on dual-energy CT with metal artifact reduction software," *Acta Radiologica*, vol. 59, no. 7, pp. 853–860, 2018.

[13] V. Alt, "Antimicrobial coated implants in trauma and orthopaedics-a clinical review and risk-benefit analysis," *Injury*, vol. 48, no. 3, pp. 599–607, 2017.

[14] J. Hardes, C. von Eiff, A. Streitbuerger et al., "Reduction of periprosthetic infection with silver-coated megaprostheses in patients with bone sarcoma," *Journal of Surgical Oncology*, vol. 101, no. 5, pp. 389–395, 2010.

[15] J. Hardes, M. P. Henrichs, G. Hauschild, M. Nottrott, W. Guder, and A. Streitbuerger, "Silver-coated megaprosthesis of the proximal tibia in patients with sarcoma," *The Journal of Arthroplasty*, vol. 32, no. 7, pp. 2208–2213, 2017.

[16] H. Wafa, R. J. Grimer, K. Reddy et al., "Retrospective evaluation of the incidence of early periprosthetic infection with silver-treated endoprostheses in high-risk patients," *The Bone & Joint Journal*, vol. 97-B, no. 2, pp. 252–257, 2015.

[17] J. Hardes, H. Ahrens, C. Gebert et al., "Lack of toxicological side-effects in silver-coated megaprostheses in humans," *Biomaterials*, vol. 28, no. 18, pp. 2869–2875, 2007.

[18] T. Schmidt-Braekling, A. Streitbuerger, G. Gosheger et al., "Silver-coated megaprostheses: review of the literature," *European Journal of Orthopaedic Surgery & Traumatology*, vol. 27, no. 4, pp. 483–489, 2017.

[19] M. Glehr, A. Leithner, J. Friesenbichler et al., "Argyria following the use of silver-coated megaprostheses: no association between the development of local argyria and elevated silver levels," *The Bone & Joint Journal*, vol. 95-B, no. 7, pp. 988–992, 2013.

[20] R. D. Burghardt, D. Kendoff, W. Klauser, H. Mau, and T. Gehrke, "A 17-year follow-up after total tibial replacement in the course of an osteosarcoma followed by total leg replacement," *Journal of Knee Surgery Reports*, vol. 1, no. 01, pp. 044–050, 2015.

14

The Treatment of Cleidocranial Dysostosis (Scheuthauer-Marie-Sainton Syndrome), a Rare Form of Skeletal Dysplasia, Accompanied by Spinal Deformities

Mehmet Bülent Balioğlu [ID],[1] **Deniz Kargın,**[2] **Akif Albayrak,**[2] and **Yunus Atıcı**[3]

[1]*Department of Orthopaedics, Istinye University Liv Hospital, Istanbul, Turkey*
[2]*Department of Orthopedics, Health Science University Baltalimani Bone Diseases Education and Research Hospital, Istanbul, Turkey*
[3]*Department of Orthopaedics, Okan University Hospital, Istanbul, Turkey*

Correspondence should be addressed to Mehmet Bülent Balioğlu; mbbalibey@gmail.com

Academic Editor: Ali F. Ozer

Cleidocranial dysostosis is a skeletal dysplasia inherited in an autosomal dominant manner and may lead to complications such as scoliosis and kyphosis, concurrent with various orthopedic involvements. Since concurrent spinal deformities are of progressive nature, surgical treatment may be necessary. In addition to other orthopedic problems, possible accompanying complications such as atlanto-axial subluxation, myelopathy, syringomyelia, congenital spine deformities, spondylosis, and spondylolisthesis should be kept in mind while planning for the treatment of scoliosis and kyphosis. Lengthening the use of growth-friendly systems (growing rod) in patients, like ours, with an early onset of symptoms, and performing posterior instrumentation and fusion once the spinal growth is complete will yield successful results with no complications in the middle and the long term. Further multicenter studies with more comprehensive assessments are required to find solutions to spinal problems related to this rare skeletal dysplasia.

1. Introduction

Cleidocranial dysostosis is a skeletal dysplasia inherited in an autosomal dominant manner and is characterized by intramembranous bone formation. It causes abnormalities in the clavicle, cranium, and pelvis. The disorder was first described by Marie and Sainton in 1898 [1, 2] and is also known as cleidocranial dysplasia, Scheuthauer-Marie-Sainton syndrome, mutational dysostosis, osteodental dysplasia, generalized dysostosis, pelvicocleidocranial dysplasia, and cleidocranial-pubic dysostosis [3].

Cleidocranial dysostosis is a condition inherited in an autosomal dominant manner in which 1/3 of the patients show spontaneous mutation and 2/3 show familial variation [4]. The responsible gene RUNX2 (Runt-related transcription factor 2) is a cloned gene located on the short arm of Chromosome 6 (6p21) [5–8]. RUNX2 activates osteoblast differentiation as an osteoblastic-specific transcription factor and a regulator of osteoblast differentiation [6, 9]. It also controls the differentiation of precursor cells in osteoblasts. The cells secrete bone matrix and thus form a bone. In addition, RUNX2 plays a key role in the regulation of chondrocyte differentiation during endochondral bone formation. This new "principal gene" may explain the underlying mechanisms of bone formation in addition to the pathobiology of cleidocranial dysostosis [10].

Characteristic findings of cleidocranial dysostosis include hypoplasia or the absence of the clavicle, brachycephalic skull, hypoplasia in the middle of the face, delayed closure of the fontanelles, and slight to moderate shortness in stature.

Although the most important abnormalities are seen in bone reformations through intramembranous ossification in the clavicle, cranium, and the pelvis, endochondral bone growth is also mildly impaired and causes a mild form of dwarfism [2, 4]. Delay in the eruption of permanent teeth and the presence of supernumerary teeth is a significant cause of morbidity [10] which in turn requires numerous oral surgeries and a long-term dental treatment [1]. As a result of the inadequate ossification of the contours of the embryonic vertebral arch, spinal deformities such as spina bifida, scoliosis, kyphosis/kyphoscoliosis, spondylolysis, spondylolisthesis, hemivertebra, posterior wedging of vertebrae, and cervical ribs may develop and these conditions may be seen together with the absence of the posterior thoracic vertebral arch or syringomyelia [1, 4, 10, 11]. Cleidocranial dysostosis has an estimated prevalence of 1/1,000,000 (Table 1). However, due to lack of diagnosis, its prevalence is estimated to be higher with no differences being reported between genders or ethnicities [1].

In order to better understand this rare skeletal dysplasia and the spinal deformities that accompany it, we present in this study the treatment outcomes in two patients with cleidocranial dysostosis and a review of the literature.

2. Case Report

We performed posterior fusion and instrumentation due to progressive scoliosis in two adolescent female patients diagnosed with cleidocranial dysostosis following genetic screening. Both patients had a positive family history of the condition. In addition to the spinal deformities, we thoroughly examined the concurrent orthopedic and dental problems of the patients. The mean age of the patients was 12 (range: 11 to 13) years at the time of surgery and the mean follow-up period was 11 (range: 6 to 16) years. The clinical and radiological outcomes were retrospectively evaluated (Table 2).

In the first case (28-year-old female), the patient had the typical phenotypic characteristics of cleidocranial dysostosis (short stature, open anterior fontanelle, typical facial appearance, a wide and protruding forehead, and dental problems), bilateral pseudoarthrosis of the clavicle, slightly widened pubic symphysis, small iliac wings, bilateral shortness of the femoral neck and coxa vara, bilateral genu valgum in the lower extremity, progressive scoliosis, and a positive family history (in her father and grandmother) at presentation. Bilateral osteotomy of the proximal tibia and variation with external fixators were performed to treat the gene valgum deformity (at the age of 11). Correction of the progressive scoliosis deformity and fusion was achieved using posterior pedicle screws and hook fixation (13 years). No complications were observed throughout the regular follow-up period of 16 years (Figures 1 and 2).

The second case had short stature, bilateral growth failure in the clavicles (pseudoarthrosis on the right side and lateral aplasia on the left one), widened pubic symphysis, coxa vara, dental problems, progressive scoliosis/kyphosis, and a positive family history. At the age of 11, a growing rod was first applied on the patient for her scoliosis and kyphosis.

TABLE 1: Distinguishing characteristics of cleidocranial dysostosis.

Distinguishing characteristics of cleidocranial dysostosis	
Heredity	Autosomal dominant
Responsible gene and chromosome	RUNX2 gene/6p21 chromosome
Stature	Shortness of stature (K > E)
Prevalence	<1 million
Appearance of the face	Protruding frontal and parietal bones, depressed nasal bridge Tooth eruption problems Incomplete fusion of the mandibular symphysis Small face Slightly widened eyes High and narrow palate
Skull	Wormian bones Open fontanelles in children No cranial nerve palsy Wide head
Clavicle	Partially present or totally absent Irritation of the brachial plexus irritation (rare)
Scapula	Small, wings may be noticeable Winging may be painful or symptomatic
Thorax, sternum and shoulders	Narrow thorax and pectus excavatum Low shoulders Sternum anomalies
Hands and feet	Delayed ossification in the carpal and tarsal bones Terminal phalanges are short, pointed, hypoplastic, or absent Presence of epiphyses on both the proximal and distal ends of the 2–5 metatarsals and metacarpals Second metacarpal bone is usually long
The pelvis and hips	Wide pubic symphysis Wide triradiate cartilage and sacroiliac joints Small iliac wings Coxa vara, short femoral neck Hip dysplasia (rare)
The spine and intraspinal structures	Spina bifida occulta (thoracic and lumbar) Scoliosis Lumbar spondylolysis (24%) and spondylolisthesis Hemi vertebrae, posterior wedging Syringomyelia Myelopathy due to atlanto-axial subluxation (rare)
Other conditions	Susceptibility to Wilms tumor

The rod was lengthened two times in two years. At 13 years of age, the patient was applied pedicle screws at all levels of the posterior spine and Ponte osteotomy and fusion to the deformity apices. Six years after the first spinal surgery and four years after the fusion, the patient developed no complications. Adequate spinal correction and patient satisfaction were achieved (Figures 3 and 4).

TABLE 2: Distinguishing features in cleidocranial dysostosis patients.

Initials	Age (yrs) Sex	Follow-up (yrs)	Clinical and radiological findings	Treatment	Scoliosis (°)		Kyphosis (°)		Complication
					Preop	Follow-up	Preop	Follow-up	
BY	13 (F)	16	Typical appearance in the face and head, tooth eruption problems, short stature, scoliosis, coxa vara, wide pubic symphysis, deformity of the lower extremity, clavicular hypoplasia, osteopenia	Posterior pedicle screw fixation and fusion with hook constructs of T2-L3	52/60	37/38	50	37	—
ET	11 (F)	6	Small face and anteriorly protruding forehead, clavicular hypoplasia, tooth problems, kyphoscoliosis, wide pubic symphysis, coxa vara	Posterior T3-L3 growing rod, following gradual lengthening Posterior pedicle screw fixation of T2-L2, Ponte osteotomy, fusion	74	19	70	34	PJK (25°) development following growing rod application. Fixed with posterior fusion of the next level above

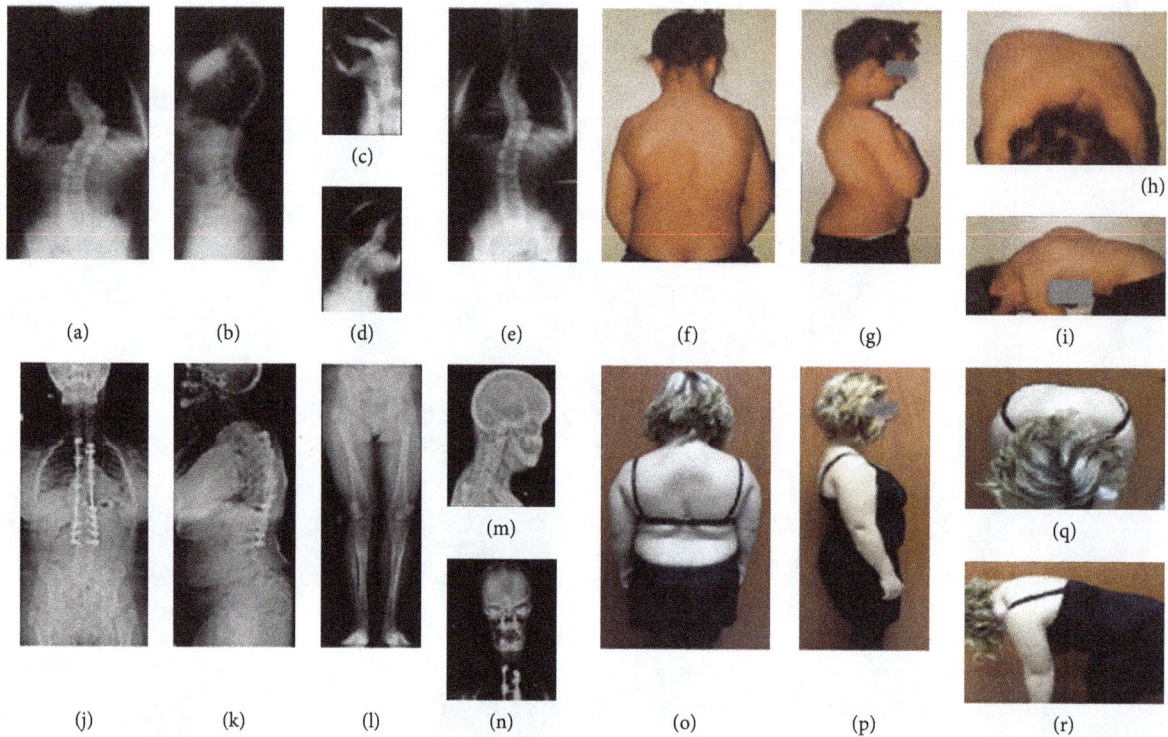

FIGURE 1: (a–i) CCD in an adolescent patient (B.Y.) accompanied by bilateral pseudoarthrosis of the clavicle, small face, protruding forehead, open anterior fontanelles, tooth eruption problems, short stature, and coxa vara. Posterior instrumentation and fusion was performed for scoliosis (posterior T2-L3 pedicle screw and fusion with hook construct). (j–r) Orthoroentgenograms and clinical appearance of the patient on postoperative 16th year.

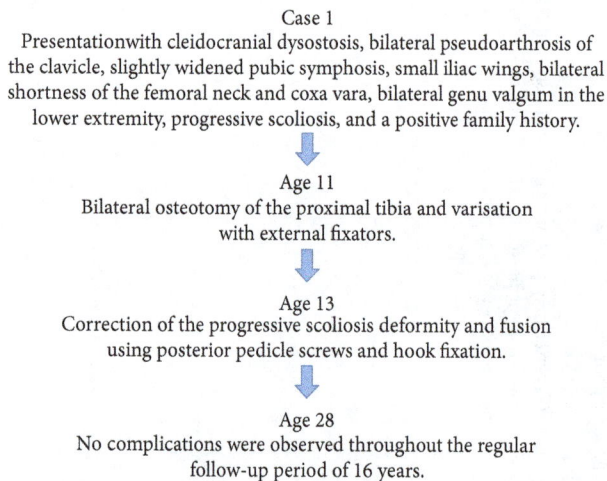

Case 1
Presentation with cleidocranial dysostosis, bilateral pseudoarthrosis of the clavicle, slightly widened pubic symphosis, small iliac wings, bilateral shortness of the femoral neck and coxa vara, bilateral genu valgum in the lower extremity, progressive scoliosis, and a positive family history.

⬇

Age 11
Bilateral osteotomy of the proximal tibia and variasion with external fixators.

⬇

Age 13
Correction of the progressive scoliosis deformity and fusion using posterior pedicle screws and hook fixation.

⬇

Age 28
No complications were observed throughout the regular follow-up period of 16 years.

FIGURE 2: Timeline of the disorder and treatment for case 1.

3. Discussion

Cleidocranial dysostosis is a skeletal dysplasia inherited in an autosomal dominant manner and is characterized by abnormal formation of the endomembranous bone. The middle 1/3 of the clavicle, the cranium, and the pelvis are the most affected areas. Dental abnormalities are a common finding in patients [4]. Coxa vara is common due to metaphyseal disorders, and the deformity is usually of moderate degree and can self-heal with growth. In general, a genu varum deformity accompanies the condition and femoral and/or tibial osteotomy may be required [12].

Cleidocranial dysostosis is a condition inherited in an autosomal dominant manner in which 1/3 of the patients show spontaneous mutation and 2/3 show familial variation [4]. The responsible gene RUNX2 (Runt-related transcription factor 2) is a cloned gene located on the short arm of Chromosome 6 (6p21) [5–7]. RUNX2 activates the osteoblast differentiation as an osteoblastic-specific transcription factor and a regulator of osteoblast differentiation [6, 9]. It also controls the differentiation of precursor cells in osteoblasts. The cells secrete bone matrix and thus form a bone. In addition, RUNX2 plays a key role in the regulation of chondrocyte differentiation during endochondral bone formation. This new "principal gene" may explain the underlying mechanisms of bone formation in addition to the pathobiology of cleidocranial dysostosis [10].

The condition typically manifests itself within the first two years of life. Although it has an estimated prevalence of 1/1,000,000, an incidence of 0.5 cases per 100,000 live births and more than 1000 cases until the year 2004 have been reported. Lachman described 38 cases based on his personal experience [3]. The affected children have a small face but a big head (the skull is bigger than usual but the face is smaller), the eyes are slightly wider, the palate is high and narrow, deciduous teeth emerge normally but the eruption of permanent teeth are delayed and imperfect

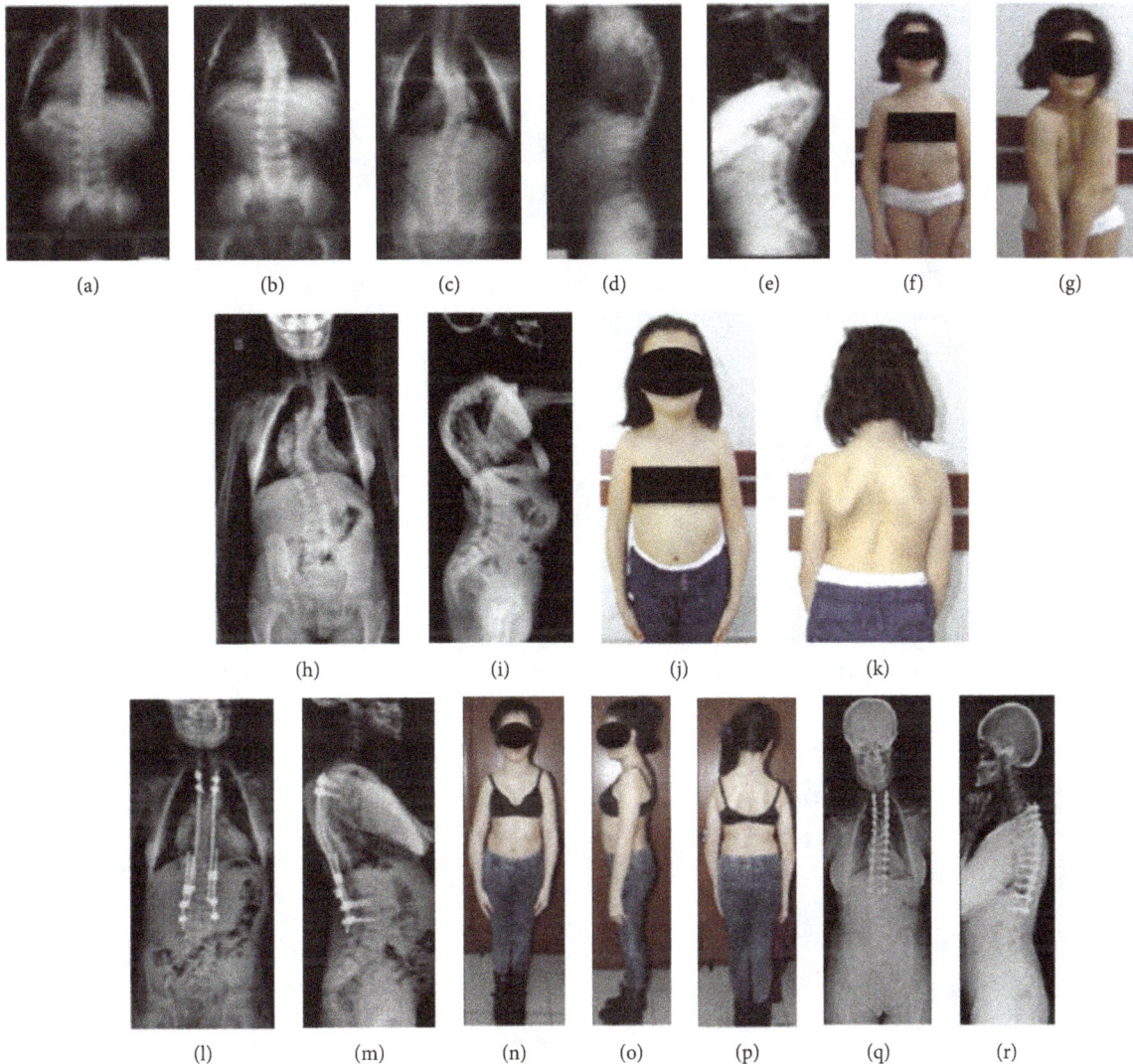

FIGURE 3: (a–g) Clavicular hypoplasia, widened pubic symphysis, bilateral coxa vara, progressive scoliosis, and kyphosis marked by growth and grade 1 spondylolisthesis in our female patient (E.T.) with CCD. Hypermobile shoulders typically coming close together before the chest, due to concurrent bilateral clavicular hypoplasia. (h–k) Radiological and clinical appearances of scoliosis and kyphosis. (l, m) Growing rod applied (from the posterior, between T2 and L3) at 11 years of age and later was lengthened two times in two years. (n–r) Clinical and radiological images from the second year follow-up of the 13-year-old patient, and Ponte osteotomy and fusion to the deformity apices (fixation with pedicle screws at all levels between T2 and L2 and Ponte osteotomy and fusion to the deformity apices).

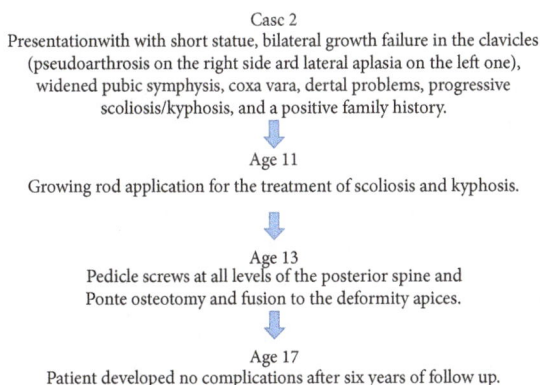

Case 2

Presentationwith with short statue, bilateral growth failure in the clavicles (pseudoarthrosis on the right side ard lateral aplasia on the left one), widened pubic symphysis, coxa vara, dertal problems, progressive scoliosis/kyphosis, and a positive family history.

↓

Age 11

Growing rod application for the treatment of scoliosis and kyphosis.

↓

Age 13

Pedicle screws at all levels of the posterior spine and Ponte osteotomy and fusion to the deformity apices.

↓

Age 17

Patient developed no complications after six years of follow up.

FIGURE 4: Timeline of the disorder and treatment for case 2.

and supernumerary teeth are present (65%) [2, 3], and the shoulders are low and the thorax looks narrow, thus leading to respiratory problems in the newborn [3, 13]. Anomalies in the sternum are due to abnormal intramembranous ossification and pectus excavatum is a prevailing condition [2]. One or both of the clavicles may show growth deficiencies and they may be totally absent [4]. The most common defect is the absence of the lateral end of the clavicle, followed by the growth failure of the middle 1/3 of the clavicle. The defect can be palpated. As a result of hypermobility in bilateral cases, the shoulders may come in contact with each other before the chest (Figure 5). The scapula may look smaller and the wings may be noticeable [2]. Patients with cleidocranial dysostosis are short, the mean height in adult males is between

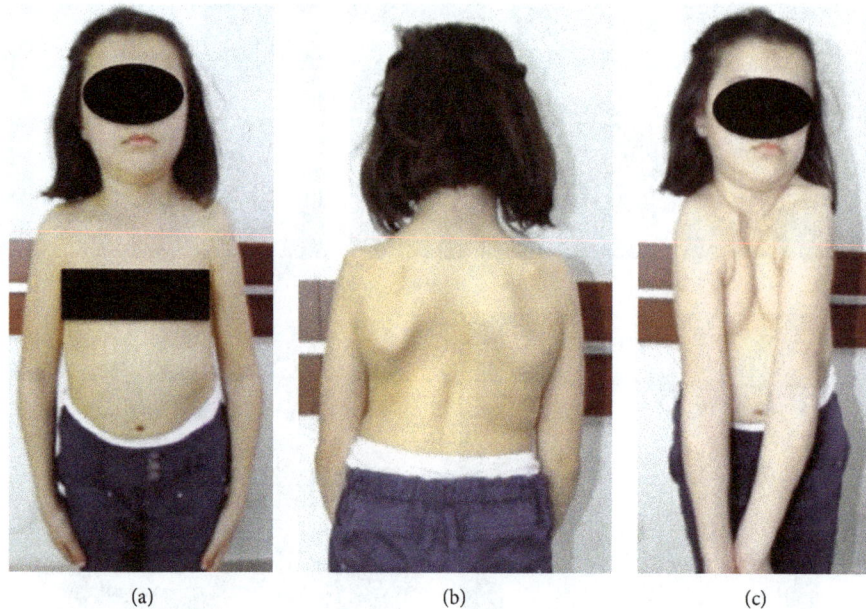

(a)   (b)   (c)

FIGURE 5: (a) Anterior and (b) posterior appearance of the clavicular winging in a 6.5-year-old girl with cleidocranial dysostosis. (c) Hypermobile shoulders typically coming close together before the chest, due to concurrent bilateral clavicular hypoplasia.

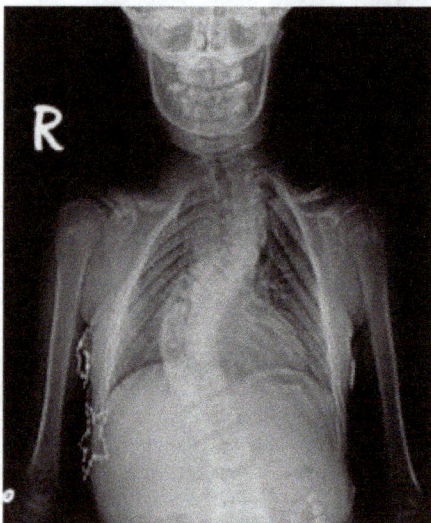

FIGURE 6: Radiograph of the same bilateral clavicular hypoplasia patient at age 11, showing poor growth of the middle 1/3 of the right clavicle and the absence of the lateral end of the left clavicle. Narrowing of the chest can be seen.

the 5th and 50th percentile of height for their age, whereas in females dwarfism is more apparent and the mean height is below the 5th percentile of height of their peers [10]. Progressive scoliosis or syringomyelia may be observed [3, 10, 11]. Susceptibility to Wilms tumor has been also reported [14].

Orthopedic problems may include the absence of the clavicular end or hypoplasia of the muscles originating from or inserting into the clavicle, particularly the anterior part of the deltoid and sternocleidomastoid muscle. Hypoplasia and the absence of the clavicle can be clearly seen in the radiographs

(Figure 6). The absence of the clavicle can be seen even in prenatal ultrasonography [15, 16]. The irritation of the brachial plexus is rare and may occur with pain and numbness. Excision of the clavicular fragment may lead to decompression of the brachial plexus. Scapular winging may be painful or symptomatic. Scapulothoracic arthrodesis has been described as the method of treatment for those cases [17].

Multiple Wormian bones and poor mineralization of the cranium are noticeable on cranial radiographs. Closure of the sutures is significantly delayed and the anterior fontanelle widens. In some patients, the anterior fontanelle never closes. Nasal, lacrimal, and malar bones may be hypoplastic or undeveloped, and the zygoma develops poorly. The maxilla may be small and the mandibular symphysis may be unfused (Figure 7) [2].

The pelvis shows bilateral involvement. The pubic symphysis remains wide (Figure 8) [18]. Fusion may be incomplete or thin in ramus. The sacroiliac joint may be wider than usual. The iliac wings are small. Coxa vara may accompany cleidocranial dysostosis and the femoral neck is significantly short (Figure 8). Coxa vara is treated with the valgus osteotomy of the proximal femur. Indications for surgery are the same as those in developmental coxa vara (a head-neck angle of less than 90°, Hilgenreiner's epiphyseal angle of 60° or more, or progression of the deformity). Following osteotomy, the acetabular bone remodeling may be observed in young patients. Pelvic osteotomy is recommended to enhance the covering of the hip in older children [19]. Dislocation of the hip is rarely encountered [2].

Ossification is delayed in the carpal and tarsal bones. Terminal phalanges may be short, pointed, hypoplastic, or totally absent. Both the proximal and distal ends of the 2–5 metatarsals and metacarpals have epiphyses. The second metacarpal bone is usually long [2].

(a)   (b)

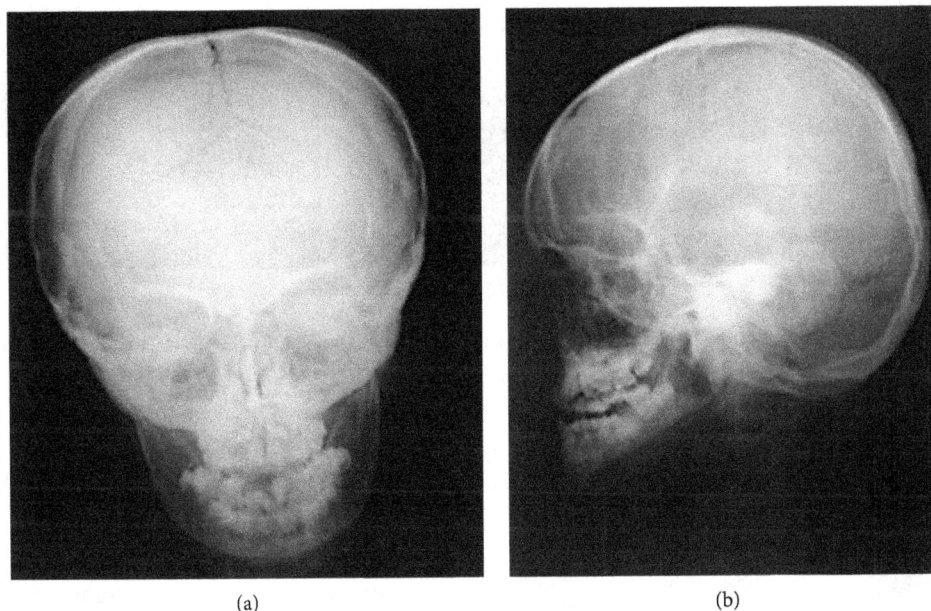

FIGURE 7: (a, b) Delayed closure of the sutures, widening of the anterior fontanelle, Wormian bones, sclerotic skull base, numerous supernumerary teeth, and malocclusion can be seen in the cranial radiographs (11 years).

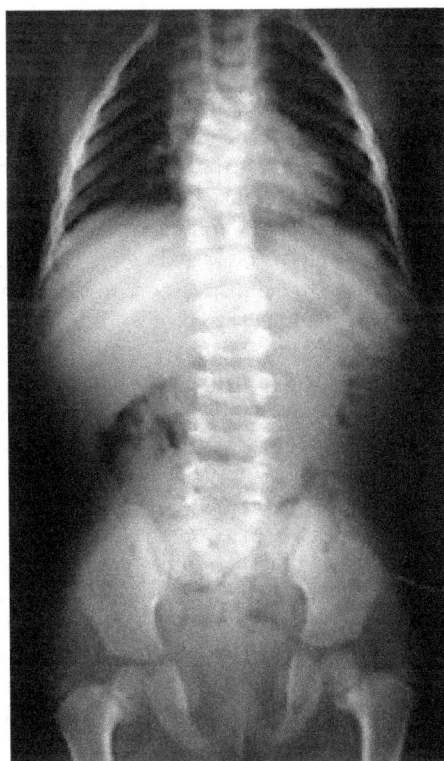

FIGURE 8: Widened pubic symphysis, bilateral coxa vara, and widened triradiate cartilage and sacroiliac joints can be seen in the pelvic radiographs (6.5 years).

Spina bifida occulta may develop in the thoracic and lumbar spine due to inadequate development of the posterior vertebral elements (Figure 9) [10], progressive scoliosis and kyphosis of the spine may be encountered (Figure 10) [9], and lumbar spondylolysis may occur in 24% of the patients concurrently (Figure 11) [10, 20]. The treatment of scoliosis in these patients is similar to that of idiopathic scoliosis (Figures 1 and 3) [2]. Syringomyelia has been also associated with the condition [21].

Cleidocranial dysostosis may be confused with pyknodysostosis due to the hypoplasia of the clavicle; however, osteosclerosis is not seen in patients with cleidocranial dysostosis but with pyknodysostosis [22, 23].

Differential diagnosis of congenital clavicle pseudoarthrosis may be necessary especially in the first years of life. Congenital clavicle pseudoarthrosis is almost always seen on the right side; only 10% of the patients show bilateral involvement. Dextrocardia may be encountered concurrently; the condition is congenital and the heart is usually pointed out toward the middle 1/3 of the clavicle [19].

Inadequate ossification of the contours of the embryonic vertebral arch may lead to spinal deformities such as spina bifida, scoliosis, kyphosis/kyphoscoliosis, hemivertebra and posterior wedging of vertebrae, and cervical ribs, and these conditions may be seen together with the absence of the posterior thoracic vertebral arch or syringomyelia [10, 21, 24]. A MRI scan of the spinal cord is recommended for syringomyelia and concurrent anomalies [21]. Spondylosis, spondylolisthesis, and spina bifida occulta may accompany the condition [10, 11]. Scoliosis may develop as a consequence to the imbalance of the shoulder girdle muscles and vertebral dysplasia [1, 11, 25]. Codsi et al. [24] suggested that the unilateral absence of the clavicle had a positive relationship with the rapid progression of scoliosis and that unilateral absence of the clavicle in immature children may lead to rapid progression of the curvature [1, 24]. In addition, the majority of the patients may encounter respiratory complications [1].

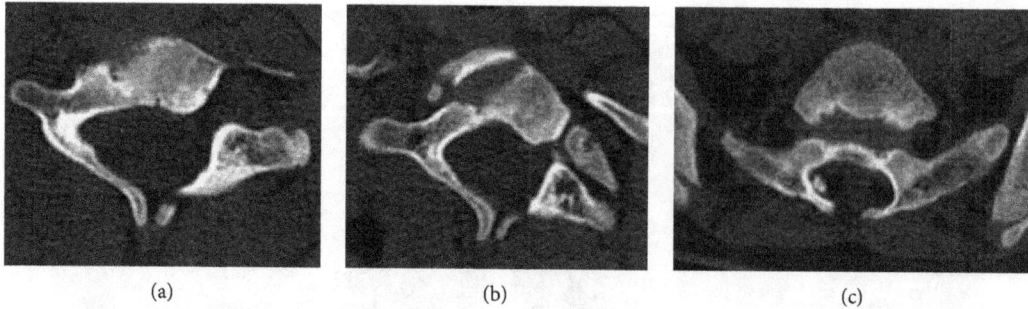

(a)   (b)   (c)

FIGURE 9: CT images showing spina bifida occulta in the (a) cervical, (b) thoracic, and (c) sacral spine of the patient (12 years).

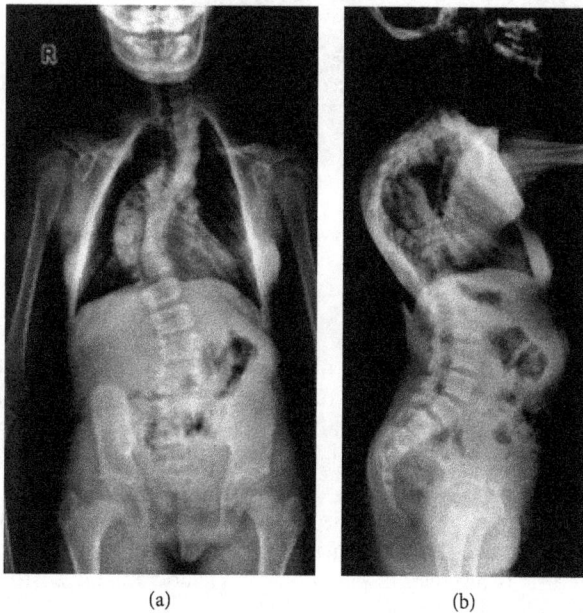

(a)   (b)

FIGURE 10: Progressive (a) scoliosis and (b) kyphosis in the spine (12 years).

The surgical treatment in idiopathic scoliosis is also recommended for scoliosis. Codsi et al. performed posterior spinal instrumentation on a girl with rapid progression of scoliosis, hypoplasia of the posterior elements of the thoracic spine, and posterior fusion anomalies in C4–6. No complications were reported after five years of follow-up [24]. In a multicenter study, Cooper et al. [1] found significant increases in genu valgum, pes planus, sinus infections, upper respiratory tract problems, recurrent otitis media, and hearing loss of 90 individuals with cleidocranial dysostosis and their 56 next of kin, identified by genetic and dental examinations. The author also reported scoliosis in 16 patients (17%) from the cleidocranial dysostosis group and one patient from the control group (1.8%). Only three of the 16 patients had used braces; none of them required surgery, and the incidence of scoliosis was much higher than that in controls and the general population. Trigui et al. studied the different clinical aspects of cleidocranial dysostosis and orthopedic problems in two cases and reported that dental anomalies, coxa vara, and scoliosis needed regular follow-up and, in case of worsening of the symptoms,

these problems should be treated [26]. Al Kaissi et al. [11] observed progressive scoliosis and kyphosis in five of seven patients with cleidocranial dysostosis and defined spinal deformities as problems leading to progressive and major orthopedic problems. The authors also stated that the spinal deformity may progress in continuation of the cartilaginous spinal structure. Injuries to the craniocervical region in cleidocranial dysostosis patients can lead to a wide range of complications from nondisplaced avulsion fractures of the occipital condyle to complete atlanto-occipital or atlanto-axial dislocations which may lead to morbid or fatal outcomes. Therefore, a thorough examination and evaluation of the patients with scoliosis deformity has been recommended [11]. In their retrospective study of 13 patients with deformities associated with rare disorders, Soultanis et al. performed posterior instrumentation and fusion on an 18-year-old male cleidocranial dysostosis patient with a rigid thoracic curve (85°) and spina bifida in the lower cervical and superior thoracic spine and reported that the patient was stable after seven years of follow-up [27]. Kobayashi et al. [28] published the clinical course and treatment outcomes of a 27-year-old female patient with cleidocranial dysostosis and spastic myelopathy due to atlanto-axial subluxation. The patient was operated two times for cervical myelopathy and atlanto-axial subluxation and had undergone a laminectomy of the atlas and C1-C2 fusion via a transpharyngeal approach and cervico-occipital fusion using Luque rod systems. The patient developed solid fusion at the postoperative seventh month and the MRI scan confirmed that the spinal cord was no longer decompressed; however, atrophy was still present. After two years of follow-up, the patient showed no neurological progress and still had spasticity. Although myelopathy due to atlanto-axial subluxation is rarely encountered in patients, it should be kept in mind during the follow-up and treatment of this disorder.

The limitation of our study was that we were able to evaluate only two patients. As the condition is a rare one, further multicenter studies are required in order to perform a more comprehensive assessment.

In conclusion, cleidocranial dysostosis may lead to complications such as scoliosis and kyphosis concurrent with various orthopedic involvements due to skeletal dysplasia. Since concurrent spinal deformities are of progressive nature, as in our cases, surgical treatment may be necessary. In addition to other orthopedic problems,

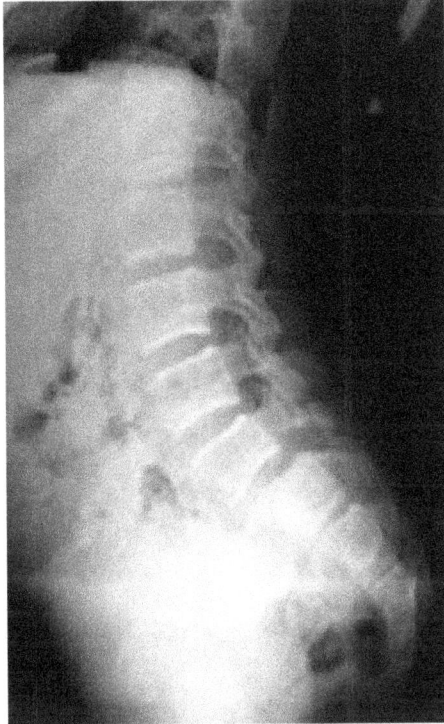

FIGURE 11: Concurrent lumbar spondylolysis (6.5 years).

possible accompanying complications such as atlanto-axial subluxation, myelopathy, syringomyelia, congenital spine deformities, spondylosis and spondylolisthesis, respiratory problems, and postoperative complications should be kept in mind while planning for the treatment of scoliosis and kyphosis. Through lengthening using growth-friendly systems (growing rod) in patients, like ours, with an early onset of symptoms, and once the spinal growth is complete, performing posterior instrumentation and fusion, as we did in both our cases, will yield successful results with no complications in the middle and long term. Further multicenter studies with more comprehensive assessments are required to find solutions to spinal problems related to this rare skeletal dysplasia.

Conflicts of Interest

The authors declare that there are no conflicts of interest regarding the publication of this paper.

References

[1] S. C. Cooper, C. M. Flaitz, D. A. Johnston, B. Lee, and J. T. Hecht, "A natural history of cleidocranial dysplasia," *American Journal of Medical Genetics*, vol. 104, no. 1, pp. 1–6, 2001.

[2] J. A. Herring, "Skeletal dysplasias," in *Tachdjian's Pediatric Orthopaedics*, J. A. Herring, Ed., pp. e449–e451, Elsevier, Philadelphia, PA, USA, 5th edition, 2014.

[3] R. S. Lachman, "Skeletal dysplasias," in *Taybi and Lachman, Radiology of Syndromes, Metabolic Disorders and Skeletal Dysplasias*, R. S. Lachman, Ed., pp. 913–915, Mosby, Philadelphia, PA, USA, 5th edition, 2007.

[4] K. Machol, R. Mendoza-Londono, and B. Lee, "Cleidocranial dysplasia spectrum disorder," in *GeneReviews®*, M. P. Adam, H. H. Ardinger, R. A. Pagon, S. E. Wallace, B. LJH, K. Stephens, and A. Amemiya, Eds., University of Washington, Seattle, WA, USA, 2006, (updated 2017).

[5] F. R. Dietz and K. D. Mathews, "Update on the genetic bases of disorders with orthopaedic manifestations," *The Journal of Bone and Joint Surgery-American Volume*, vol. 78, no. 10, pp. 1583–1598, 1996.

[6] B. Lee, K. Thirunavukkarasu, L. Zhou et al., "Missense mutations abolishing DNA binding of the osteoblast-specific transcription factor OSF2/CBFA1 in cleidocranial dysplasia," *Nature Genetics*, vol. 16, no. 3, pp. 307–310, 1997.

[7] S. Mundlos, F. Otto, C. Mundlos et al., "Mutations involving the transcription factor CBFA1 cause cleidocranial dysplasia," *Cell*, vol. 89, no. 5, pp. 773–779, 1997.

[8] Y. Qian, Y. Zhang, B. Wei et al., "A novel Alu-mediated microdeletion in the RUNX2 gene in a Chinese patient with cleidocranial dysplasia," *Journal of Genetics*, vol. 97, no. 1, pp. 137–143, 2018.

[9] P. Ducy, R. Zhang, V. Geoffroy, A. L. Ridall, and G. Karsenty, "Osf2/Cbfa1: a transcriptional activator of osteoblast differentiation," *Cell*, vol. 89, no. 5, pp. 747–754, 1997.

[10] S. Mundlos, "Cleidocranial dysplasia: clinical and molecular genetics," *Journal of Medical Genetics*, vol. 36, no. 3, pp. 177–182, 1999.

[11] A. A. Kaissi, F. B. Chehida, V. Kenis et al., "Broad spectrum of skeletal malformation complex in patients with cleidocranial dysplasia syndrome: radiographic and tomographic study," *Clinical Medicine Insights: Arthritis and Musculoskeletal Disorders*, vol. 6, article CMAMD.S11933, 2013.

[12] M. Trigui, S. Pannier, G. Finidori, J. P. Padovani, and C. Glorion, "Coxa vara in chondrodysplasia prognosis study of 35 hips in 19 children," *Journal of Pediatric Orthopedics*, vol. 28, no. 6, pp. 599–606, 2008.

[13] K. L. Tan and L. K. A. Tan, "Cleidocranial dysostosis in infancy," *Pediatric Radiology*, vol. 11, no. 2, pp. 114–116, 1981.

[14] J. H. M. Merks, H. N. Caron, and R. C. M. Hennekam, "High incidence of malformation syndromes in a series of 1,073 children with cancer," *American Journal of Medical Genetics Part A*, vol. 134A, no. 2, pp. 132–143, 2005.

[15] L. H. Hamner 3rd, E. L. Fabbri, and P. C. Browne, "Prenatal diagnosis of cleidocranial dysostosis," *Obstetrics and Gynecology*, vol. 83, 5, Part 2, pp. 856–857, 1994.

[16] J. Hassan, W. Sepulveda, J. Teixeira, C. Garrett, and N. M. Fisk, "Prenatal sonographic diagnosis of cleidocranial dysostosis," *Prenatal Diagnosis*, vol. 17, no. 8, pp. 770–772, 1997.

[17] S. G. Krishnan, R. J. Hawkins, J. D. Michelotti, R. Litchfield, R. B. Willis, and Y. K. Kim, "Scapulothoracic arthrodesis: indications, technique, and results," *Clinical Orthopaedics and Related Research*, vol. 435, no. 6, pp. 126–133, 2005.

[18] J. G. Gamble, S. C. Simmons, and M. Freedman, "The symphysis pubis anatomic and pathologic considerations," *Clinical Orthopaedics and Related Research*, vol. 203, pp. 261–272, 1986.

[19] M. F. Richie and C. E. Johnston 2nd, "Management of developmental coxa vara in cleidocranial dysostosis," *Orthopedics*, vol. 12, no. 7, pp. 1001–1004, 1989.

[20] B. L. Jensen, "Somatic development in cleidocranial dysplasia," *American Journal of Medical Genetics*, vol. 35, no. 1, pp. 69–74, 1990.

[21] D. D. Dore, G. D. MacEwen, and M. I. Boulos, "Cleidocranial dysostosis and syringomyelia: review of the literature and case report," *Clinical Orthopaedics and Related Research*, vol. 214, no. 1, pp. 229–234, 1987.

[22] A. Greenspan, "Sclerosing bone dysplasias: a target-site approach," *Skeletal Radiology*, vol. 20, no. 8, pp. 561–583, 1991.

[23] J. A. Herring, "Skeletal dysplasias," in *Tachdjian's Pediatric Orthopaedics*, J. A. Herring, Ed., pp. e446–e449, Elsevier, Philadelphia, PA, USA, 5th edition, 2014.

[24] M. J. Codsi, R. M. Kay, P. Masso, and D. L. Skaggs, "Unilateral absence of the clavicle with rapidly progressive scoliosis in an 8-year old," *The American Journal of Orthopedics*, vol. 29, no. 5, pp. 383–386, 2000.

[25] G. Taglialavoro, D. Fabris, and S. Agostini, "A case of progressive scoliosis in a patient with craniocleidopelvic dysostosis," *Italian Journal of Orthopaedics and Traumatology*, vol. 9, no. 4, pp. 507–513, 1983.

[26] M. Trigui, K. Ayadi, M. O. Elhassan, M. Zribi, I. Chabchoub, and H. Keskes, "Cleidocranial dysplasia: report of 2 cases and literature review," *Archives de Pédiatrie*, vol. 18, no. 6, pp. 672–677, 2011.

[27] K. C. Soultanis, A. H. Payatakes, V. T. Chouliaras et al., "Retracted article. Rare causes of scoliosis and spine deformity: experience and particular features," *Scoliosis*, vol. 2, no. 1, p. 15, 2007.

[28] S. Kobayashi, K. Uchida, H. Baba et al., "Atlantoaxial subluxation-induced myelopathy in cleidocranial dysplasia. Case report," *Journal of Neurosurgery: Spine*, vol. 7, no. 2, pp. 243–247, 2007.

15

Ipsilateral Acetabular Fracture with Displaced Femoral Head and Femoral Shaft Fracture: A Complex Floating Hip Injury

Raja Bhaskara Rajasekaran ⓘ**, Dheenadhayalan Jayaramaraju,**
Dhanasekara Raja Palanisami, Ramesh Perumal, and Rajasekaran Shanmuganathan

Department of Orthopaedics & Trauma, 313 Mettupalayam Road, Ganga Medical Centre & Hospitals Pvt. Ltd., Coimbatore, India

Correspondence should be addressed to Raja Bhaskara Rajasekaran; rajalibra299@gmail.com

Academic Editor: Narender Kumar Magu

Floating hip injuries involving the acetabulum, femoral head, and the femoral shaft are a very rare presentation. A complex floating hip injury comprising of an ipsilateral acetabular fracture associated with a displaced femoral head fracture and a femoral shaft fracture following a high-velocity road traffic accident presented to us where all the fractures were addressed with internal fixation during the primary surgery. Postoperatively, the patient suffered a dislocation of the femoral head which eventually went on to avascular necrosis at 5 months from the initial presentation. Then, the patient underwent a total hip replacement with an acetabular reconstruction following which he went on to have a good functional outcome. Our experience in dealing with such a complex case shows that it is difficult to set a protocol for such injuries and they need to be addressed on a case-to-case basis depending on the complexity of the injury.

1. Introduction

A "floating hip" injury—a fracture of the pelvis or acetabulum with a concomitant fracture of the femur—is a very rare presentation with an incidence of about 1 in 10,000 fractures [1–3]. The combination of an ipsilateral acetabular fracture with a displaced femoral head fracture and a femoral shaft fracture is an even rarer presentation. Only two cases of such injuries have been described so far and there is paucity in literature regarding the management of such cases [4]. Here, we present such a case following a road traffic accident and the challenges we faced while addressing all the fractures.

2. Case Report

A 52-year-old farmer was referred to us 7 hours after he had met with a high-velocity road traffic accident. He was resuscitated as per the ATLS protocol at the hospital where he was initially treated and when he arrived at the casualty department of our hospital, he was conscious and all his vital parameters were within normal limits. He also gave the

history that he was under treatment for segmental myoclonus which was characterised by semirhythmic involuntary muscle contractions.

His radiographs showed a left-sided posterior acetabular wall fracture (AO type 6 2 A1). He also had an ipsilateral femoral neck fracture with the femoral head displaced anteriorly (Figures 1(a) and 1(b)) and also an associated middle-third fracture of the shaft of the femur (Figure 1(c)). He also had an extra-articular distal femur fracture on the opposite side (AO type 3 3 A1). On arrival, his serum lactate level was 1.9 mmol/l indicating that he had been adequately resuscitated.

He was taken for definitive surgery 9 hours after arrival. The patient was positioned in the lateral position and a posterolateral approach was planned to address the acetabular and femoral head fractures. Upon dissection, the femoral head (Figure 2(a)) was found to have buttonholed and displaced anteriorly through the capsule which was found to be torn. The posterior wall of the acetabulum was addressed using two contoured reconstruction plates (Figure 2(b)). Using the trochanteric flip osteotomy, better access to the

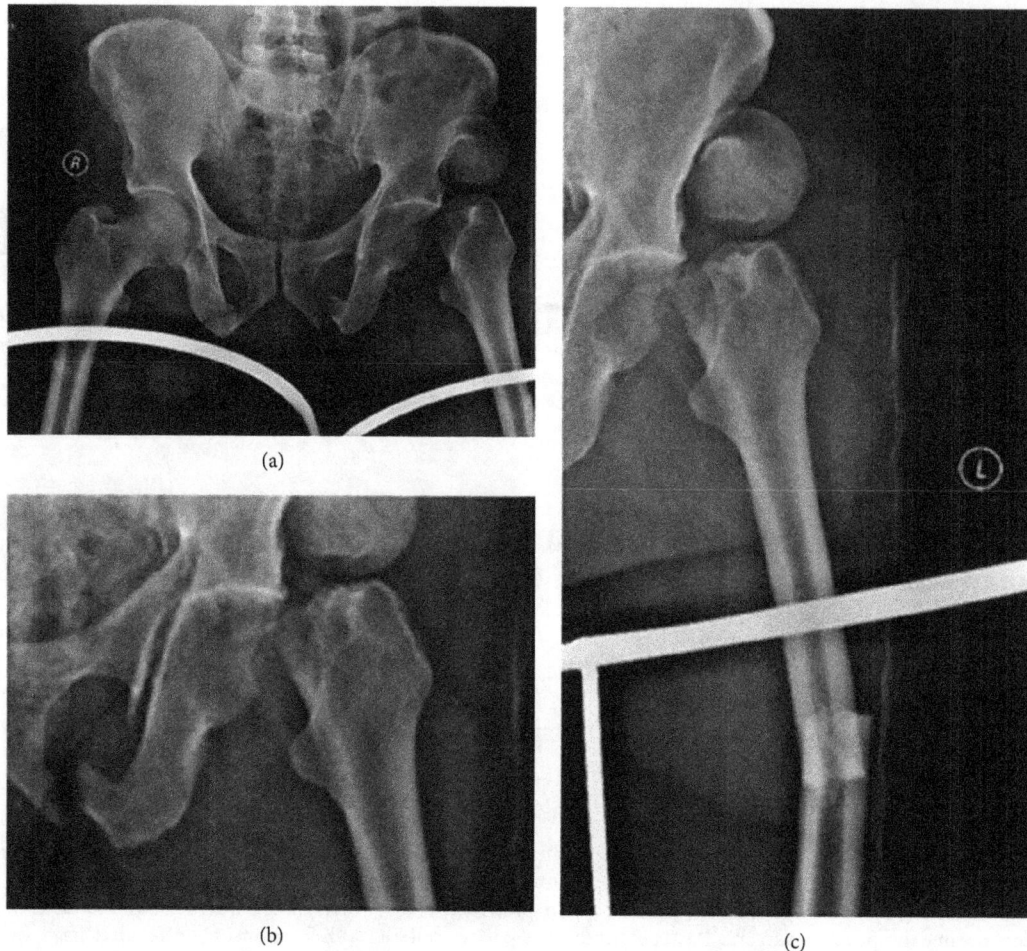

FIGURE 1: Radiographs of the pelvis (a), showing a posterior wall acetabulum fracture (b) with a displaced femoral head and a concomitant femur shaft fracture (c).

femoral neck was achieved and the femoral head was reduced anatomically and secured with K-wires. Then the femoral shaft fracture was reduced by opening the fracture site and held with a clamp. The femoral head fracture and the shaft fracture were fixed with an antegrade femoral nail with two screws securing the femoral head (Figures 2(c) and 2(d)). The flip osteotomy was fixed using a tension band wire and the joint was reduced. The torn capsule was sutured. Closure was done in layers. The operating time was 4 hours and the intraoperative blood loss was 600 ml. Three days following this surgery, the contralateral distal femur fracture was addressed using a titanium locking plate. The postoperative period was uneventful.

Three weeks after the initial surgeries, the patient experienced an episode of rhythmic contractions of the lower limbs at his home. He presented to us with an anterior dislocation of the left hip joint (Figures 3(a) and 3(b)). An open surgery was done to reduce the left hip joint (Figure 3(c)). Considering the displacement of the femoral head at the time of initial presentation, the chances of avascular necrosis of the femoral head was explained to the patient. The patient was also on follow-up treatment with a neurologist to manage the myoclonus problem.

Four weeks after the surgery to relocate the femoral head, non-weight-bearing mobilization was initiated. As expected,

avascular necrosis of the femoral head occurred (Figure 4(a)) and we waited for union of the femoral shaft to occur as any procedure to address the femoral head would require removal of the intramedullary nail.

Eight months after the initial surgery and after union of the femoral shaft fracture, the patient was planned for total hip replacement surgery. Through a posterior approach, the antegrade femoral nail was removed. The acetabulum was reconstructed using a cage, and an uncemented hydroxyapatite-coated stem was used for the femur (Figure 4(b)). A ceramic on a polybearing surface was used. Postoperatively, there was no shortening of the limb. Immediate full weight-bearing mobilization was started using walker support. One year following the hip replacement surgery and 22 months following the initial trauma, the patient was ambulatory without any support and able to do all activities with an LEFS (lower extremity functional score) of 72. The radiographs showed complete union of all the fractures and there was no loosening of the femoral prosthesis.

3. Discussion

Floating hip injuries are a rare presentation [1, 2, 4]. Moreover, a case with a similar presentation to the one discussed

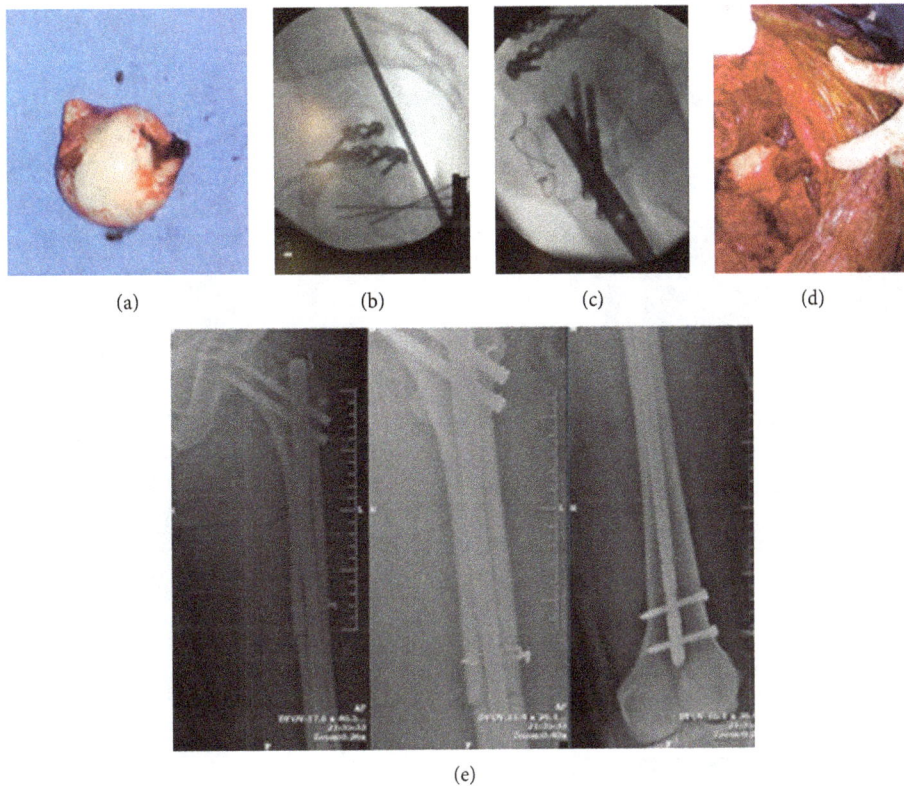

FIGURE 2: Intraoperative images of the displaced femoral head (a) which was reduced and fixed following the acetabulum fixation (b, c, d). Postoperative radiograph (e).

in our report is even more rare. To our knowledge, only two case reports of concomitant acetabular fracture with femoral head and femur shaft fracture have been published before. However, our case is unique with regard to the femoral head being extruded out and displaced out of the capsule. The management of such cases is difficult due to their low incidence and paucity in literature regarding their management [4–7].

Whenever one comes across a patient with the associated fractures as shown in our case, two main issues need to be planned before surgery. The first issue is with regard to which fracture will be addressed first, and the second issue is with regard to the implant to be used. Literature has shown that different surgeons have addressed different fractures in varying sequences. While Kregor [6] suggested prioritising the acetabular fracture first in fixation, Liebergall et al. [1] stated that fixing the femur first would help in easy reduction and traction while fixing the acetabulum. There has also been a disparity in the choice of implants between authors, with some authors suggesting a single implant and other authors suggesting separate implants for separate fractures [5–7]. We feel that these decisions have to be made based on a case-to-case basis.

In our case, since the femoral head and the acetabulum could be approached using a posterior approach, we employed it and since a single implant (antegrade femoral nail) would help in addressing all the fractures, we used it. Hence, we suggest that the management plan and the choice of implant for such complex injuries need to be planned from

a case-to-case basis. The morphology and the complexity of the fracture influence the decision making, surgical approach, and the choice of implant.

Two case reports of similar type of injuries have been reported earlier. Duygulu et al. [8] managed their case with an antegrade nail for the femoral neck and shaft fractures followed by acetabular fixation, whereas Irifune et al. [9] employed screws to fix the femoral neck and a retrograde nail for the femur shaft fracture followed by the acetabular fixation. However, our case presented with a more complex fracture of the femoral neck which was different from the other two cases. The complexity of our injury was severe and such injuries have shown to be associated with a high chance of avascular necrosis (AVN) of the femoral head [10]. In our case, the AVN was addressed at the later stage with a total hip replacement. The plan of doing a total hip replacement at the initial stage was not possible in our case due to the concomitant fracture of the femur shaft.

To the best of our knowledge, such a complex case of a floating hip injury has not been reported. Though the chances of avascular necrosis was high in our case due to the fracture pattern of the femoral head, we decided to address the fracture with the same implant fixing the femur shaft as it was the best option for managing this fracture. Unfortunately, our patient had a hip dislocation following a myoclonus episode which was addressed appropriately by an open reduction of the joint. Eventually following AVN and after fracture union of the shaft, total hip replacement was done which led to a good functional outcome.

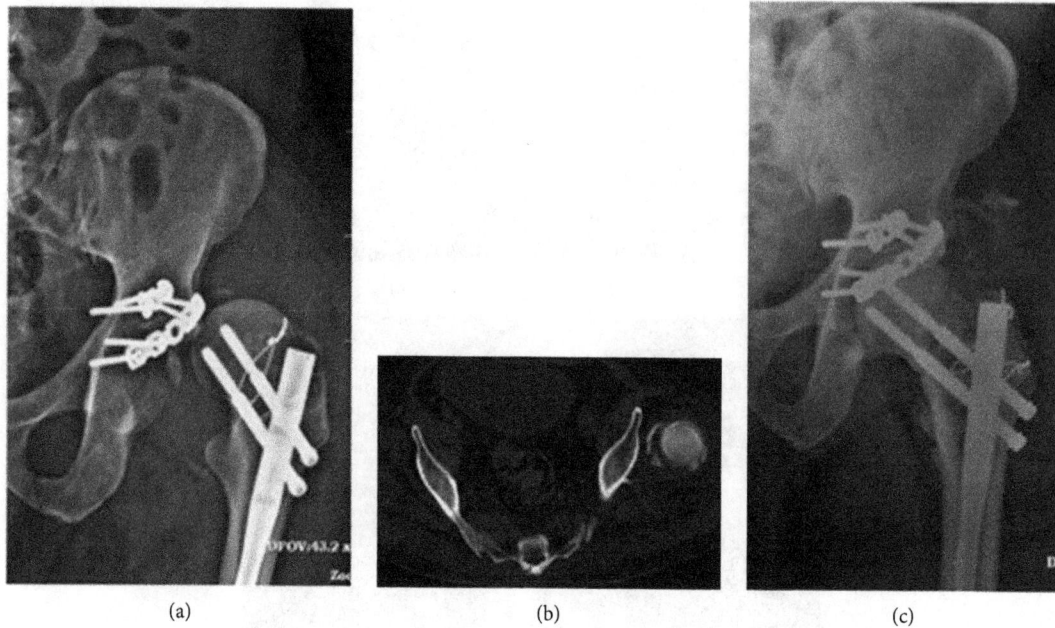

(a)   (b)   (c)

FIGURE 3: Anterior dislocation of the hip joint (a, b) following an episode of myoclonus which was managed by open reduction (c).

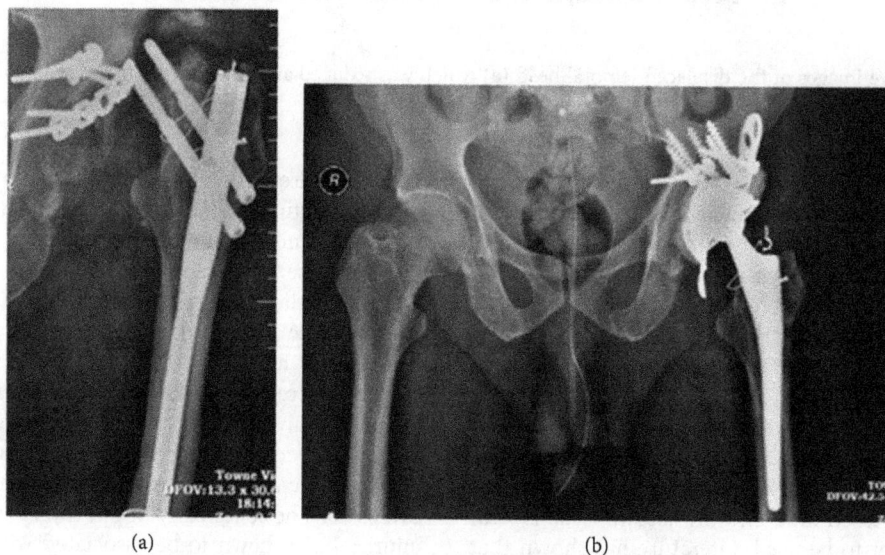

(a)   (b)

FIGURE 4: Avascular necrosis of the left femoral head (a) which was managed by implant removal and left total hip replacement (b) after union of the femur shaft fracture.

4. Conclusion

Ipsilateral acetabular fractures with femoral neck and femoral shaft fractures are very rare and a surgical challenge. Each case needs to be planned and addressed differently based on the complexity of the fracture, and our case report throws light on tackling this complex injury.

Disclosure

Level of evidence is Level IV case report.

Conflicts of Interest

The authors declare that there is no conflict of interests regarding the publication of this paper.

References

[1] M. Liebergall, R. Mosheiff, O. Safran, A. Peyser, and D. Segal, "The floating hip injury: patterns of injury," *Injury*, vol. 33, no. 8, pp. 717–722, 2002.

[2] E. J. Müller, K. Siebenrock, A. Ekkernkamp, R. Ganz, and G. Muhr, "Ipsilateral fractures of the pelvis and the femur—

floating hip?," *Archives of Orthopaedic and Trauma Surgery*, vol. 119, no. 3-4, pp. 179–182, 1999.

[3] T. A. Burd, M. S. Hughes, and J. O. Anglen, "The floating hip: complications and outcomes," *The Journal of Trauma: Injury, Infection, and Critical Care*, vol. 64, no. 2, pp. 442–448, 2008.

[4] A. Iotov, N. Tzachev, D. Enchev, and A. Baltov, "Operative treatment of the floating hip," *Journal of Bone and Joint Surgery British Volume*, vol. 88-B, Supplement I, p. 160, 2006.

[5] T. Suzuki, M. Shindo, and K. Soma, "The floating hip injury: which should we fix first?," *European Journal of Orthopaedic Surgery and Traumatology*, vol. 16, no. 3, pp. 214–218, 2006.

[6] P. J. Kregor and D. Templeman, "Associated injuries complicating the management of acetabular fractures: review and case studies," *Orthopedic Clinics of North America*, vol. 33, no. 1, pp. 73–95, 2002.

[7] C.-W. Oh, J.-K. Oh, B.-C. Park et al., "Retrograde nailing with subsequent screw fixation for ipsilateral femoral shaft and neck fractures," *Archives of Orthopaedic and Trauma Surgery*, vol. 126, no. 7, pp. 448–453, 2006.

[8] F. Duygulu, M. Calis, M. Argun, and A. Guney, "Unusual combination of femoral head dislocation associated acetabular fracture with ipsilateral neck and shaft fractures: a case report," *The Journal of Trauma: Injury, Infection, and Critical Care*, vol. 61, no. 6, pp. 1545–1548, 2006.

[9] H. Irifune, S. Hirayama, N. Takahashi, and E. Narimatsu, "Ipsilateral acetabular and femoral neck and shaft fractures," *Case Reports in Orthopedics*, vol. 2015, Article ID 351465, 4 pages, 2015.

[10] S. Milenkovic, M. Mitkovic, J. Saveski et al., "Avascular necrosis of the femoral head in the patients with posterior wall acetabular fractures associated with dislocations of the hip," *Acta Chirurgica Iugoslavica*, vol. 60, no. 2, pp. 65–69, 2013.

16

Spinal Metastasis of Well-Differentiated Liposarcoma Component in Retroperitoneal Dedifferentiated Liposarcoma Treated by Minimally Invasive Surgery

Jiro Ichikawa [ID],[1] Tetsuro Ohba,[1] Hiroaki Kanda,[2] Koji Fujita,[1] Shigeto Ebata,[1] and Hirotaka Haro[1]

[1]*Department of Orthopaedic Surgery, Graduate School of Medicine, University of Yamanashi, 1110 Shimokato, Chuo, Yamanashi 409-3898, Japan*
[2]*Department of Pathology, The Cancer Institute of the Japanese Foundation for Cancer Research (JFCR), 3-8-31 Ariake, Koto-ku, Tokyo 135-8550, Japan*

Correspondence should be addressed to Jiro Ichikawa; jichi@sb4.so-net.ne.jp

Academic Editor: Akio Sakamoto

Case. Generally, well-differentiated liposarcoma (WDL) has recurrence potential but lacks metastatic potential. We present a rare case of spinal metastasis of WDL component in retroperitoneal dedifferentiated liposarcoma (DDL) treated by tumor curettage and L1 laminectomy followed by percutaneous pedicle screw fixation. Histological examination showed metastasis of the WDL component of DDL. The patient was ambulatory until death. *Conclusion.* To our knowledge, no case of spinal metastasis of WDL component in retroperitoneal DDL has been reported. We should carefully consider characteristics of DDLs during treatment. Minimally invasive surgery may be a powerful tool in patients with spinal metastasis.

1. Introduction

Retroperitoneal sarcomas (RPS) are rare, accounting for approximately 12% of all soft tissue sarcomas [1]. Liposarcoma is the most frequent histological subtype, and well-differentiated liposarcoma (WDL) and dedifferentiated liposarcoma (DDL) account for 90% of retroperitoneal liposarcomas [2]. Although WDL lacks metastatic potential, WDL that has differentiated into DDL has metastatic capacity [3]. We report the first case of spinal metastasis of WDL component in retroperitoneal DDL and successful treatment by minimally invasive surgery (MIS).

2. Case Presentation

A 65-year-old woman was admitted to our hospital because of low back pain and left posterior thigh and calf pain. When symptoms of sciatica began 2 months previously, she underwent radiography and magnetic resonance imaging (MRI) of the lumbar spine at another hospital. These showed a vertebral tumor in the lumbar spine. Both the patellar tendon and the Achilles tendon reflex were normal. The sensory exam was also normal. Although the left tibialis anterior (TA) muscle and extensor hallucis longus (EHL) muscle were manual muscle testing (MMT) grade 3, muscles other than the TA and EHL were MMT grade 5. Laboratory blood tests revealed hypoalbuminemia, anemia, and increased alkaline phosphatase and C-reactive protein. She had undergone resection of retroperitoneal DDL 5 years previously (Figure 1(a)) and repeated resection for recurrence 3 years previously. Recurrence occurred again 1 year previously, and spinal metastasis of WDL component occurred in the L2 vertebrae 8 months previously (Figure 1(b)) and gradually increased (Figure 1(c)) in computed tomography (CT), but she did not undergo additional treatment (Figures 1(d) and 1(e)). MRI showed a mass with high signal intensity on both T1-weighted images and T2-weighted images and no enhancement on gadolinium-

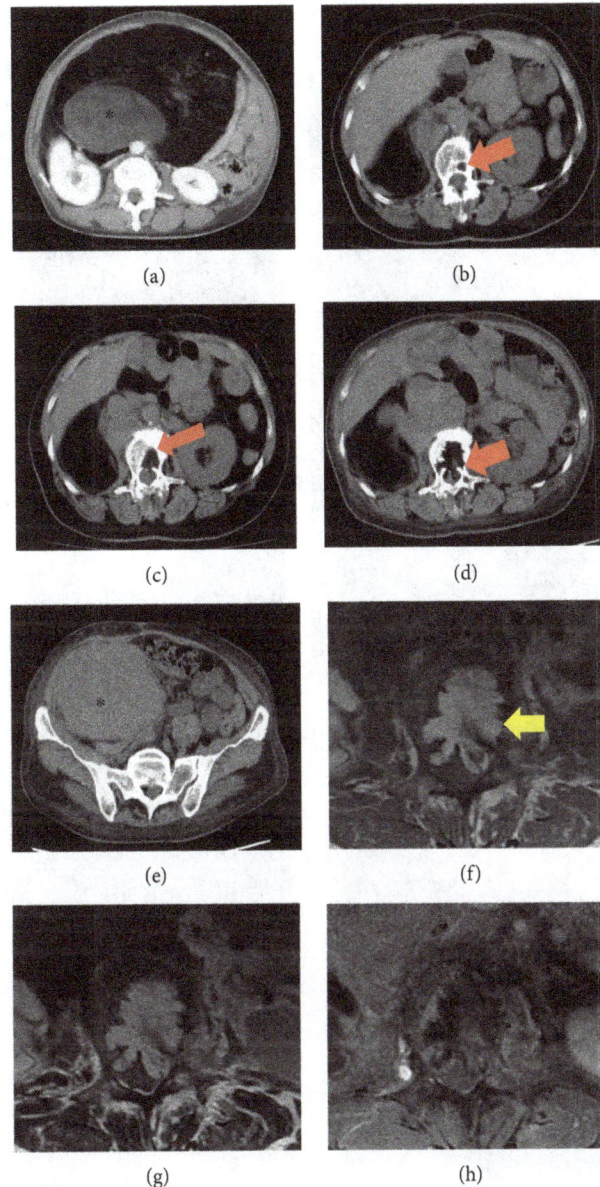

FIGURE 1: Abdominal computed tomography (CT). (a) Enhanced CT prior to the first surgery showed a large retroperitoneal mass in the second lumbar vertebra level, which consisted of both lipomatous (yellow asterisk) and nonlipomatous (red asterisk) components. Plain CT at 8 months (b) and 3 months (c) before our first visit showed metastatic lipomatous component (red arrow) involved in the vertebral body. (d, e) CT findings at our first visit showed both lipomatous (yellow asterisk) and nonlipomatous (red asterisk) components; in addition, the metastatic lipomatous component in the vertebral body had increased and destroyed the vertebral body. Magnetic resonance image of the lumbar spine. Axial T1-weighted (f), T2-weighted (g), and enhanced T1-weighted images (h) showed the mass with a similar intensity to fat and widespread from the vertebral body to the canal space (yellow arrow).

enhanced T1-weighted images (Figures 1(f)–1(h)). The revised Tokuhashi score [4] was 11/15, and the Spinal Instability Neoplastic Score (SINP) was 10/18 [5]. Therefore, we diagnosed the vertebral tumor as the metastasis of WDL component in DDL and planned surgery for symptomatic improvement. Tumor curettage and L1 laminectomy followed by percutaneous pedicle screw fixation from the Th11 to L3 using intraoperative 3-D CT computer navigation were performed (Figures 2(a) and 2(b)). Histological examination showed mixed well-differentiated and well-dedifferentiated liposarcoma in the primary lesion

(Figures 3(a), 3(c), and 3(e)). Lipoblasts containing hyperchromatic nuclei were apparent in the well-differentiated area. Myxoid liposarcoma was ruled out in the dedifferentiated area. Positive staining for MDM2 (Figures 3(b), 3(d), and 3(f)) and CDK4 (data not shown) by immunohistochemistry and negativity of DDIT3 or FUS by FISH (data not shown) confirmed dedifferentiated liposarcoma. She could walk and had no pain in her back and no signs of palsy. However, the retroperitoneal mass subsequently increased, and she died 1.5 years after surgery.

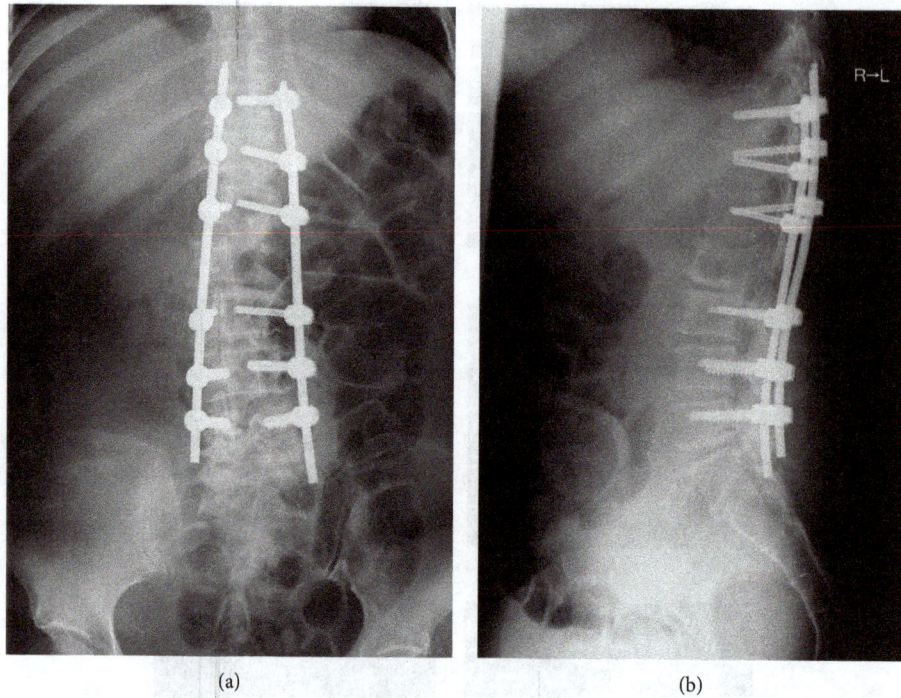

(a)   (b)

FIGURE 2: Postoperative radiograph of the anteroposterior view (a) and lateral view (b).

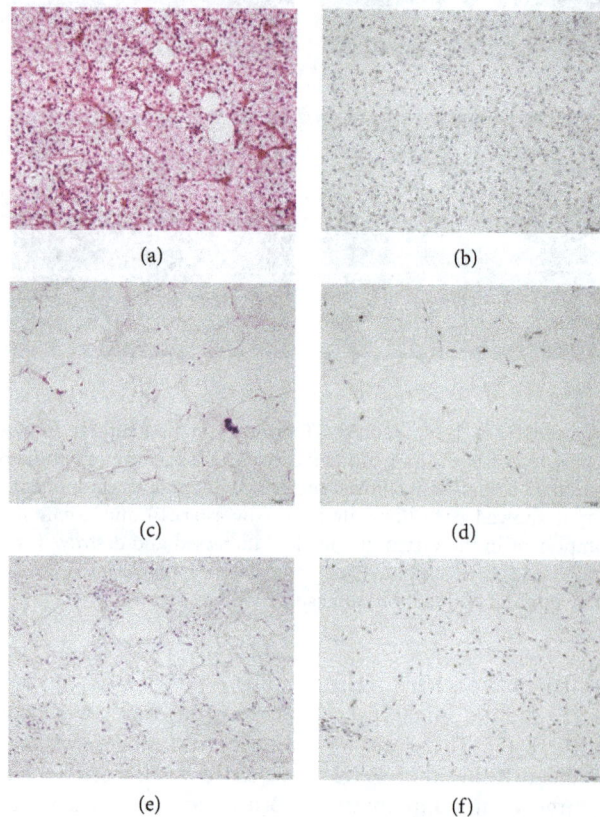

(a)   (b)

(c)   (d)

(e)   (f)

FIGURE 3: Histology of the primary site-dedifferentiated liposarcoma (a, b) and well-differentiated liposarcoma components (c, d) and the metastasis (e, f). (a, c, e) Hematoxylin-eosin stain. (b, d, f) Immunohistochemistry of MDM2. There was a mixed well-differentiated and dedifferentiated component in the primary lesion (a, c). Only the well-differentiated component was seen in the spine metastasis (e). Bar = 50 μm.

3. Discussion

Histologically, liposarcoma is classified into four subtypes: well-differentiated, dedifferentiated, myxoid/round, and pleomorphic [6]. Evans et al. described DDL as high-grade and nonlipogenic sarcoma, juxtaposed with WDL [7]. Although the preferred site of myxoid, round, and pleomorphic liposarcoma is the extremities, WDL and DDL are common in the retroperitoneum, accounting for more than 90% of retroperitoneal liposarcomas [2, 8]. WDL and DDL show high-level amplification of CDK4 and MDM2, which are useful for differential diagnosis from other adipocytic tumors [9]. In our case, CDK4 and MDM2 expression in both the primary site and the metastatic site was confirmed by immunohistochemistry.

Histologically, WDL and DDL are quite different. WDL, which potentiates not metastasis but recurrence, is defined as an intermediate tumor, on the borderline of benign and malignant [6]. DDL generally shows high-grade sarcoma but can show low grade and a low ratio of dedifferentiation. Because the correlation of histological grade, ratio of dedifferentiation, and prognosis has been controversial, we should take care in making treatment decisions [10].

In the treatment of RPS, wide resection has been recommended and leads to better survival and local control [2, 11]. Wide resection is often impossible in RPS, because RPS have no characteristic symptoms; their size is much larger than the extremities, and they are usually found in important organs, including the kidney, colon, spleen, ureter, and common iliac artery and vein. However, wide resection often fails; the local 3- and 5-year recurrence rates are 31% and 47%, respectively. However, the 3- and 5-year survival rates of WDL are both 92%. In DDL, local recurrence rates at 3 and 5 years were reported as 43% and 60%, respectively [2, 8], and the survival rate was reported as 39% at 3 years and 61% at 5 years. Although the survival rate for DDL is much lower than that for WDL, it is higher than those for other sarcomas [12].

Adjuvant therapy, including chemotherapy and radiotherapy, should be considered because of the high incidence of recurrence and metastasis. Although the regimen of ifosfamide and doxorubicin has been reported in patients with DDL, the efficiency was low, and the development of new regimens and anticancer drugs is awaited [13]. Although radiotherapy and chemotherapy do not affect survival, both post- or preoperative radiotherapies can reduce recurrence, and preoperative radiotherapy is favored because of the low risk of radiation-induced toxicity [14]. Considering that our patient experienced recurrence twice, radiotherapy may have been advisable.

The number of patients with bone metastasis, including in the spine, has been increasing, because the number of patients with cancer has been increasing. Additionally, the prognosis of these patients has improved because of improvements in early diagnosis, surgery, chemotherapy, and radiotherapy. For surgical decisions about spinal metastasis, the revised Tokuhashi score has often been used, as has the recently developed SINP score. Although the revised Tokuhashi score is dependent on primary cancer type and patient condition, the SINP score is dependent on the stability of the spine, regardless of the primary cancer or patient condition. In our case, a revised Tokuhashi score of 11 indicated that treatment was dependent on the patient, and a SINP score of 10 indicated that the operation was favored because of spinal instability. Considering that our patient had only one metastasis and her muscle weakness and sciatica worsened, we decided to perform surgery. The option of MIS allowed us to opt for surgical treatment without the frequent accompanying adverse effects. We recently reported on the clinical efficacy and safety of minimally invasive percutaneous fixation surgery with intraoperative 3-D CT computer navigation [15]. Radiotherapy, including intensity-modulated radiation therapy and stereotactic radiosurgery, has been developed, such that the combination of MIS and radiotherapy has become standard [16]. In addition, the use of bone-modifying agents, including denosumab and zoledronate, may result in better local control.

While it is important to carefully evaluate the clinical behavior of the primary cancer as well as the patient's condition, the extent of surgical indication in spinal metastasis should be considered because of the development of multidisciplinary therapies and surgical techniques.

Consent

Written informed consent was obtained from the patient for the publication of this case report and any accompanying images.

Conflicts of Interest

The authors report no conflict of interest concerning the materials or methods used in this study or findings specified in this paper.

Authors' Contributions

Jiro Ichikawa, Tetsuro Ohba, and Hiroaki Kanda are responsible for the conception and design. All the authors are responsible for to the acquisition of data. Jiro Ichikawa, Tetsuro Ohba, Hiroaki Kanda, and Hirotaka Haro drafted the article.

References

[1] J. C. Gutierrez, E. A. Perez, D. Franceschi, F. L. Moffat Jr., A. S. Livingstone, and L. G. Koniaris, "Outcomes for soft-tissue sarcoma in 8249 cases from a large state cancer registry," *The Journal of Surgical Research*, vol. 141, no. 1, pp. 105–114, 2007.

[2] S. Singer, C. R. Antonescu, E. Riedel, and M. F. Brennan, "Histologic subtype and margin of resection predict pattern of recurrence and survival for retroperitoneal liposarcoma," *Annals of Surgery*, vol. 121, no. 3, pp. 52–65, 2003.

[3] K. Thway, R. L. Jones, J. Noujaim, S. Zaidi, A. B. Miah, and C. Fisher, "Dedifferentiated liposarcoma: updates on morphology, genetics, and therapeutic strategies," *Advances in Anatomic Pathology*, vol. 23, no. 1, pp. 30–40, 2016.

[4] Y. Tokuhashi, Y. Ajiro, and N. Umezawa, "Outcome of treatment for spinal metastases using scoring system for

preoperative evaluation of prognosis," *Spine*, vol. 34, no. 1, pp. 69–73, 2009.

[5] D. R. Fourney, E. M. Frangou, T. C. Ryken et al., "Spinal instability neoplastic score: an analysis of reliability and validity from the spine oncology study group," *Journal of Clinical Oncology*, vol. 29, no. 22, pp. 3072–3077, 2011.

[6] C. D. M. Fletcher, K. K. Unni, and F. Mertens, "World Health Organization. Classification of tumours," in *Pathology and Genetics of Tumours of Soft Tissue and Bone*, pp. 35–46, IARC Press, Lyon, 2002.

[7] H. L. Evans, E. H. Soule, and R. K. Winkelmann, "Atypical lipoma, atypical intramuscular lipoma, and well differentiated retroperitoneal liposarcoma: a reappraisal of 30 cases formerly classified as well differentiated liposarcoma," *Cancer*, vol. 43, no. 2, pp. 574–584, 1979.

[8] H. G. Smith, D. Panchalingam, J. A. Hannay et al., "Outcome following resection of retroperitoneal sarcoma," *British Journal of Surgery*, vol. 102, no. 13, pp. 1698–1709, 2015.

[9] K. Thway, R. Flora, C. Shah, D. Olmos, and C. Fisher, "Diagnostic utility of p16, CDK4, and MDM2 as an immunohistochemical panel in distinguishing well-differentiated and dedifferentiated liposarcomas from other adipocytic tumors," *The American Journal of Surgical Pathology*, vol. 36, no. 3, pp. 462–469, 2012.

[10] W. H. Henricks, Y. C. Chu, J. R. Goldblum, and S. W. Weiss, "Dedifferentiated liposarcoma: a clinicopathological analysis of 155 cases with a proposal for an expanded definition of dedifferentiation," *The American Journal of Surgical Pathology*, vol. 21, no. 3, pp. 271–281, 1997.

[11] S. Bonvalot, M. Rivoire, M. Castaing et al., "Primary retroperitoneal sarcomas: a multivariate analysis of surgical factors associated with local control," *Journal of Clinical Oncology*, vol. 27, no. 1, pp. 31–37, 2009.

[12] M. Toulmonde, S. Bonvalot, P. Méeus et al., "Retroperitoneal sarcomas: patterns of care at diagnosis, prognostic factors and focus on main histological subtypes: a multicenter analysis of the French sarcoma group," *Annals of Oncology*, vol. 25, no. 3, pp. 735–742, 2014.

[13] J. A. Livingston, D. Bugano, A. Barbo et al., "Role of chemotherapy in dedifferentiated liposarcoma of the retroperitoneum: defining the benefit and challenges of the standard," *Scientific Reports*, vol. 7, no. 1, article 11836, 2017.

[14] G. Molina, M. A. Hull, Y. L. Chen et al., "Preoperative radiation therapy combined with radical surgical resection is associated with a lower rate of local recurrence when treating unifocal, primary retroperitoneal liposarcoma," *Journal of Surgical Oncology*, vol. 114, no. 7, pp. 814–820, 2016.

[15] T. Ohba, S. Ebata, K. Fujita, H. Sato, and H. Haro, "Percutaneous pedicle screw placements: accuracy and rates of cranial facet joint violation using conventional fluoroscopy compared with intraoperative three-dimensional computed tomography computer navigation," *European Spine Journal*, vol. 25, no. 6, pp. 1775–1780, 2016.

[16] N. Kumar, R. Malhotra, A. S. Zaw et al., "Evolution in treatment strategy for metastatic spine disease: presently evolving modalities," *European Journal of Surgical Oncology*, vol. 43, no. 9, pp. 1784–1801, 2017, Review.

17

Opening Wedge Osteotomy for Valgus Deformity of the Little Finger after Proximal Phalangeal Fracture in Children

Souichi Ohta ⓘⒹ, Ryosuke Ikeguchi, Hiroki Oda, Hirofumi Yurie, Hisataka Takeuchi, and Shuichi Matsuda

Department of Orthopaedic Surgery, Kyoto University, Kyoto, Japan

Correspondence should be addressed to Souichi Ohta; sota@kuhp.kyoto-u.ac.jp

Academic Editor: Ali F. Ozer

In the treatment of posttraumatic valgus deformity of the pediatric little finger, it is usually difficult to achieve accurate correction of angular and rotational deformity using closing wedge osteotomy. We report two cases of valgus deformity of the little finger (both 11-year-old female patients) successfully treated using opening wedge osteotomy followed by intramedullary semirigid fixation with a single Kirschner wire. A wire tip inserted from the retrocondylar fossa of the proximal phalangeal head was advanced along the radial side of the intramedullary cortex after gradual opening of the osteotomy site. If needed, further fine adjustment of the rotational alignment can be performed even after K-wire insertion. Postoperatively, the gap between the little and ring fingers in the fully extended and adducted position and the finger overlapping in the fully flexed position were completely resolved. The flexibility of the pediatric bone and sagittal clearance between the wire and the inner wall of the proximal phalangeal medullary cavity allow fine adjustment of the rotational alignment even after wire insertion.

1. Introduction

A valgus deformity of the little finger sometimes occurs after conservative treatment or neglect of the proximal phalangeal neck fracture. Because of remaining ulnar tilt of the proximal phalangeal distal articular surface with or without rotation, the distal part of the little finger cannot touch the ulnar side of the ring finger in the fully extended and adducted finger position, although the proximal parts of the fingers can touch. The ring and little fingers overlap when the patient makes a fist, causing functional impairment [1].

To resolve the problems associated with such valgus deformity, closing wedge osteotomy is usually performed with fixation using a plate and screws or two Kirschner wires (K-wires) [2–4]. However, it is difficult to accomplish the exact resection of wedge bone and fixation according to preplanned correction angles. In contrast, an opening wedge osteotomy needs only one cutting line and careful opening of

the wedge while making the opposite side cortex the center of rotation of angulation [5]. As pediatric bones have a more elastic cortex and thicker periosteum than adult bones, opening wedge osteotomy is suitable for the treatment of pediatric bone deformity; moreover, children have superior bone healing potential and do not necessarily need bone grafting into the opening gap at the osteotomy site. After opening the osteotomy site, we performed intramedullary fixation with a single K-wire. This semirigid fixation allows further fine adjustment of the rotational alignment even after K-wire insertion. Herein, we report two cases of pediatric little finger posttraumatic valgus deformity successfully treated with opening wedge osteotomy followed by intramedullary fixation with a single K-wire.

2. Case Reports

2.1. Surgical Procedure. A midlateral skin incision of approximately 1 cm was made over the distal ulnar side of the

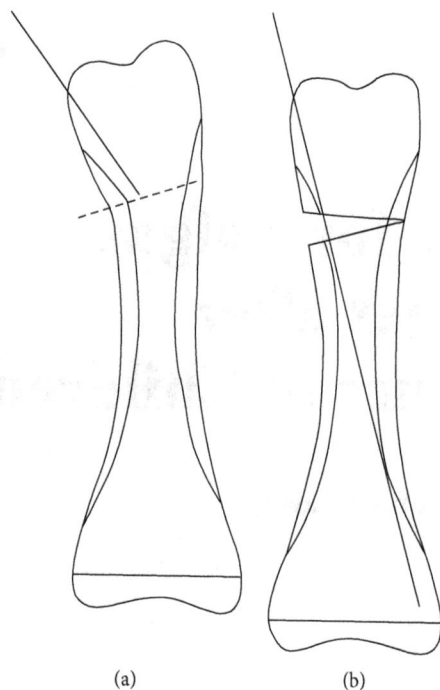

(a)   (b)

FIGURE 1: Surgical procedure. (a) Insert a K-wire until just distal to the preplanned osteotomy line (a dotted line). (b) Advance the tip of the K-wire along the radial side of the intramedullary cortex after gradual opening of the osteotomy site.

proximal phalanx. The ulnar lateral band was moved aside dorsally, and the distal ulnar side of the proximal phalanx was exposed subperiosteally. An image intensifier was used to confirm the preplanned osteotomy line at the distal metaphysis of the proximal phalanx. The osteotomy line does not need to be the same as the fracture line, as long as the center lines of the reconstructed proximal phalanx and the middle phalanx of the same digit coincide. The osteotomy line in the metaphysis was preplanned to be parallel with a line tangential to the distal articular surfaces on an anteroposterior view on plain radiography. Multiple drilling was made at the preplanned osteotomy line using a 1 mm diameter wire. A 1.2 mm K-wire was then inserted through the retrocondylar fossa of the proximal phalangeal head, and the K-wire tip was advanced until just distal to the preplanned osteotomy line (Figure 1(a)). The insertion angle between the K-wire and the distal ulnar cortex of the phalangeal head was approximately 20°. Osteotomy was performed with a small thin osteotome, leaving the most radial cortex of the osteotomy site intact. The osteotomy site was then gradually opened until the preplanned angle was achieved, and the tip of the K-wire was advanced along the radial side of the intramedullary cortex to a point just distal to the epiphyseal line (Figure 1(b)). The distal tip of the exposed K-wire was bent, truncated, and buried under the skin. Bone grafting was not performed. After closing the surgical incision, the little finger was loosely buddy taped with the ring finger to allow active range of motion (ROM) exercises. At postoperative 4 weeks, we removed the K-wire after radiographic confirmation of callus formation at the osteotomy site.

2.2. Case 1: An 11-Year-Old Female. At 9 years of age, the patient fractured the proximal phalanx of the right little finger during kendo (Japanese fencing) training. At the time of the injury, she felt pain but did not consult any medical institution. When the pain resolved, the patient noticed valgus deformity of the little finger in extension and difficulty in gripping caused by finger overlapping.

Two years after the injury, she consulted our clinic due to functional and cosmetic impairments. There was a gap between the ring and little fingers in the fully extended and adducted position. The patient could not make a fist because of the overlapping of the little finger over the ring finger (Figure 2). The ROM of the finger joints was normal, except for the metacarpophalangeal (MCP) joint of the little finger (right: 40–45°; left: 40–70°). Plain radiography showed that the angle between the proximal growth plate and the distal articular surface of the proximal phalanx was 29° on the affected side compared with 5.5° on the contralateral noninjured side (Figure 3). Bilateral middle brachyphalangia of the little fingers was also detected. Surgery was performed as described above.

At postoperative 1 year, the valgus deformity and overlapping of the little finger had completely resolved (Figure 4). The extension contracture of the little finger MCP joint remained. The angle between the growth plate and the distal articular surface of the proximal phalanx was 4.5° (Figure 5).

2.3. Case 2: An 11-Year-Old Female. At 9 years of age, the patient fractured the proximal phalanx of the left little finger in a fall. At the time of the injury, the former doctor performed conservative therapy with cast fixation. Valgus finger deformity was noticed after fixation removal, but this was not addressed as there was no functional impairment.

At 2 years after the injury, the patient consulted our clinic due to a gap between the ring and little fingers in the fully extended and adducted position (Figure 6). There was also partial overlapping of the ring finger over the little finger in the fully flexed position. The ROM of the fingers was normal. Plain radiography showed that the angle between the proximal growth plate and the distal articular surface of the proximal phalanx was 15.3° on the affected side compared with 4.7° on the contralateral noninjured side (Figure 7). Surgery was performed as described above.

At 1 year and 2 months postoperatively, the valgus deformity and overlapping of the little finger had completely resolved (Figure 8). The angle between the growth plate and the distal articular surface of the proximal phalanx was 5.0°.

3. Discussion

We described two cases of pediatric little finger valgus deformity successfully treated using opening wedge osteotomy and intramedullary semirigid fixation with a single K-wire.

Closing wedge osteotomy results in a good outcome in correction of an angulated phalanx [3]; however, it is not easy to perform the exact resection of the wedge bone, especially the apex of the wedge bone, according to the

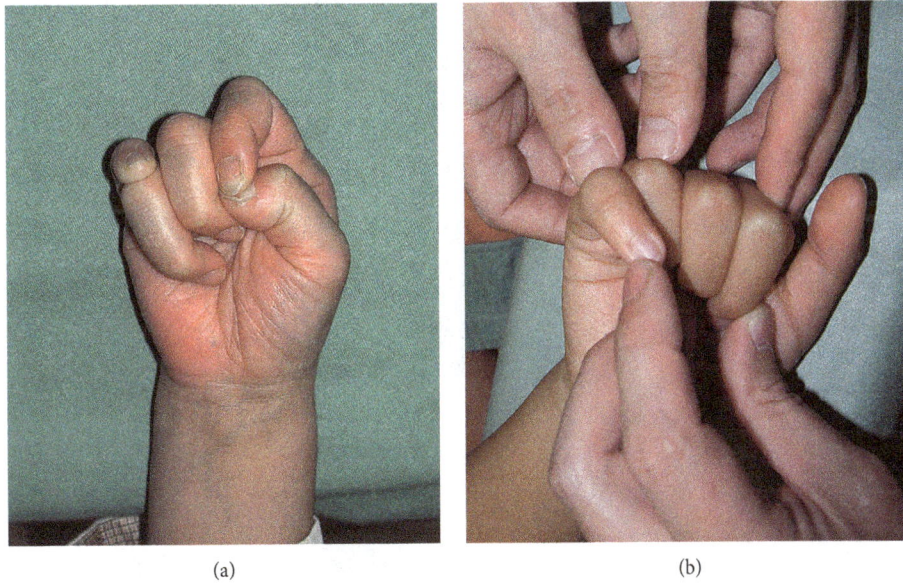

FIGURE 2: Preoperative photographs of the affected hand in Case 1. (a) Making a fist was difficult due to finger overlapping. (b) Passive finger flexion under general anesthesia revealed marked rotation of the little finger.

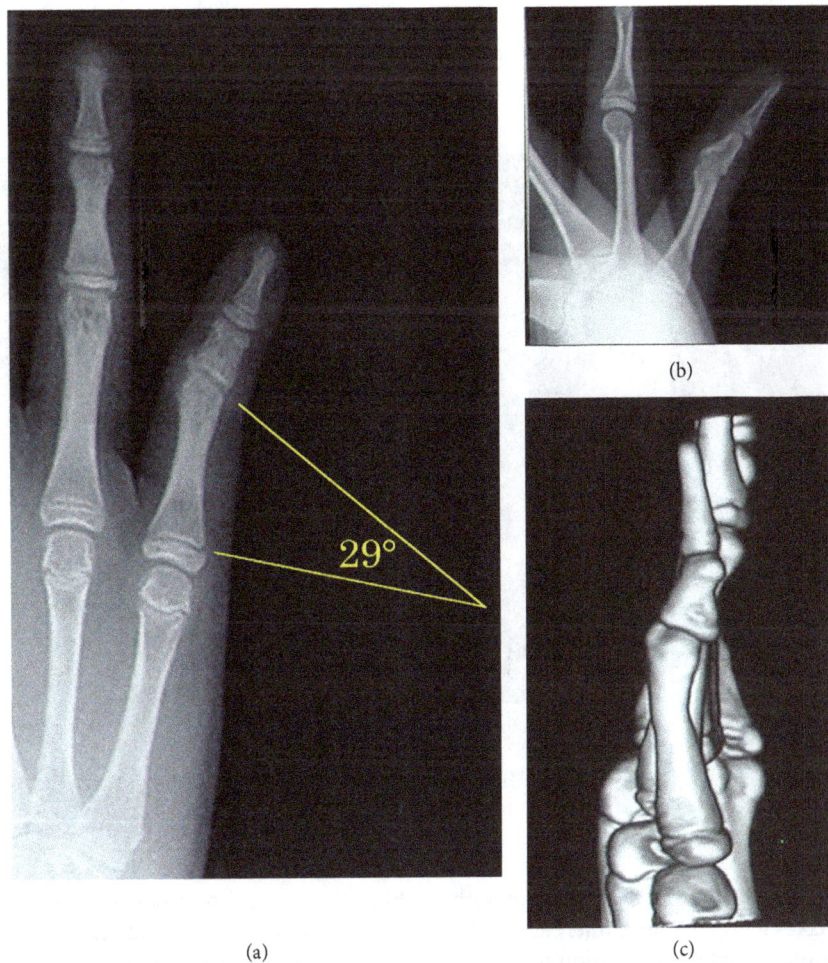

FIGURE 3: Preoperative imaging in Case 1. (a) Plain radiographic anteroposterior view of the right little finger. The distal articular surface of the proximal phalanx of the little finger was tilted in the ulnar direction. (b) Plain radiographic lateral view of the right little finger. (c) Three-dimensional computed tomography of the proximal phalanx of the right little finger.

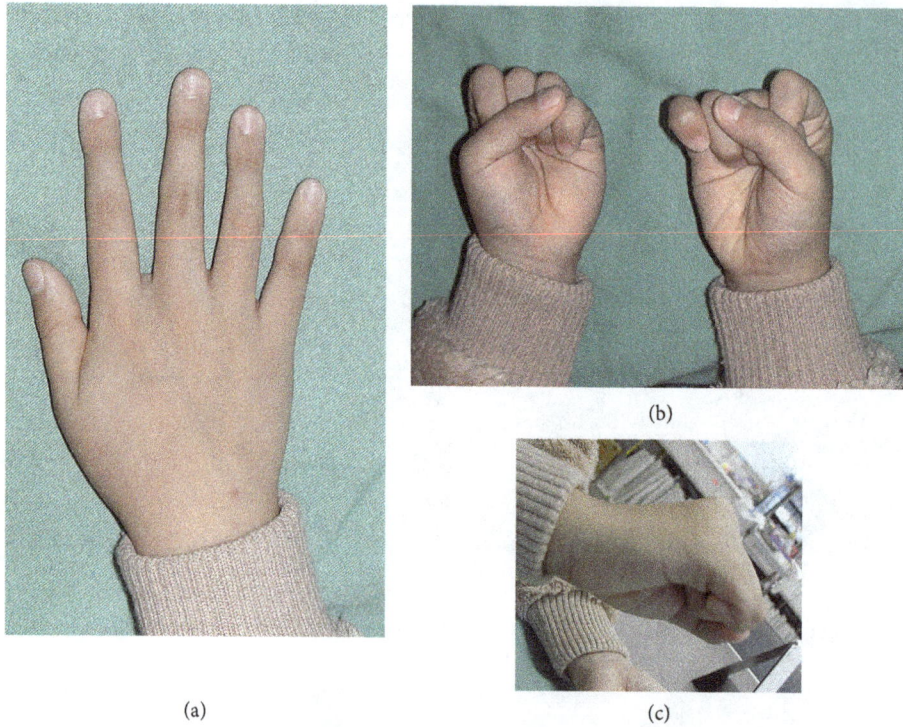

FIGURE 4: Photographs of Case 1 taken 1 year postoperatively. (a) Dorsal view. (b) Palmar view of the clenched fist. The alignment of the little finger was good. Because of the retained extension contracture of the metacarpophalangeal joint, the tip of the little finger could not touch the palm. (c) Lateral view.

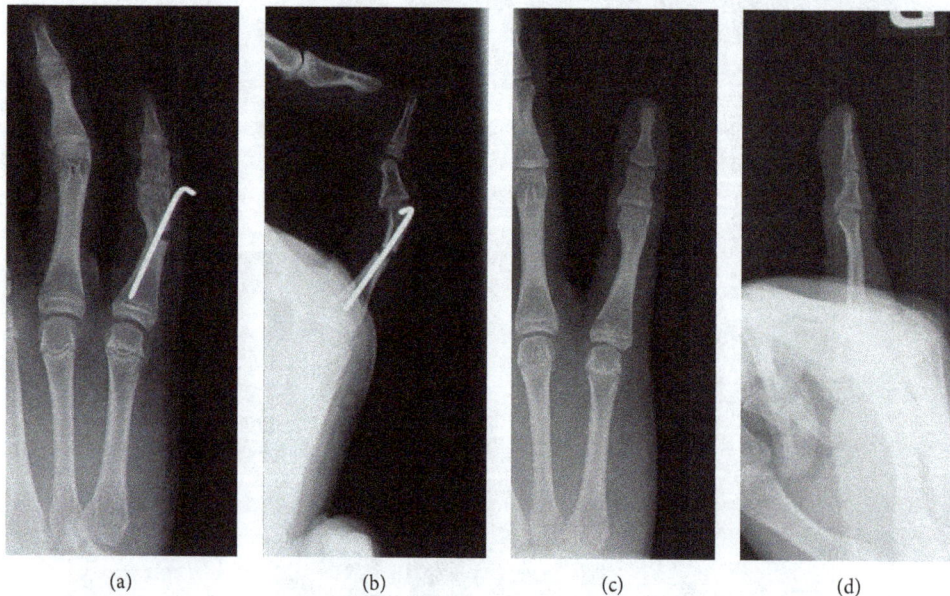

FIGURE 5: Postoperative radiographs of Case 1. (a, b) Images taken immediately after the surgery. (c, d) Images taken 1 year postoperatively.

preplanned correction angles. Moreover, rigid fixation with a plate or two K-wires makes it impossible to finely adjust the alignment after the fixation procedure. In fixation using two K-wires, the prominent radial stump of the K-wire interferes with the attaching of the little and ring fingers to each other and makes it difficult to check the exact alignment of the little finger. In our procedure, the operative field and the K-wire stump are on the ulnar side of the little finger; hence, there is nothing between the little and ring fingers, and it is easy to check the coronal alignment in the fully extended and adducted position and the rotational alignment in the fully flexed position.

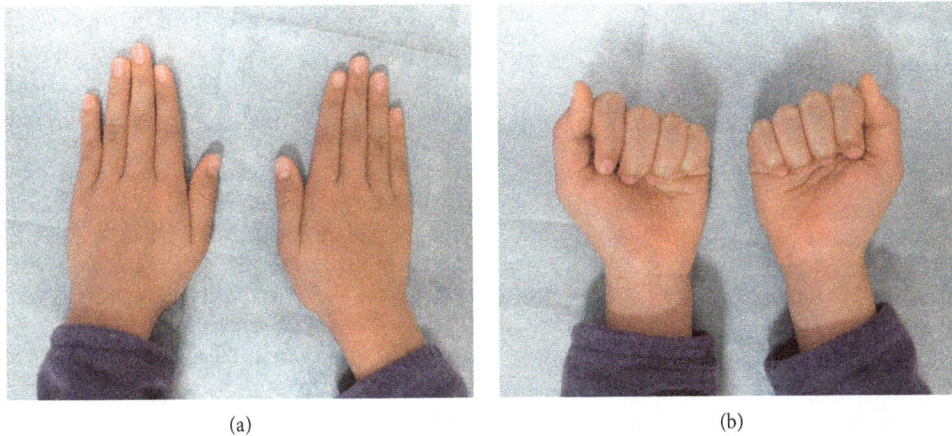

FIGURE 6: Preoperative photographs of Case 2. (a) There was a gap between the left ring and little fingers in the fully extended and adducted position. (b) The left little finger was partially covered by the ring finger in the fully flexed position.

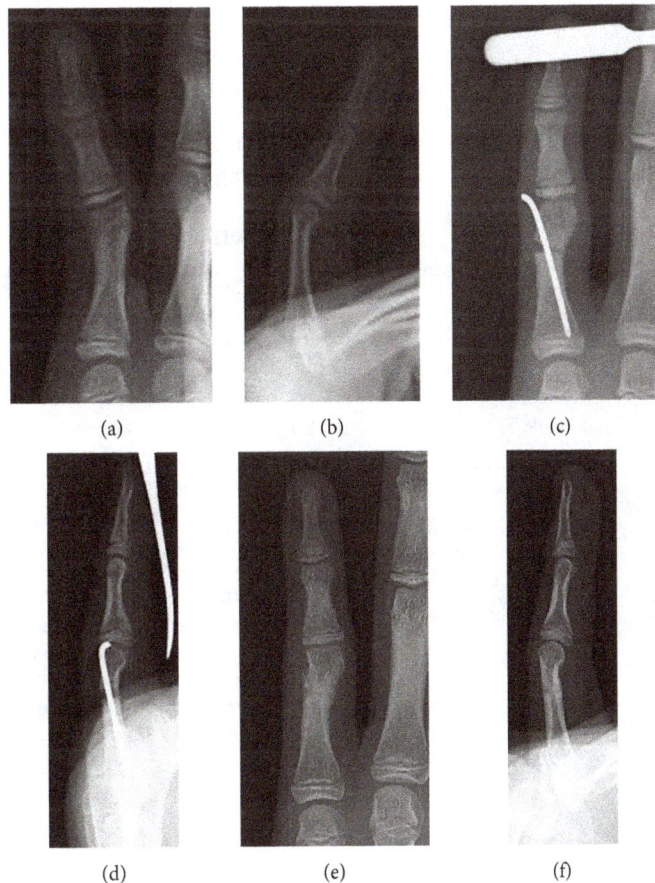

FIGURE 7: Radiographs of Case 2. (a, b) Preoperative radiography of the left little finger. (c, d) Images taken immediately after the surgery. (e, f) Images taken 3 months postoperatively.

Before the osteotomy, we inserted a K-wire from the retrocondylar fossa of the proximal phalanx at an angle of approximately 20° against the ulnar side cortex of the proximal phalangeal head. This angle is appropriate for further advancement of the K-wire after opening of the osteotomy site; the K-wire tip could be advanced while maintaining contact with the inner cortex without cortical penetration. A K-wire insertion angle of less than 10° should be avoided, as the K-wire may not maintain contact with the radial inner cortex, which will result in undercorrection in the coronal plane. Overcorrection in the coronal plane is prevented by the closely attached

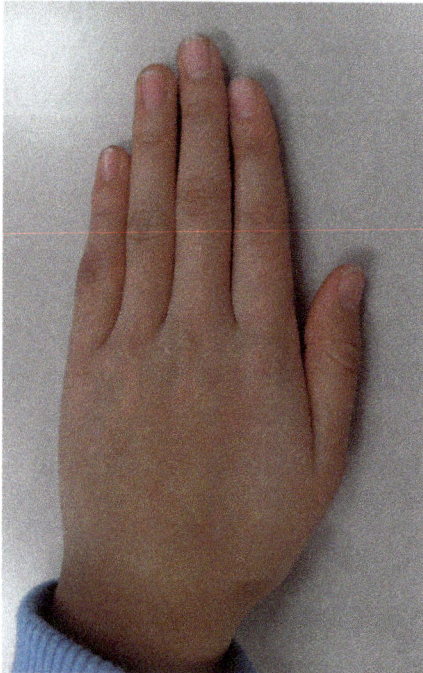

(a)

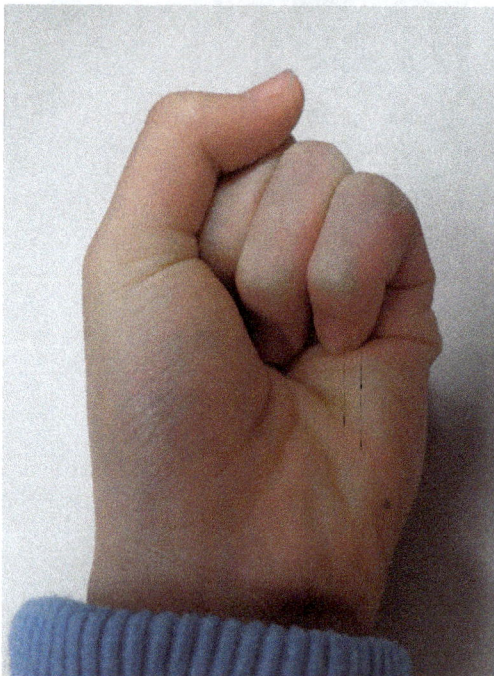

(b)

FIGURE 8: Photographs of Case 2 taken 1 year and 2 months postoperatively. The valgus deformity and overlapping of the left little finger had completely resolved.

normally aligned ring finger and the flexibility of the inserted K-wire.

Correction of the tilted distal articular surface in the coronal plane usually improves the rotational alignment of the little finger to some extent. However, further adjustment of the residual rotational alignment is sometimes needed. In our procedure, further adjustment of the

rotational alignment can be performed, even after K-wire insertion; the clearance between the K-wire and the inner wall of the proximal phalangeal medullary cavity in the sagittal plane makes it possible to finely adjust the alignment of the little finger. When fine rotational correction is needed, only gentle manual corrective force should be applied toward the desired direction. As the additional rotation angle required is usually small, further correction is accomplished without disruption of the preserved radial cortex of the osteotomy site. The corrected alignment is maintained during early active exercise with a loosely buddy-taped ring finger.

In the cutting of the bone, multiple drilling was first performed without penetrating the most radial cortex. Bone cutting was then gradually performed with a small osteotome, with pushing performed by hand. Tapping the osteotome with a hammer should be avoided, as fine tuning of the tapping power is difficult.

Opening wedge osteotomy and intramedullary semirigid fixation with a single K-wire allow fine correction of rotational alignment even after K-wire insertion and are appropriate for treating pediatric little finger posttraumatic valgus deformity.

Conflicts of Interest

The authors declare that there are no conflicts of interest regarding the publication of this article.

References

[1] B. van der Lei, J. de Jonge, P. H. Robinson, and H. J. Klasen, "Correction osteotomies of phalanges and metacarpals for rotational and angular malunion: a long-term follow-up and a review of the literature," *Journal of Trauma*, vol. 35, no. 6, pp. 902–908, 1993.

[2] U. Buchler, A. Gupta, and S. Ruf, "Corrective osteotomy for post-traumatic malunion of the phalanges in the hand," *Journal of Hand Surgery*, vol. 21, no. 1, pp. 33–42, 1996.

[3] A. I. Froimson, "Osteotomy for digital deformity," *Journal of Hand Surgery*, vol. 6, no. 6, pp. 585–589, 1981.

[4] S. Gollamudi and W. A. Jones, "Corrective osteotomy of malunited fractures of phalanges and metacarpals," *Journal of Hand Surgery*, vol. 25, no. 5, pp. 439–441, 2000.

[5] S. L. Piper, C. A. Goldfarb, and L. B. Wall, "Outcomes of opening wedge osteotomy to correct angular deformity in little finger clinodactyly," *Journal of Hand Surgery*, vol. 40, no. 5, pp. 908–913e1, 2015.

18

Solitary Osteochondroma of the Ventral Scapula Associated with Large Bursa Formation and Pseudowinging of the Scapula

Kiyohisa Ogawa ⓘ **and Wataru Inokuchi**

Department of Orthopedic Surgery, Eiju General Hospital, 2-3-23 Higashiueno, Taito-ku, Tokyo 110-8645, Japan

Correspondence should be addressed to Kiyohisa Ogawa; ogawa51@jcom.home.ne.jp

Academic Editor: Akio Sakamoto

Osteochondroma (OC) is the most common benign bone tumor and may occur on any bone in which endochondral ossification develops. Although scapular OC accounts for less than 5% of the cases of solitary OC, OC is the most common lesion among the tumors and tumor-like lesions of the scapula. OC that develops near the medial scapular border easily causes friction with the ribcage; hence, almost half the number of cases of OC associated with marked bursa formation develops in the ventral scapula. We report a case of a 27-year-old female with a painful OC of the ventral scapular surface associated with large bursa formation and pseudowinging of the scapula. After 12 years of follow-up with magnetic resonance imaging, we confirm that the accompanied bursa left at surgery disappears.

1. Introduction

Osteochondroma (OC) is the most common benign bone tumor, of which the detailed development process is still debatable. The reported incidence of OC is 33–35% of benign and 8–10% of all surgically removed bone tumors, which may be an underestimation as most OCs are asymptomatic and are never found [1, 2]. OC may occur on any bone in which endochondral ossification develops. The most common sites of OC development are the metaphyseal region of the long bones of the limbs, while flat bones are less commonly involved [2]. Symptoms often develop in relation to the size and location of the OC lesion. Pain may result from fracture, bursa formation, arthritis, and impingement of adjacent tendons, blood vessels, nerves, or the spinal cord [1, 2]. We describe a case of a 27-year-old female with a painful OC on the ventral surface of the scapula associated with a large bursa and pseudowinging of the scapula with 12 years of follow-up. Written informed consent was obtained from the patient for publication of this case report and accompanying images.

2. Case Report

A 27-year-old right-hand-dominant and otherwise healthy female student presented with a pain in the right upper scapular region that increased with shoulder motion and resting in the supine position. She reported that a painless snap in her back had occurred during sports activity 11 years previously and had disappeared 2 years later after discontinuing sports activity. The pain in the right upper scapular region had appeared 3 months earlier during continuous inputting to her personal computer and had rapidly worsened. She presented at a nearby hospital because the pain was generated during activities of daily life and prevented her from sleeping in the supine position. A physician suspected a malignant bone tumor based on radiographic and magnetic resonance imaging (MRI) findings and referred the patient to our hospital.

The patient had no relevant family or medical history. The right shoulder was slightly lower than the contralateral shoulder. There were no neurological deficits in the right shoulder or arm. There was winging of the right scapula with

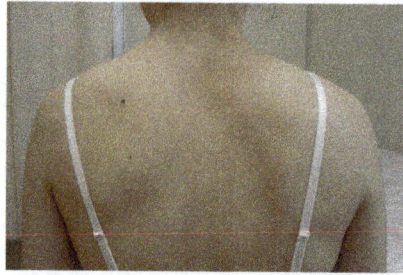

FIGURE 1: Preoperative photograph showing the deformity of the right scapula. The right scapula showed winging with the arm at the side. An upper interval between the spine and medial scapular border was widened, but the lower one was not.

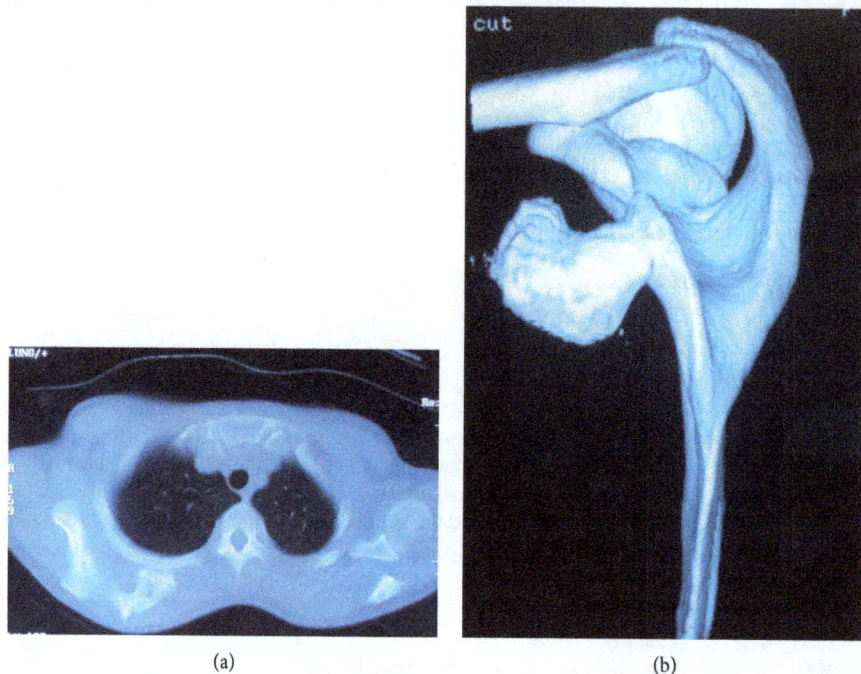

(a)

(b)

FIGURE 2: Preoperative computed tomography (CT) findings. (a) CT showed the mushroom-shaped osseous tumor composed of a cortex continuous with the scapular cortex, with a broad flat distal end that almost contacted the third rib. (b) Three-dimensional CT revealed the close relationship between the base of the osseous tumor and the superomedial scapular angle.

the arm at the side. An upper interval between the spine and the medial scapular border was widened by 70%, but the lower one was not (Figure 1). There was no atrophy of the back muscle, and contraction of the trapezius was normal. The muscle bellies of the short rotators and rotator cuff were not tender and were without defects. The limitations of the active ranges of motion were 10° for total elevation, 15° for external rotation, and two vertebrae for internal rotation. Horizontal adduction was not limited with moderate pain beyond 100°. The empty can test generated upper scapular pain. No deformity or osseous tumor was palpable in the large joints, pelvis, or ribcage. Radiographs revealed a bone mass extruding from the ventral side of the superomedial scapular angle; no abnormality was depicted in the large joints. Computed tomography showed a mushroom-shaped osseous tumor composed of a cortex continuous with the scapular cortex, with a broad flat distal end that almost contacted with the third rib, as well as a soft tissue tumor between the serratus

anterior and the ribcage (Figures 2(a) and 2(b)). MRI taken at the previous hospital revealed a cystic lesion containing a large amount of fluid that surrounded the osseous tumor and spread over the upper two-thirds of the scapula (Figures 3(a) and 3(b)). Marked rim enhancement was demonstrated on contrast-enhanced T1-weighted imagery with fat suppression. From these imaging findings, our diagnosis was a solitary OC with a large bursa; the possibility of malignant transformation was considered to be low.

We performed surgery 3 months after the patient's first visit to our hospital. Under general anesthesia, the patient was placed in the lateral decubitus position with the shoulder flexed and abducted at 110°. The upper extremity was supported on a pillow to avoid excessive horizontal adduction so that the superomedial scapular angle was situated just underneath the middle trapezius. A 10 cm longitudinal incision was made along and 3 cm medial to the medial scapular border, centering at the most proximal end of the scapular spine. The trapezius

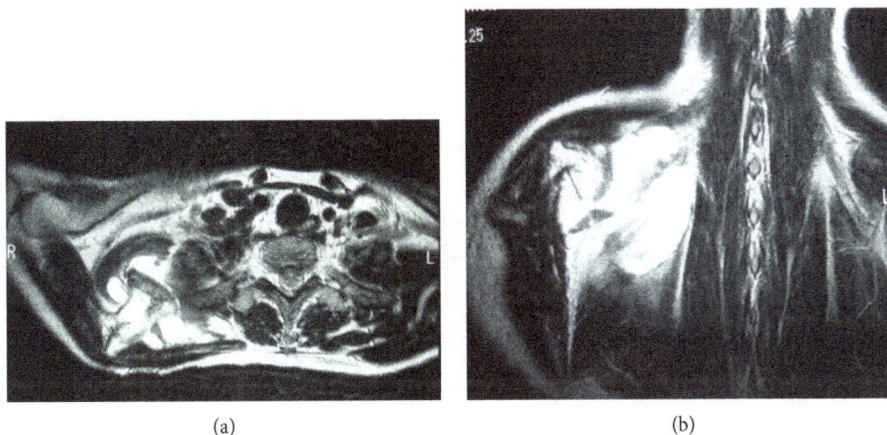

(a)   (b)

FIGURE 3: Preoperative T2-weighted magnetic resonance imaging. (a) Axial view demonstrated the cystic lesion containing a large amount of fluid that surrounded the osseous tumor. (b) Coronal view revealed that the cystic lesion spread over the upper two-thirds of the scapula.

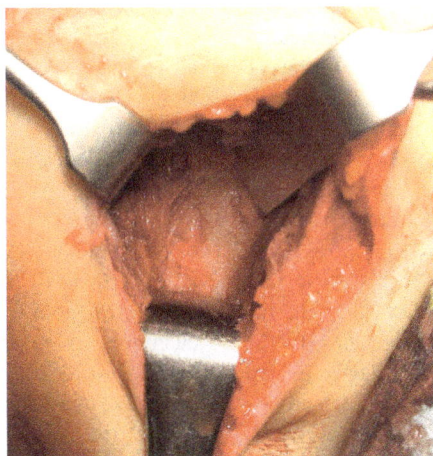

FIGURE 4: Intraoperative photograph showing the exposure of the rib. After resection of the osseous lesion, a large cystic space appeared, covered by a white thick membrane; at the bottom of this space, a 1×3 cm section of rib surface covered by edematous synovium was exposed in a defect of the thick membrane.

and rhomboid minor were divided along their fibers. The thick and edematous cyst wall exposed in the bottom of the operative field was cut, and about 100 ml of clear yellow-brown fluid flowed out. The stalk of the OC arose in the superomedial scapular angle 1 cm lateral to the medial scapular border and penetrated the subscapularis and serratus anterior muscles. The base of the lesion was cut with its periosteum along the ventral scapular surface. We cut the attached thick fibrous tissue attached around the distal stalk, which was considered to be a bursal wall. After resection of the osseous lesion, a large cystic space appeared, covered by a white thick membrane considered to be inflamed synovial tissue; at the bottom of this space a 1×3 cm section of the rib surface was exposed in the defect of the thick membrane (Figure 4). There was no free body in the space or palpable indurations on its wall. We irrigated the space, sutured the fascias of the divided muscles, and subsequently closed the skin.

Macroscopically, the typical thick perichondrium and cartilage cap were not found, although the flat distal end of the lesion was covered by spotty fibrocartilage-like tissue (Figure 5). Histological examination revealed characteristic findings of OC without any malignant changes. The distal end was covered by synovial tissue and was composed of bony trabeculae in which mostly fatty tissue and bone marrow intervened.

The postoperative course was uneventful. The patient returned to normal daily life and full activity 3 weeks postoperatively. At the time of final follow-up 12 years postoperatively, the right scapula was in the normal position, the scapulothoracic rhythm was symmetrical, and there was no limitation of active range of motion or any associated crepitus. The Constant score ratio compared with the contralateral left shoulder was 100% [3]. MRI showed no abnormality of the soft tissue or bony structures (Figure 6).

3. Discussion

OC is the most common benign bone tumor [1, 2]. It has been reported that 14% of OC are hereditary multiple OC

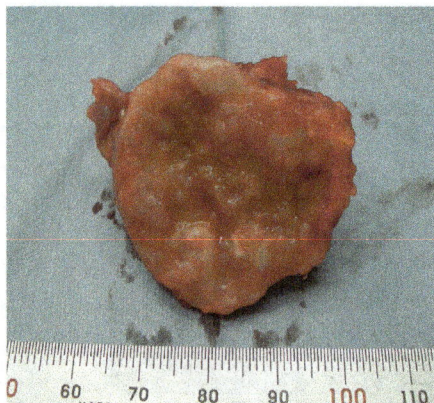

FIGURE 5: Macroscopic findings of the distal end of the osseous tumor. The distal surface was rather irregular. The typical thick perichondrium and cartilage cap were not found, although it was covered by spotty fibrocartilage-like tissue.

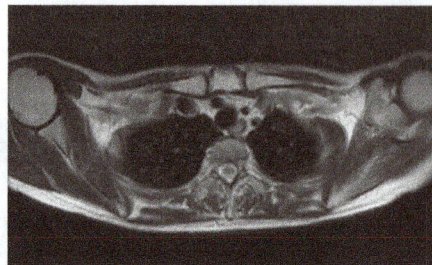

FIGURE 6: T2-weighted magnetic resonance images taken at the final follow-up 12 years postoperatively. There was no abnormality of the soft tissue or bony structures, although some asymmetry existed.

(an autosomal-dominant disorder) and 86% are solitary OC without heredity [1, 4]. Solitary OC is a common lesion estimated to occur in 1-2% of individuals [4]. The literature indicates little sex predilection [1]. The cartilaginous cap is the site of active growth, and the degree of maturity parallels the host bone. If the OC is arrested, as may occur in adults, there may be practically no cartilaginous cap. This appearance is especially likely with the rare OC associated with an overlying bursa [1]. In a minority of cases, OC may grow beyond skeletal maturity [5]. The lesion in our case was a solitary OC, as the physiological and radiographic investigations found no other bony abnormalities. The OC was considered to be arrested, as there was no cartilaginous cap histologically.

The most common sites of involvement are the metaphyseal region of the long bones of the limbs, while involvement of flat bones is less common [2]. The scapula is reportedly the site of occurrence of 1–3% of all primary bone tumors [6]. OC is the most common of the tumors and tumor-like lesions of the scapula, accounting for 17–40% [6, 7]. The majority of scapular tumors are of cartilaginous origin; this may be because the scapula develops by endochondral ossification from seven ossification centers and has a total length of physes exceeding any tubular bone [6]. Scapular lesions account for 4–4.9% of the solitary OC cases [1, 4].

The vast majority of OC are asymptomatic. Symptoms are often related to the size and location of the lesion [2]. The most common symptom is a nontender, painless cosmetic deformity related to the slowly enlarging mass. Additional complications that cause pain include fracture, bursa formation, arthritis, and impingement of the adjacent tendons, blood vessels, nerves, or spinal cord [1, 2, 4]. Approximately 60–80% of patients with OC were younger than 20 years at the time of the first excision of the OC [1, 4]. Although it is uncommon for a solitary OC to become symptomatic after skeletal maturity, there are some well-documented reports of the appearance of symptoms in adults that resulted from the following: mechanical irritation of muscle, tendon, or soft tissue; compression of a nerve; formation of a pseudoaneurysm or an adventitious bursa; fracture; infection; ischemic necrosis; or malignant

transformation [8]. In our case, the symptoms appeared after skeletal maturity.

In 1891, Orlow [9] originally described the bursa formation between an OC and the surrounding soft tissue as "exostosis bursata," although this had been recognized previously. The exact occurrence rate of bursal formation associated with OC is unknown, but Unni and Inwards [1] stated that an overlying bursa was significant enough to be described in 1.3% of their cases treated surgically. McWilliams [10] reported the first case of ventral-side scapular OC accompanied by adventitious bursa. Since this first reported case, to the best of our knowledge, there have been 20 cases of the solitary ventral-side scapular OC associated with a large bursa (including our case) reported in the English literature (Table 1). The scapula glides over the thoracic wall, cushioned from the undulating surface of the ribs by the serratus anterior and subscapularis muscles. However, the scapular superior and inferior angles, and its medial border, are relatively poorly cushioned [11]. Endochondral ossification occurs at the medial border and lateral angle of the scapula, where OC commonly develops. OC near the medial scapular border then easily causes friction with the ribcage. In the literature, 41–73% of OC associated with marked bursa formation are located on the ventral scapula [4, 12–14]. Many authors described that the scapular OC with a large bursa penetrated the subscapularis and serratus anterior muscles and that the bursae were formed along the chest wall; although Chiarelli et al. reported an OC case associated with intramuscular bursa formation in the serratus anterior [15]. It remains unknown whether the bursa associated with the OC in our case was an adventitious bursa or an inflamed consistent bursa located between the serratus anterior and the ribcage [16]. These bursae associated with OC are lined by synovium and may hemorrhage or become inflamed or infected. In addition, the bursa may contain chondral or fibrin bodies, and chondrometaplasia can occur within the synovial lining, leading to secondary synovial chondromatosis [4, 14, 17–20]. In our case, there was no free body in the bursa and no palpable induration on the bursal wall that would have indicated chondrometaplasia or secondary osteochondromatosis. Traces of direct contact between the lesion and the ribs were apparent, and the bursa was formed between the serratus anterior and the chest wall. These findings are consistent with other reports that

TABLE 1: Reported cases of solitary ventral-side scapular osteochondroma associated with a large bursa.

Year	Author(s)	Patient's age/sex/affected side*	Duration of symptoms	Scapular winging	Osteochondroma location
1914	McWilliams	18/F/L	1 year	Yes	Lower: inner
1973	Parsons	20/M/L	?	Yes	Vertebral: center
1979	El-Khoury and Bassett	23/M/R	2 months	?	Axillar: midportion
1981	Borges et al.	56/F/L	?	?	Vertebral: 3rd and 4th ribs
1991	Griffiths et al.	38/M/L	?	Yes	Near the inferior angle
1997	Jacobi et al.	17/F/R	7 weeks after injury	?	Near the inferior angle
1999	Okada et al.	33/M/R	1 month	?	Lateral: inferior
2000	Shackcloth and Page	32/M/R	6 months	?	Lateral: center
2006	Mohsen et al.	19/M/R	6 months	Yes	Vertebral: midportion
2010	Scott and Alexander	14/M/R	9 months	Yes	Near the inferior angle
2010	Aalderink and Wolf	Mid-20s/F/R	15 years	Yes	Medial: inferior
2010	Frost et al.	11/F/R	?	Yes	?
		20/M/L	?	Yes	?
		25/M/L	?	Yes	?
2012	Orth et al.	35/F/R	2-3 months	Yes	Near the superior angle
		48/F/L	2-3 years	Yes	Lateral: inferior
2014	Sivananda et al.	31/F/R	6 months	Yes	Superior angle
2015	Flugstad et al.	20/M/L	4 months	Yes	?
2016	Mohamed et al.	30/M/R	1 year		Near the inferior angle
	This study	27/F/R	3 months	Yes	Superior angle

*Patients' ages are given in years. "?" indicates that the information was not provided in the case report.

described the existence of resorption or erosion of the contacting ribs [21, 22].

Scapular winging and snapping have been well recognized as symptoms of OC development on the ventral scapula. The causes of scapular winging are numerous. Increased scapular prominence from causes other than paralysis of the serratus anterior muscle is referred to as "pseudowinging" of the scapula [23]; this pseudowinging often leads to the discovery of OC on the ventral scapula. Of the 20 reported cases of ventral scapular OC (including our case), 14 cases showed pseudowinging (Table 1). The types of winging indicate the developing location of the OC, although they are characteristically present even at rest with the arm at the side. Carlson et al. [24] analyzed the etiologies of the snapping scapula syndrome causing shoulder discomfort characterized by painful, audible, and/or palpable abnormal scapulothoracic motion in 89 reported cases. They found that the most common causes of snapping scapula syndrome were skeletal abnormalities (43% of reported cases), of which three were OC. Of 20 reported cases of ventral scapular OC (including our case), 14 cases had symptoms consistent with snapping scapula syndrome (Table 1). Therefore, snapping scapula is a common symptom in cases of ventral scapular OC, although OC is an uncommon cause of snapping scapula.

Malignant transformation of OC is well known. WHO reported that the risk of malignant transformation to secondary peripheral chondrosarcoma is estimated at about 1% for solitary and up to 5% for multiple OC [2]. Some authors reported that 27.3–36.3% of patients with multiple OC who underwent surgery had secondary chondrosarcoma, whereas only 3.2–7.6% of patients with the solitary form had malignant changes [1, 25, 26]. Nevertheless, follow-up studies in a number of patients with multiple hereditary OC revealed that malignant change occurs in less than 1% of patients [27]. Secondary chondrosarcoma in OC reportedly has a predilection for flat bones [26]. Clinically, malignant transformation should be suspected in lesions that grow or cause pain after skeletal maturity, as OC only rarely enlarges after this time [4]. The most frequent imaging findings of malignant transformation are irregularity or indistinctness of the surface of the OC, areas of lucency and inhomogeneous mineralization within the OC, and a soft tissue mass frequently containing foci of scattered, punctuate calcifications [26]. On MRI, malignant transformation should be suspected in large tumors with cartilaginous caps that are thick (>1.5–2 cm in an adult) and unmineralized [2]. However, differentiation between the fluid in the inflamed bursa and a large cartilaginous cap is difficult, as they have similar signal characteristics on MRI [5]. In our case, there were no characteristic radiographic findings that indicated malignant transformation. The existence of a thick cartilaginous cap was almost definitively ruled out preoperatively, as the interval between the distal end of the OC and the opposite ribs was 2-3 mm. Histopathological examination confirmed that there were no malignant findings and no cartilaginous cap.

In the approach for OC on the ventral side of the superomedial scapular angle, the superior fibers of the trapezius must be separated. This approach carries a risk of harm to the spinal accessory nerve, which travels an average of 2.7 cm lateral to the superomedial scapular angle [16]. To minimize this risk, we placed the patient in the lateral decubitus position with the shoulder flexed and abducted at 110°, so that the superomedial scapular angle was situated just underneath the middle fibers of the trapezius. An operative field large enough to remove the OC was gained, but it was impossible to observe the whole interior of the associated bursa. We left the bursa untouched to avoid damaging the long thoracic and dorsal scapular nerves that travel closely along the bursal wall. Of the 19 previously reported cases of ventral scapular OC, complete resection of the bursa was performed in eight cases and partial resection was done in two. Regarding treatment of the bursa, there are two different opinions: one that total resection has to be performed [13] and one that aggressive resection of the bursa is unnecessary as the bursa should not recur once there is no longer irritation of the underlying ribs [22]. Some authors have reported success with no or partial resection of the bursa [22, 28, 29]. The bursa accompanying OC involves inflammation caused by mechanical irritation, which produces excess synovial fluid. When the mechanical irritation disappears, the inflammation resolves and the bursal tissue should be normalized. In our case, MRI taken at the time of final follow-up 12 years postoperatively showed no abnormality of soft tissue. Therefore, the bursa itself may resolve when there is no osteochondral free body and indurations in the bursal wall. Arthroscopic excision recently developed for symptomatic OC is effective if the OC is definitely benign [29].

Consent

Written informed consent was obtained from the patient for the publication of this case report and accompanying images.

Conflicts of Interest

The authors declare that there are no conflicts of interest regarding the publication of this paper.

References

[1] K. K. Unni and C. Y. Inwards, *Dahlin's Bone Tumors: General Aspects and Data on 10,165 Cases*, Wolters Kluwer/Lippincott Williams & Wilkins, Philadelphia, PA, USA, 6th edition, 2010.

[2] J. V. M. G. Bovee, D. Heymann, and W. Wuyts, "Osteochondroma," *WHO Classification of Tumours of Soft Tissue and Bone*, C. D. M. Fletcher, J. A. Bridge, P. C. W. Hogendoorn, and F. Mertens, Eds., pp. 250-251, International Agency for Research on Cancer, Lyon, France, 2013.

[3] C. R. Constant and A. H. Murley, "A clinical method of functional assessment of the shoulder," *Clinical Orthopaedics and Related Research*, no. 214, pp. 160-164, 1987.

[4] M. D. Murphey, J. J. Choi, M. J. Kransdorf, D. J. Flemming, and F. H. Gannon, "Imaging of osteochondroma: variants and complications with radiologic-pathologic correlation," *Radiographics*, vol. 20, no. 5, pp. 1407-1434, 2000.

[5] K. C. Lee, A. M. Davies, and V. N. Cassar-Pullicino, "Imaging the complications of osteochondromas," *Clinical Radiology*, vol. 57, no. 1, pp. 18-28, 2002.

[6] J. Brtková, A. Nidecker, H. Zídková, and G. Jundt, "Tumours and tumour-like lesions of scapula," *Acta medica (Hradec Králové)*, vol. 42, no. 3, pp. 103-110, 1999.

[7] Z. Khan, A. M. Gerrish, and R. J. Grimer, "An epidemiological survey of tumour or tumour like conditions in the scapula and periscapular region," *SICOT-J*, vol. 2, p. 34, 2016.

[8] J. C. Krieg, J. A. Buckwalter, K. K. Peterson, G. Y. El-Khoury, and R. A. Robinson, "Extensive growth of an osteochondroma in a skeletally mature patient. A case report," *Journal of Bone and Joint Surgery*, vol. 77, no. 2, pp. 269-273, 1995.

[9] L. W. Orlow, "Die Exostosis bursata und ihre Entstehung," *Deutsche Zeitschrift für Chirurgie*, vol. 31, no. 3-4, pp. 293-308, 1891, in German.

[10] C. A. McWilliams, "Subscapular exostosis with adventitious bursa," *Journal of the American Medical Association*, vol. 63, no. 17, pp. 1473-1474, 1914.

[11] T. A. Parsons, "The snapping scapula and subscapular exostoses," *The Journal of Bone and Joint Surgery*, vol. 55, no. 2, pp. 345-349, 1973.

[12] H. J. Griffiths, R. C. Thompson Jr., H. R. Galloway, L. I. Everson, and J. S. Suh, "Bursitis in association with solitary osteochondromas presenting as mass lesions," *Skeletal Radiology*, vol. 20, no. 7, pp. 513-516, 1991.

[13] C. A. Jacobi, K. Gellert, and J. Zieren, "Rapid development of subscapular exostosis bursata," *Journal of Shoulder and Elbow Surgery*, vol. 6, no. 2, pp. 164-166, 1997.

[14] K. Okada, K. Terada, R. Sashi, and N. Hoshi, "Large bursa formation associated with osteochondroma of the scapula: a case report and review of the literature," *Japanese Journal of Clinical Oncology*, vol. 29, no. 7, pp. 356-360, 1999.

[15] G. M. Chiarelli, L. Massari, E. Grandi, L. Lupi, S. Bighi, and G. L. Limone, "Bursal degeneration of the serratus magnus muscle in a solitary exostosis of the scapula," *La Chirurgia Degli Organi di Movimento*, vol. 72, no. 4, pp. 371-374, 1988, in Italian.

[16] G. R. Williams Jr., M. Shakil, J. Klimkiewicz, and J. P. Iannotti, "Anatomy of the scapulothoracic articulation," *Clinical Orthopaedics and Related Research*, vol. 359, pp. 237-246, 1999.

[17] J. W. Milgram and R. D. Keagy, "Bursal osteochondromatosis: a case report," *Clinical Orthopaedics and Related Research*, no. 144, pp. 269-271, 1979.

[18] G. Y. El-Khoury and G. S. Bassett, "Symptomatic bursa formation with osteochondromas," *American Journal of Roentgenology*, vol. 133, no. 5, pp. 895-898, 1979.

[19] A. M. Borges, A. G. Huvos, and J. Smith, "Bursa formation and synovial chondrometaplasia associated with osteochondromas," *American Journal of Clinical Pathology*, vol. 75, no. 5, pp. 648-653, 1981.

[20] M. Mehta, L. M. White, T. Knapp, R. A. Kandel, J. S. Wunder, and R. S. Bell, "MR imaging of symptomatic osteochondromas with pathological correlation," *Skeletal Radiology*, vol. 27, no. 8, pp. 427-433, 1998.

[21] P. Sivananda, B. K. Rao, P. V. Kumar, and G. S. Ram, "Osteochondroma of the ventral scapula causing scapular static winging and secondary rib erosion," *Journal of Clinical and Diagnostic Research*, vol. 8, no. 5, pp. LD03-LD05, 2014.

[22] N. A. Flugstad, J. R. Sanger, and D. A. Hackbarth, "Pseudowinging of the scapula caused by scapular osteochondroma: review of literature and case report," *Hand*, vol. 10, no. 2, pp. 353-356, 2015.

[23] L. H. Cooley and J. S. Torg, ""Pseudowinging" of the scapula secondary to subscapular osteochondroma," *Clinical Orthopaedics and Related Research*, no. 162, pp. 119-124, 1982.

[24] H. L. Carlson, A. J. Haig, and D. C. Stewart, "Snapping scapula syndrome: three case reports and an analysis of the literature," *Archives of Physical Medicine and Rehabilitation*, vol. 78, no. 5, pp. 506-511, 1997.

[25] R. C. Garrison, K. K. Unni, R. A. McLeod, D. J. Pritchard, and D. C. Dahlin, "Chondrosarcoma arising in osteochondroma," *Cancer*, vol. 49, no. 9, pp. 1890–1897, 1982.

[26] A. R. Ahmed, T. S. Tan, K. K. Unni, M. S. Collins, D. E. Wenger, and F. H. Sim, "Secondary chondrosarcoma in osteochondroma: report of 107 patients," *Clinical Orthopaedics and Related Research*, vol. 411, pp. 193–206, 2003.

[27] H. A. Peterson, "Multiple hereditary osteochondromata," *Clinical Orthopaedics and Related Research*, no. 239, pp. 222–230, 1989.

[28] M. S. Mohsen, N. K. Moosa, and P. Kumar, "Osteochondroma of the scapula associated with winging and large bursa formation," *Medical Principles and Practice*, vol. 15, no. 5, pp. 387–390, 2006.

[29] K. Aalderink and B. Wolf, "Scapular osteochondroma treated with arthroscopic excision using prone positioning," *American Journal of Orthopedics*, vol. 39, no. 2, pp. E11–E14, 2010.

[30] M. J. Shackcloth and R. D. Page, "Scapular osteochondroma with reactive bursitis presenting as a chest wall tumour," *European Journal of Cardio-Thoracic Surgery*, vol. 18, no. 4, pp. 495-496, 2000.

[31] D. A. Scott and J. R. Alexander, "Relapsing and remitting scapular winging in a pediatricpatient," *American Journal of Physical Medicine & Rehabilitation*, vol. 89, no. 6, pp. 505–508, 2010.

[32] N. L. Frost, S. A. Parada, M. W. Manoso, E. Arrington, and P. Benfanti, "Scapular osteochondromas treated with surgical excision," *Orthopedics*, vol. 33, no. 11, p. 804, 2010.

[33] P. Orth, K. Anagnostakos, E. Fritsch, D. Kohn, and H. Madry, "Static winging of the scapula caused by osteochondroma in adults: a case series," *Journal of Medical Case Reports*, vol. 6, p. 363, 2012.

19

Posttraumatic Proximal Radioulnar Synostosis after Closed Reduction for a Radial Neck and Olecranon Fracture

Patrick R. Keller [iD],[1] Heather A. Cole [iD],[1] Christopher M. Stutz,[2] and Jonathan G. Schoenecker [iD][1,3,4,5,6]

[1]Department of Orthopaedics and Rehabilitation, Vanderbilt University Medical Center, 4202 Doctors' Office Tower, 2200 Children's Way, Nashville, TN 37232-9565, USA

[2]Texas Scottish-Rite Children's Hospital for Children, 2222 Welborn Ave., Dallas, TX 75219, USA

[3]Department of Pathology, Vanderbilt University Medical Center, 4202 Doctors' Office Tower, 2200 Children's Way, Nashville, TN 37232-9565, USA

[4]Department of Pharmacology, Vanderbilt University Medical Center, 4202 Doctors' Office Tower, 2200 Children's Way, Nashville, TN 37232-9565, USA

[5]Department of Pediatrics, Vanderbilt University Medical Center, 4202 Doctors' Office Tower, 2200 Children's Way, Nashville, TN 37232-9565, USA

[6]Vanderbilt Center for Bone Biology, Vanderbilt University Medical Center, 4202 Doctors' Office Tower, 2200 Children's Way, Nashville, TN 37232-9565, USA

Correspondence should be addressed to Jonathan G. Schoenecker; jon.schoenecker@vanderbilt.edu

Academic Editor: Georg Singer

Posttraumatic proximal radioulnar synostosis (PPRUS) is a severe complication of radial head and neck fractures known to occur after severe injury or operative fixation. Cases of PPRUS occurring after minimally displaced, nonoperatively treated radial neck injuries are, by contrast, extremely rare. Here, we present a pediatric case of PPRUS that developed after a nonoperatively treated minimally displaced radial neck fracture with concomitant olecranon fracture. While more cases are needed to establish the association between this pattern of injury and PPRUS, we recommend that when encountering patients with a minimally displaced radial neck fracture and a concomitant elbow injury, the rare possibility of developing proximal radioulnar synostosis should be considered.

1. Introduction

Fractures of the proximal radius are among the most problematic of elbow injuries due to the high incidence of complications including nerve injury, osteonecrosis, stiffness, and decreased range of motion [1]. Posttraumatic synostosis of the proximal radioulnar joint (PRUJ) is recognized as a severe complication of radial head and neck fractures because it severely limits range of motion. It is most commonly associated with displaced radial neck injury and/or operative intervention [1–22], especially after percutaneous fixation or open reduction and internal fixation

maneuvers are performed [1]. Thus, in keeping with current standard of practice [1], radial neck fractures with <30° angulation and less than 3-4 millimeters of translation are usually best treated with closed reduction and casting. For these cases, closed reduction and casting almost universally provides an optimal reduction and avoids major complications, including PPRUS [2, 3, 23–25]. However, though extremely rare, cases of PPRUS after minimally displaced nonoperatively treated radial neck injury have occurred. In our review of the literature, there was only one case report of PPRUS that developed after closed reduction and immobilization for a radial neck fracture with concomitant elbow

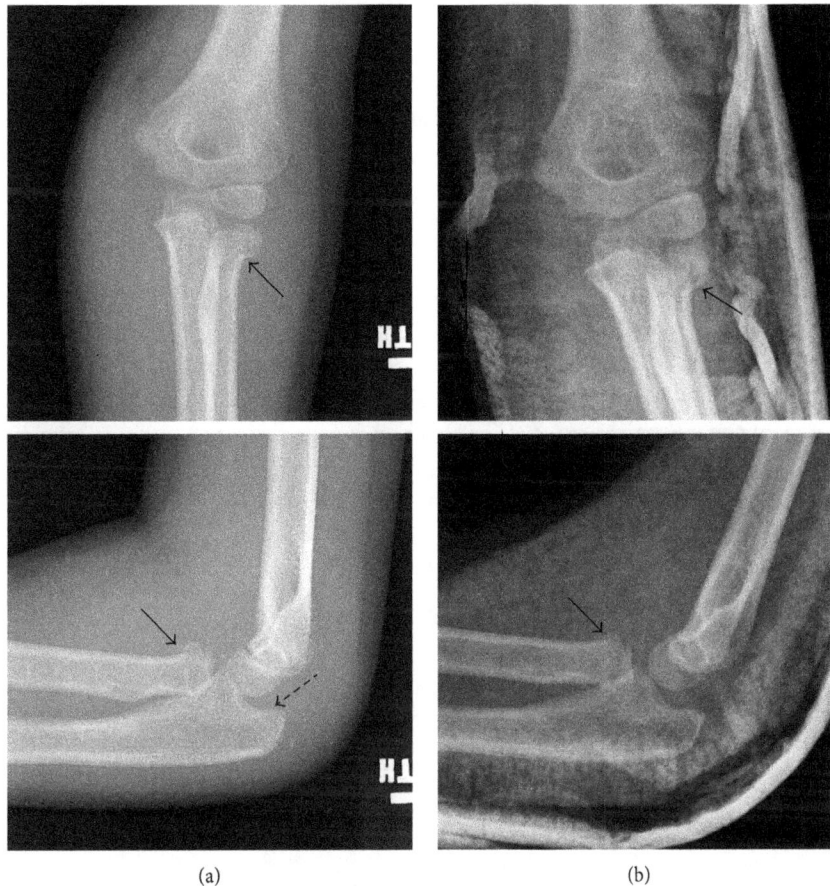

(a)   (b)

FIGURE 1: Left elbow before (a) and after (b) attempted closed reduction. Initial injury AP and lateral radiographs (a) demonstrate a radial neck fracture with 20–30° angulation (solid arrows in (a)) and a nondisplaced olecranon fracture (hatched arrow in (a)). Post-closed reduction AP and lateral radiographs (b) are partially obscured by plaster splint but demonstrate no change in alignment of radial neck (solid arrows in (b) compared to (a)).

dislocation. Here, we present a novel case of PPRUS following a minimally displaced, nonoperatively treated radial neck fracture with concomitant olecranon fracture in a pediatric patient.

2. Case

The patient was an 8-year-old right-handed girl who fell from eight feet onto her outstretched and supinated left upper extremity. She immediately experienced elbow pain and swelling. In the emergency department, she was unable to move her elbow without significant pain. Initial radiographs showed a left radial neck fracture and a non-displaced olecranon fracture (Figure 1(a)). Elbow range of motion was 40° shy of full extension to 110° of flexion, supination 15° shy of neutral and pronation of 30°. Reduction of the radial neck fracture was attempted via closed reduction under fluoroscopic guidance. Follow-up radiographs showed <30° angulation and 1 mm of translation of the radial head (Figure 1(b)). Her left arm was placed in a well-padded posterior A-frame splint. She was sent home in the splint and returned to clinic one week later. One week after injury, radiographs were taken and then her splint was removed. A long arm cast was placed (Figure 2

(a)). Two weeks after injury, left elbow radiographs showed no change in alignment (Figure 2(b)).

Three weeks after injury, the cast was removed and physical examination revealed full extension with 90° of flexion and a pronosupination arc of 40°, both limited by pain. Radiographs demonstrated minimal displacement of the olecranon fracture, but no change in radial neck fracture alignment (Figure 3(a)). She was prescribed range of motion exercises with the assistance of a physical therapist. Four weeks after injury, physical examination revealed pronosupination between −10° and 20°, with almost full pronation. She was without pain. Radiographs demonstrated healing radial neck and olecranon fractures (Figure 3(b)). Eleven weeks after injury, physical examination revealed extension to 90°, flexion to 30°, supination 15° from neutral, and pronation to 20° from neutral, all limited by pain. In addition to continued healing of fractures, radiographs demonstrated a new finding of synostosis at the PRUJ (Figure 3(c)). Continued physical therapy was recommended, and the family was informed that surgical resection of the synostosis may be needed to improve her range of motion. She was lost to follow-up for almost two years, at which point she returned to our clinic.

Two years after injury, physical examination of the elbow revealed 135° of flexion and full extension, but complete loss

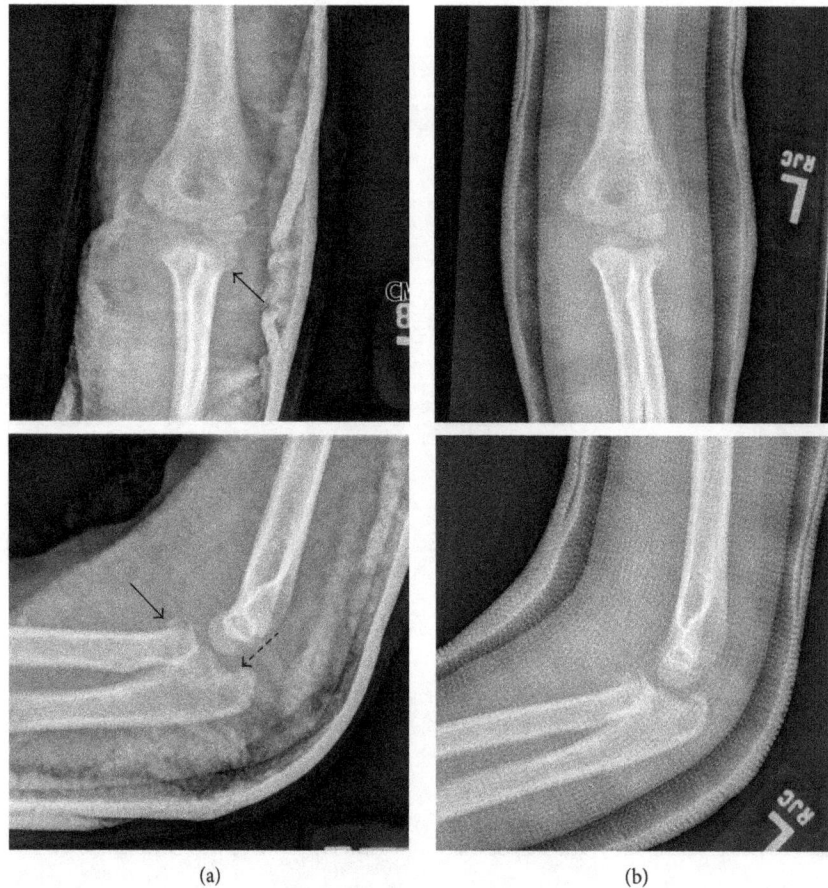

(a)   (b)

FIGURE 2: Left elbow radiographs one (a) and two (b) weeks after injury. One-week AP and lateral radiographs (a) are partially obscured by splint material but demonstrate radial neck fracture with less than 30° of angulation (solid arrows in (a)) and a nondisplaced olecranon fracture (hatched arrow in (a)). Splint was removed and cast placed at one week. Two-week AP and lateral radiographs (b) are partially obscured by overlying cast material but demonstrate no changes from prior radiographs.

of pronosupination with the forearm fixed in 10° of supination. Radiographs demonstrated healed radial neck and olecranon fractures, and an extensive bony synostosis at the PRUJ (Figures 4(a) and 4(b)). At that time, surgical treatment of the synostosis was offered, but the patient was again lost to follow-up for six months. Two years six months after injury, she again returned to our clinic, and physical examination was unchanged from prior. CT scan (Figure 5) confirmed extensive bony synostosis at the proximal radioulnar joint. She was again offered a multitude of treatment options, including surgical resection, and family chose nonsurgical management with physical therapy. She has not returned to our clinic since.

3. Discussion

While past studies have described risk factors for and the incidence of PPRUS as it occurs after displaced injury or operative fixation for radial neck fractures [1–3, 10, 11, 14, 16–19, 22], this same information is lacking in regard to minimally displaced, nonoperatively treated injury. Our review of literature suggests that in cases of radial neck fracture treated by closed reduction, two factors increase risk of PPRUS: (i) increased radial head

angulation or displacement [13] and (ii) concomitant elbow injuries [4].

Regarding the risk factor of increased severity of fracture, literature suggests that PPRUS tends to develop in displaced radial neck fractures (>45° angulation or >3-4 mm translation), especially in injuries that have been treated operatively [3, 11, 24, 26]. This feature of radial neck fractures is well known and has been recognized since the early 20th century. In 1933, Dr. John Bohrer described radial head and neck fractures in twenty adults and nine children, all of whom were treated conservatively. He found that PPRUS occurred only when there was "marked displacement" or "severe injury with displacement or comminution of the head of the radius." By contrast, in cases of "slight displacement" or "slight trauma," he observed "excellent results" [13]. Other studies, by and large, support the conclusion that minimally displaced nonoperatively treated radial neck fractures do not typically develop PPRUS [12, 27, 28]. This is in contrast to our patient who, although she sustained a minimally displaced nonoperatively treated injury, did have a concomitant elbow injury.

Much less is known about minimally displaced radial neck fractures that both (i) were treated conservatively and (ii) had associated elbow injuries (e.g., elbow dislocation or

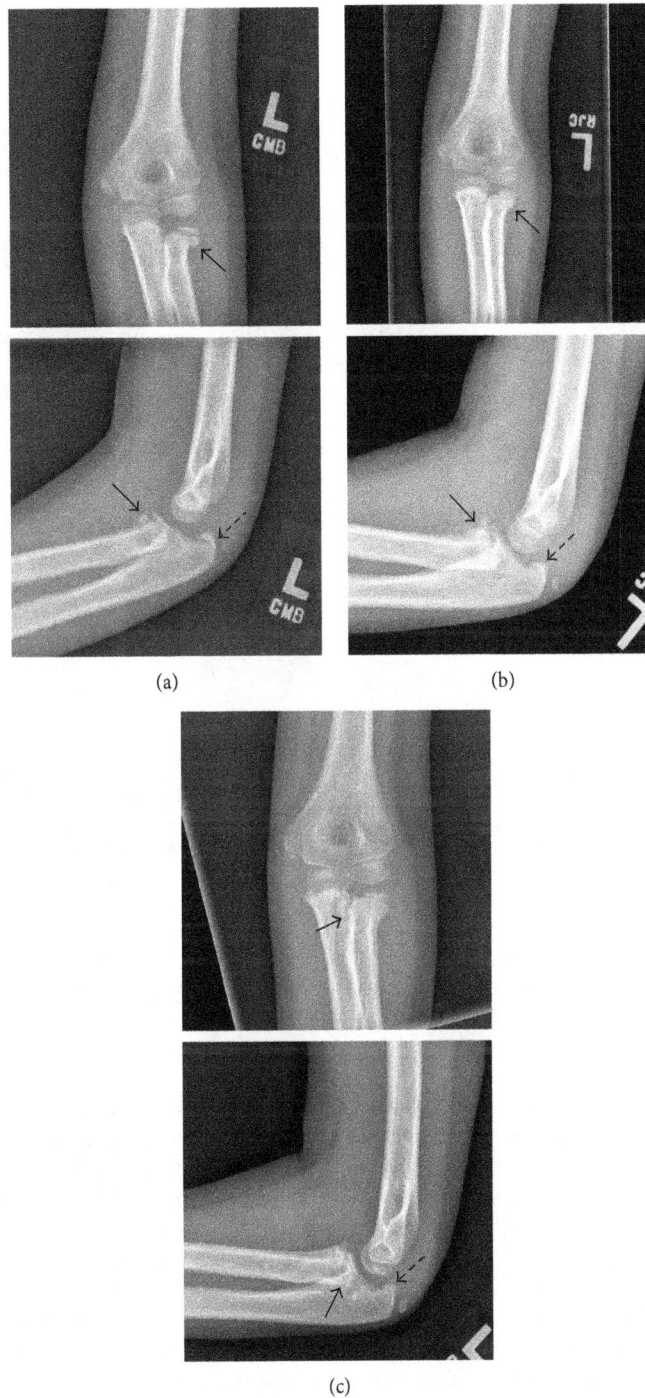

FIGURE 3: Left elbow radiographs three (a), four (b), and eleven (c) weeks after injury. Cast was removed at three weeks. Three-week AP and lateral radiographs (a) demonstrate a radial neck fracture with mild medial displacement and no change in alignment from prior (solid arrows in (a)) and a now-displaced olecranon fracture (hatched arrow in (a)). Four-week AP and lateral radiographs (b) demonstrate increased periosteal reaction about the radial neck fracture (solid arrows in (b)) with no change in alignment from prior and a healing olecranon fracture (hatched line in (b)). Eleven-week AP and lateral radiographs (c) demonstrate increased callus formation and synostosis about the medial aspect of the radial neck fracture (solid arrows in (c)) and a healed olecranon fracture (hatched arrow in (c)).

ulnar fracture). In one case series, Jones et al. [4] described a young girl who, after sustaining a radial neck fracture with associated elbow dislocation, was treated with closed reduction and immobilization for two weeks and then developed PPRUS. The displacement of her radial neck fracture was not described. Because of that, there is no way of discerning whether PPRUS was secondary to the associated elbow dislocation, the severity of the radial neck fracture, or

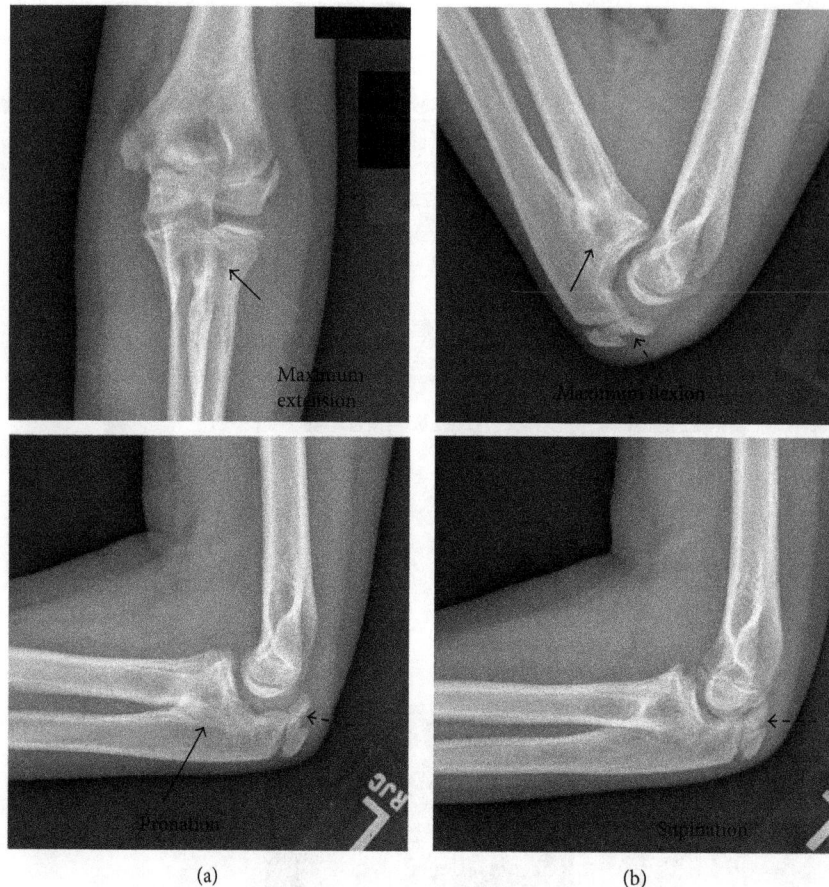

FIGURE 4: Left elbow radiographs at two years after injury. Maximum extension and pronation (a) and flexion and supination (b) are shown. On physical examination, she had full range of motion in extension and flexion, but pronosupination was entirely lost. All radiographs show synostosis of the proximal radioulnar joint (solid arrows in (a) and (b)) and fracture deformity from the previously healed proximal radial fracture. The olecranon fracture is healed (hatched arrows in (a) and (b)).

a combination of both. However, our case report adds to the literature an example of PPRUS from a minimally displaced radial neck fracture that occurred in the setting of concomitant elbow injury (proximal ulnar fracture in our case), thus supporting the latter interpretation (combination) of increased risk in the Jones et al. case.

Our hypothesis is that in cases of minimally displaced nonoperatively treated proximal radius fracture with concomitant elbow injury, PPRUS forms because of disruption of periosteum from the transmission of energy from the wrist, to the radial neck, through the PRUJ, and finally to the ulna. In our patient's case, her pattern of injury can be classified as a Monteggia variant fracture; such fractures are characterized by an olecranon fracture with an associated radial neck fracture [2]. The most common mechanism of injury for Monteggia variant fractures is from fall on an outstretched supinated arm [3, 25]. Valgus torque is exerted on the elbow joint which, when combined with the force that is transmitted from the wrist up through the radial shaft, drives the radial head into the capitellum [2, 5, 20]. Because the radius and ulna articulate proximally in only one place, the PRUJ, injury to the radius will transmit the force to the ulna through the PRUJ. This increases the likelihood of

injury to the periosteum at the PRUJ, predisposing the patient to development of PPRUS. This mechanism is supported by studies that have shown that injury (e.g., from trauma or surgery) stimulates pluripotential mesenchymal stem cells to differentiate into osteoblasts, which then lay osteoid which becomes heterotopic lamellar bone [18]. Further, injuries to the interosseous membrane of the forearm have the potential to serve as the nidus for heterotopic ossification and subsequent synostosis at any point along the membrane [19, 29].

This hypothesis does not exist in a vacuum, however, as several other etiologic mechanisms of PPRUS have been proposed in the past. These include arthrosis of the elbow joint space, ossification of elbow ligaments (including the annular and collateral ligaments), disruption of the joint capsule leading to capsular fibrosis [20], soft tissue contracture, ectopic calcification of surrounding soft tissue structures (including myositis ossificans of the brachialis muscle), failure of fracture healing [18], and bone fragments that inadvertently remain in the interosseous membrane [19]. It is possible that one or more of these other etiologic factors played a role in our patient's case. Thus, more case reports are needed to further develop and test our hypothesis.

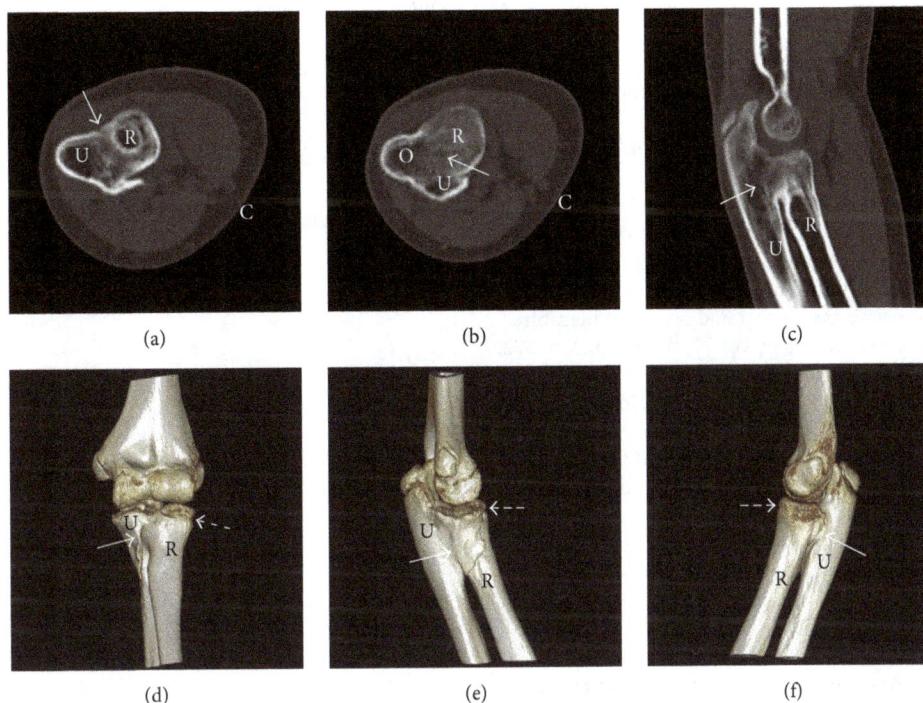

FIGURE 5: Left elbow CT scans (a–c) and CT 3D reconstruction (d–f) at two years six months after injury. Axial (a, b) and sagittal (c) CT views demonstrate synostosis of the proximal radioulnar joint, as do anterior (d), medial (e), and lateral (f) CT 3D reconstruction views (solid white arrows in all). The radial head fracture is healed (hatched white arrows in (d)–(f)). U = ulna; R = radius; O = olecranon; C = cubital fossa.

4. Conclusion

Our case is a radiographically confirmed report of association between a minimally displaced, nonoperatively treated proximal radius injury and development of PPRUS over subsequent weeks. Critically, this occurred in a patient whose radial neck fracture (i) was minimally displaced, (ii) had a concomitant olecranon fracture, and (iii) was treated nonoperatively. This suggests that proximal radioulnar synostosis may be a rare part of the natural history of minimally displaced radial neck fractures in children, especially in cases of associated elbow injury. Therefore, we recommend that when encountering patients who sustain a radial neck fracture with associated elbow injuries, the clinician should consider the rare possibility of the patient developing proximal radioulnar synostosis and obtain closer follow-up with radiography and range of motion. Further work should strive to better establish the pattern of injury described herein, and whether certain types of concomitant elbow injuries in the setting of radial neck fracture are more associated with PPRUS than others.

Conflicts of Interest

The authors declare that they have no conflicts of interest.

References

[1] P. M. Waters and D. S. Bae, *Pediatric Hand and Upper Limb Surgery: A Practical Guide*, Chapter 31, Lippincott Williams & Wilkins, Philadelphia, PA, USA, 2012.

[2] N. E. Green and M. F. Swiontkowski, *Skeletal Trauma in Children*, Chapter 9, Elsevier Health Sciences, Amsterdam, Netherlands, 2008.

[3] B. H. M. Tan and A. Mahadev, "Radial neck fractures in children," *Journal of Orthopaedic Surgery*, vol. 19, no. 2, pp. 209–212, 2011.

[4] M. E. Jones, M. A. Rider, J. Hughes, and M. A. Tonkin, "The use of a proximally based posterior interosseous adipofascial flap to prevent recurrence of synostosis of the elbow joint and forearm," *Journal of Hand Surgery*, vol. 32, no. 2, pp. 143–147, 2007.

[5] D. Ceroni, J. Campos, A. Dahl-Farhoumand, J. Holveck, and A. Kaelin, "Neck osteotomy for malunion of neglected radial neck fractures in children: a report of 2 cases," *Journal of Pediatric Orthopaedics*, vol. 30, no. 7, pp. 649–654, 2010.

[6] J. P. Cullen, V. D. Pellegrini, R. J. Miller, and J. A. Jones, "Treatment of traumatic radioulnar synostosis by excision and postoperative low-dose irradiation," *Journal of Hand Surgery*, vol. 19, no. 3, pp. 394–401, 1994.

[7] J. B. Jupiter and D. Ring, "Operative treatment of post-traumatic proximal radioulnar synostosis," *Journal of Bone & Joint Surgery*, vol. 80, no. 2, pp. 248–257, 1998.

[8] M. Henket, P. J. van Duijn, J. N. Doornberg, D. Ring, and J. B. Jupiter, "A comparison of proximal radioulnar synostosis excision after trauma and distal biceps reattachment," *Journal of Shoulder and Elbow Surgery*, vol. 16, no. 5, pp. 626–630, 2007.

[9] D. Ring, J. B. Jupiter, and L. Gulotta, "Atrophic nonunions of the proximal ulna," *Clinical Orthopaedics and Related Research*, vol. 409, pp. 268–274, 2003.

[10] G. Bauer, M. Arand, and W. Mutschler, "Post-traumatic radioulnar synostosis after forearm fracture osteosynthesis,"

Archives of Orthopaedic and Trauma Surgery, vol. 110, no. 3, pp. 142–145, 1991.

[11] D. R. Roy, "Radioulnar synostosis following proximal radial fracture in child," *Orthopaedic Review*, vol. 15, no. 2, pp. 89–94, 1986.

[12] K. G. Vince and J. E. Miller, "Cross-union complicating fracture of the forearm part II: children," *Journal of Bone & Joint Surgery*, vol. 69, no. 5, pp. 654–661, 1987.

[13] J. V. Bohrer, "Fractures of the head and neck of the radius," *Annals of Surgery*, vol. 97, no. 2, p. 204, 1933.

[14] V. K. Singh and G. S. Vargaonkar, "An iatrogenic proximal radioulnar synostosis: a case report and review of literature," *Chinese Journal of Traumatology*, vol. 17, no. 6, pp. 370–372, 2014.

[15] M. Sugimoto, K. Masada, H. Ohno, and T. Hosoya, "Treatment of traumatic radioulnar synostosis by excision, with interposition of a posterior interosseous island forearm flap," *Journal of Hand Surgery: British & European Volume*, vol. 21, no. 3, pp. 393–395, 1996.

[16] S. Kamineni, N. G. Maritz, and B. F. Morrey, "Proximal radial resection for posttraumatic radioulnar synostosis: a new technique to improve forearm rotation," *Journal of Bone and Joint Surgery-American Volume*, vol. 84, no. 5, pp. 745–751, 2002.

[17] J. M. Failla, P. C. Amadio, and B. F. Morrey, "Post-traumatic proximal radio-ulnar synostosis. Results of surgical treatment," *Journal of Bone & Joint Surgery*, vol. 71, no. 8, pp. 1208–1213, 1989.

[18] A. L. C. Lindenhovius and J. B. Jupiter, "The posttraumatic stiff elbow: a review of the literature," *Journal of Hand Surgery*, vol. 32, no. 10, pp. 1605–1623, 2007.

[19] P. Dohn, F. Khiami, E. Rolland, and J.-N. Goubier, "Adult post-traumatic radioulnar synostosis," *Orthopaedics & Traumatology: Surgery & Research*, vol. 98, no. 6, pp. 709–714, 2012.

[20] K. Tucker, "Some aspects of post-traumatic elbow stiffness," *Injury*, vol. 9, no. 3, pp. 216–220, 1978.

[21] S. Pfanner, P. Bigazzi, C. Casini, C. De Angelis, and M. Ceruso, "Surgical treatment of posttraumatic radioulnar synostosis," *Case Reports in Orthopedics*, vol. 2016, Article ID 5956304, 4 pages, 2016.

[22] S. G. Bergeron, N. M. Desy, M. Bernstein, and E. J. Harvey, "Management of posttraumatic radioulnar synostosis," *Journal of the American Academy of Orthopaedic Surgeons*, vol. 20, no. 7, pp. 450–458, 2012.

[23] J. E. Tibone and M. Stoltz, "Fractures of the radial head and neck in children," *Journal of Bone and Joint Surgery*, vol. 63, no. 1, p. 100, 1981.

[24] S. D'souza, R. Vaishya, and L. Klenerman, "Management of radial neck fractures in children: a retrospective analysis of one hundred patients," *Journal of Pediatric Orthopedics*, vol. 13, no. 2, pp. 232–238, 1992.

[25] A. Majed and A. M. Baco, "Late diagnosis and treatment of a paediatric radial neck fracture," *Injury Extra*, vol. 37, no. 9, pp. 322–324, 2006.

[26] R. Breit, "Post-traumatic radioulnar synostosis," *Clinical Orthopaedics and Related Research*, vol. 174, pp. 149–152, 1983.

[27] E. D. Mcbride and J. Charles Monnet, "Epiphysial fractures of the head of the radius in children," *Clinical Orthopaedics*, vol. 16, pp. 264–271, 1960.

[28] D. E. Garland, R. C. Jones, and R. W. Kunkle, "Upper extremity fractures in the acute spinal cord injured patient," *Clinical Orthopaedics and Related Research*, vol. 233, pp. 110–115, 1988.

[29] T. D. J. Botting, "Posttraumatic radio-ulna cross union," *Journal of Trauma and Acute Care Surgery*, vol. 10, no. 1, pp. 16–24, 1970.

20

Acetabular Reconstruction Using a Trabecular Metal Cup with a Novel Pelvic Osteotomy Technique for Severe Acetabular Bone Defect

Keizo Wada ⓘD, Tomohiro Goto ⓘD, Tomoya Takasago, Takahiko Tsutsui ⓘD, and Koichi Sairyo ⓘD

Department of Orthopaedics, Institute of Biomedical Sciences, Tokushima University Graduate School, Tokushima, Japan

Correspondence should be addressed to Keizo Wada; wadahank@hotmail.com

Academic Editor: Paul E. Di Cesare

Case. A 79-year-old woman with an extreme bone defect after failed cementless total hip arthroplasty underwent revision arthroplasty with a novel technique that involved cutting the anterior iliac bone and sliding it distally to reconstruct the anterior acetabular wall. A three-dimensional printed bone model enabled understanding the details of the bone defect. The clinical outcome at 3 years after surgery was favorable. *Conclusion.* The advantages of this technique are twofold, namely, stable fixation of the cup sandwiched between the anterior and posterior walls and reconstruction of the anterior wall using living bone, which allows bone ingrowth into the cup.

1. Introduction

Acetabular reconstruction surgery after failed total hip arthroplasty (THA) with severe bone loss is a challenging procedure. Various surgical techniques have been introduced for acetabular reconstruction; however, the outcomes of these techniques are not necessarily reliable [1–3], particularly in the case of severe bone loss or pelvic discontinuity (i.e., a Paprosky 3A or 3B defect) [4]. Stable initial fixation of the implant with precise preoperative planning, assessment of the condition of the residual bone and bone defects, and preservation of as much bone stock as possible are key to achieving a favorable outcome. In this report, we describe the use of a novel technique for pelvic osteotomy assisted by placement of a trabecular metal cup for acetabular reconstruction surgery in a patient with catastrophic bone loss after failed THA. Preoperative planning using a three-dimensional (3D) printed bone model was extremely useful for understanding the relationship between the implant and the host bone.

2. Case Presentation

The patient was an elderly woman with osteoarthritis secondary to developmental dysplasia of the right hip who underwent THA using a VerSys® MidCoat Hip System femoral stem and a Trilogy® Acetabular System cup (Zimmer Biomet, Warsaw, IN) at the age of 76 years. Three years later, she developed right groin pain with gradually progressing difficulty in walking. She visited her local hospital and was referred to our hospital for further treatment. Her body weight was 46 kg, and height was 143 cm. She had a medical history of hypertension and asthma, which were controlled by medication. Physical examination revealed a slightly limited range of motion at the right hip (100 degrees of flexion, 0 degrees of extension, 20 degrees of abduction, 10 degrees of adduction, 45 degrees of external rotation, and 10 degrees of internal rotation). Her right leg was approximately 3 cm shorter than the left leg.

Anteroposterior pelvic radiography revealed migration of the acetabular cup into the pelvis with destruction of the

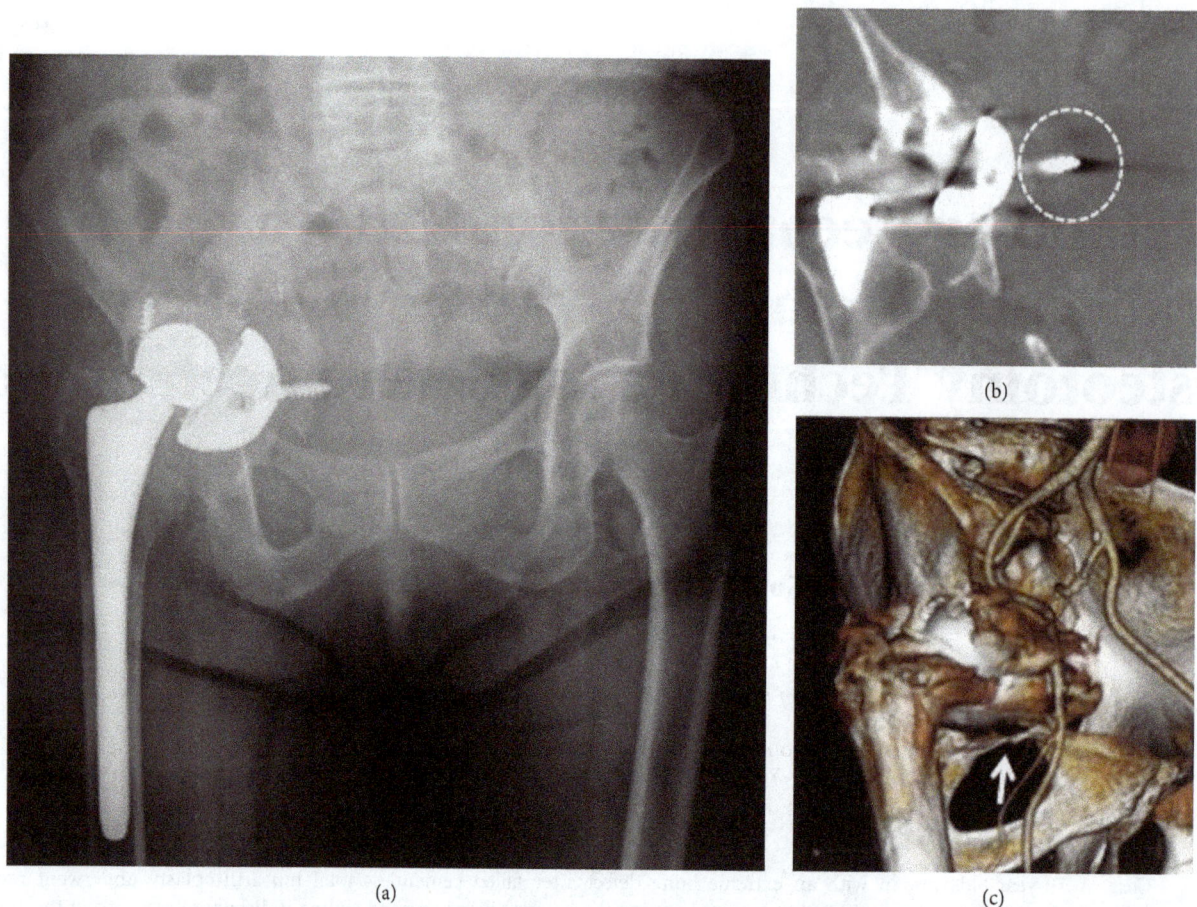

FIGURE 1: Preoperative plain radiographic (a) and computed tomographic (b, c) images of the pelvis. Coronal computed tomographic image shows a screw pressing the bladder wall (white dotted circle). White arrow indicates a fracture of the superior aspect of the obturator foramen.

medial wall of the acetabulum (Figure 1(a)). Computed tomography (CT) showed extensive destruction of bone at the anterior and medial aspects of the acetabulum and a migrated cup screw compressing the bladder wall (Figure 1(b)). The migrated cup was also pushed anteriorly and in contact with the femoral vessels (Figure 1(c)). The remaining bone at the superior aspect of the obturator foramen was fractured, and osteolysis was observed in the posterior column. There were no abnormal findings on the femoral side, and there was no evidence of infection on pre-operative culture of joint fluid. A 3D printed bone model was created from a 2 mm slice CT image using Biotec Bones (Zimmer Biomet, Warsaw, IN) to assess the condition of the residual bone at the acetabulum and to allow detailed preoperative planning, including simulation of the iliac osteotomy, acetabular reaming, and implanting of a trial cup to check the relationship between the cup and the host bone (Figure 2). We planned to cut the ilium longitudinally and slide it distally to reconstruct the anterior column of the acetabulum (Figure 2(b)). The acetabulum was gently reamed, and the cup was inserted into the acetabulum, supported by the reconstructed anterior column of the ilium (Figure 2(c)).

Reconstruction surgery was performed using a trabecular metal cup (Zimmer Biomet, Warsaw, IN) with pelvic osteotomy and bone grafting using a bridging plate from the pubis to the ilium. First, we removed the migrated cup and screws from inside the pelvis using an ilioinguinal approach in the supine position. Next, we cut the anterior part of the iliac bone and slid it distally and fixed it at the iliac crest with screws and small reconstruction plates (Figures 2(b) and 3(b)). An additional long reconstruction plate bridging the pubis and the iliac bone was inserted to support the medial wall of the acetabulum (Figure 3(b)). The patient was then shifted into the left lateral position for cup placement and bone grafting using a direct lateral approach. A bulk and impacted morselized bone allograft (measuring two and a half times the volume of the femoral head) was used to fill the anterior, medial, and superior aspects of the acetabular bone defect. The acetabulum was then carefully reamed to 68 mm in diameter. Finally, a 68 mm sized trabecular metal cup was placed and fixed to the residual posterior column using 3 screws. The amount of blood loss was 920 ml, and the operation time was 8 hours and 41 minutes. The postoperative course was uneventful. There was no complication around the iliac crest. Partial weight bearing was started from 8 weeks postoperatively, and full weight bearing was allowed at 12 weeks postoperatively. The patient could perform active knee flexion at 2 weeks and straight leg raising at 4 weeks postoperatively. At the most recent follow-up 3 years after surgery, the patient was walking with a T-cane and was

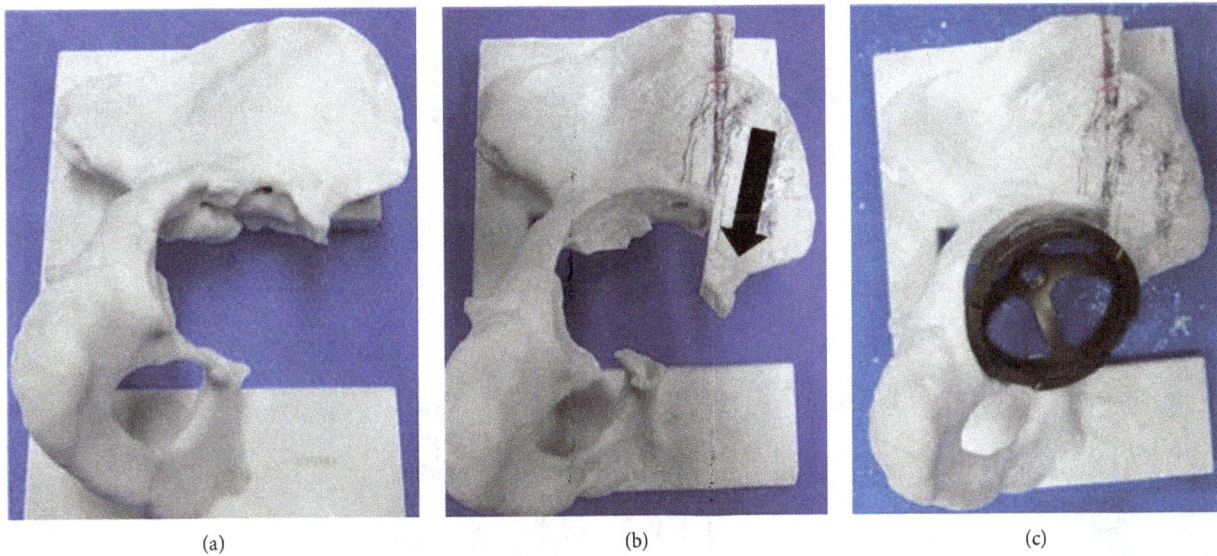

FIGURE 2: Images from the bone model used for preoperative planning. (a) A bone defect is seen at the acetabulum. (b) We rehearsed the iliac osteotomy and slid the ilium distally (black arrow). (c) The trial cup was placed in the acetabulum.

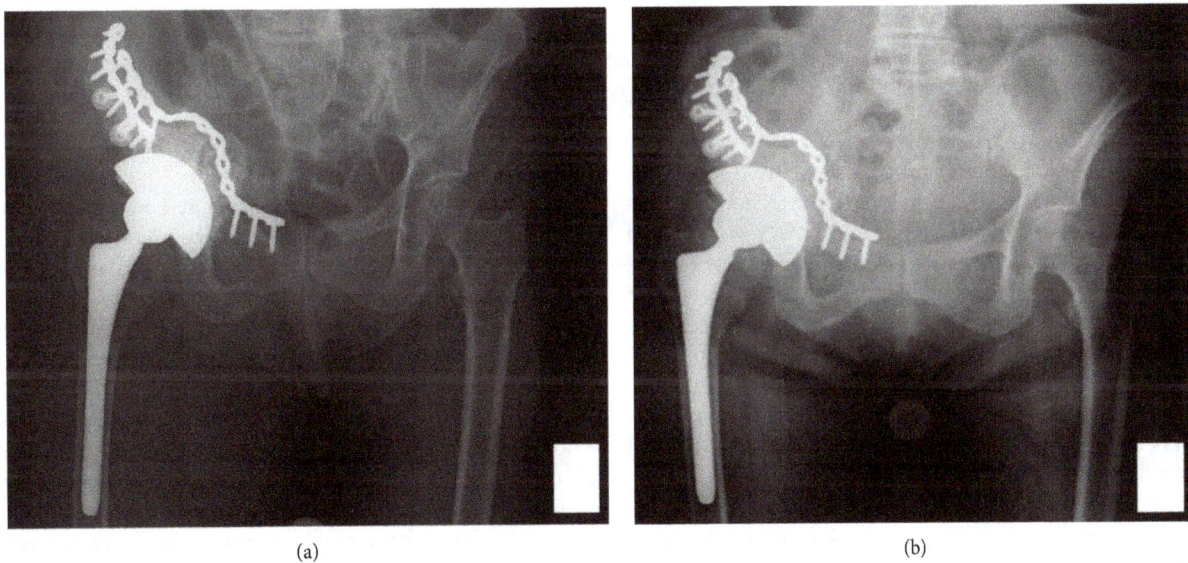

FIGURE 3: Postoperative radiograph at immediately after surgery (a) and at final follow-up (b).

independent in activities of daily living with no infection or dislocation of the hip. A plain radiograph at final follow-up showed her limb length discrepancy was 5 mm and revealed no evidence of implant migration (Figure 3). Bone union at the osteotomy site was observed on postoperative plain radiographs and CT images, and there was no evidence of aseptic loosening of the cup (Figure 4).

3. Discussion

We were able to achieve an excellent clinical outcome using a novel technique of pelvic osteotomy for acetabular reconstruction surgery in a patient with catastrophic bone loss after failed THA. The advantages of this technique are twofold, that is, stable fixation of the cup sandwiched between the anterior and posterior walls and reconstruction of the anterior wall using living bone, which allow ingrowth of bone into the cementless cup.

There are two main concepts in acetabular reconstruction: one is to achieve rigid containment and recover bone stock using metal mesh or reinforcement devices with bone grafting to stabilize the cemented cup and the other is to achieve bone ingrowth using a cementless cup with or without bone grafting or augmentation devices. Surgical techniques representative of the former concept include a cemented cup with a reinforcement plate [5, 6], a cage [7], or impaction bone grafting [8, 9]. The success of these techniques depends on achieving adequate initial stability followed by a biological response of graft incorporation and remodeling. In a patient with a massive bone defect, a large

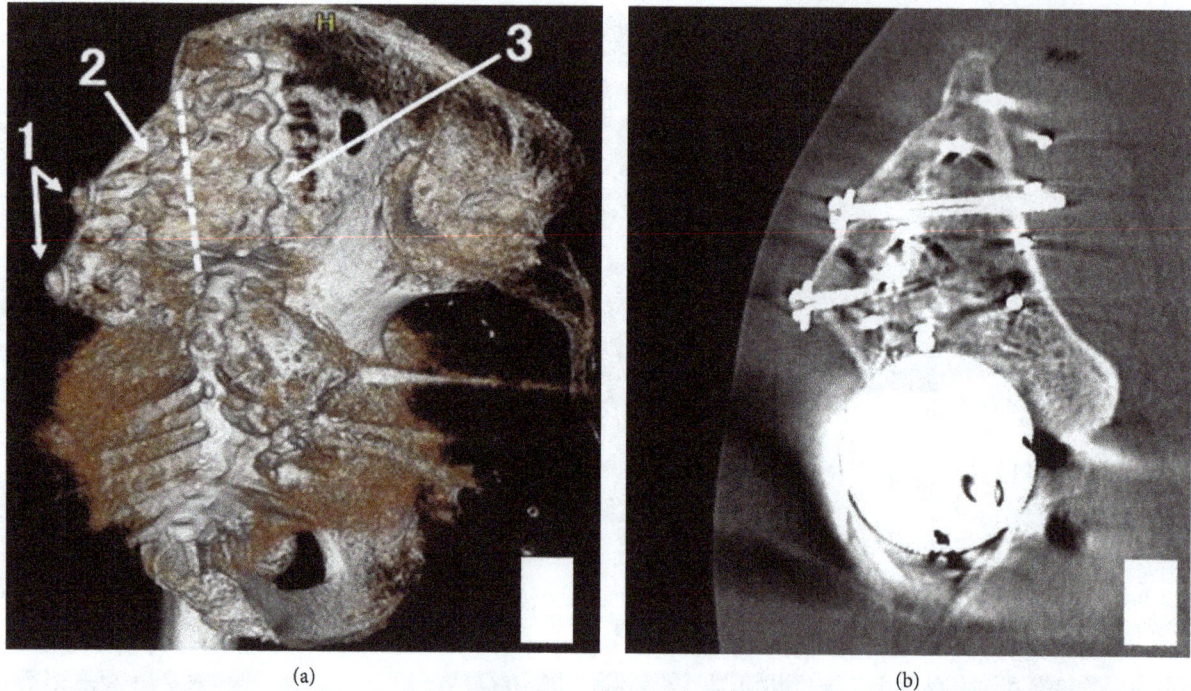

(a)   (b)

FIGURE 4: Reconstructed computed tomographic image (a). The dotted line indicates the osteotomy line of the iliac bone. The slid bone is fixed by two screws (1) and a small plate (2), and (3) indicates the reconstruction plate. Cross-sectional computed tomographic image (b).

bone graft is needed, and incorporation or remodeling of the grafted bone takes quite a long time. Therefore, we need to be cautious about the long-term results when using these techniques in patients with severe bone defects [8, 9]. Moreover, when using reinforcement devices, such as the Ganz ring or Kerboull-type acetabular device, the bone at the obturator foramen must be restored for fixation of the distal hook of the device. In our patient, the residual bone at the superior aspect of the obturator foramen was very poor and fractured, so stable fixation could not be achieved using these reinforcement devices.

Trabecular metal component systems (Zimmer Biomet) are reported which may have increased biocompatibility and allow enhanced bone ingrowth and fixation [10]. Currently, a trabecular metal cup with augmentation is probably the most reasonable option for patients with severe bone loss; however, the preoperative 3D printed model revealed that the largest trabecular metal cup available did not extend from the posterior column to the pubis, and the contact area between living bone and the implant would have been too small even if metal augmentation was used. Therefore, we considered that it would be better to reconstruct the anterior wall of the acetabulum using living bone, which could provide anterior support for the implant and allow ingrowth of biological bone in the cup.

The technique described here has several potential risks. The first concern is the possibility of postoperative muscle weakness caused by sliding of the anterior part of the ilium distally, which involves the anterior superior and inferior iliac spines. Theoretically, this could lead to muscle weakness by shortening of the quadriceps and sartorius muscles. However, postoperative muscle recovery was only slightly delayed

in our patient; she was able to perform active knee flexion at 2 weeks and active straight leg raising at 4 weeks after surgery and subsequently gained full recovery of muscle strength at the hip. The second concern is that the mechanical strength of the refixed anterior part of the ilium might be weak. We anticipated that even partial bone ingrowth or bone union would be needed to withstand the mechanical stress of weight bearing so did not allow our patient to bear weight until 8 weeks after the surgery. However, a long period of non-weight bearing is generally needed in patients with large bone defects when using the other reconstruction methods. The third issue is that this surgical method was invasive. Therefore, close attention needs to be paid to the patient's general physical status and a comprehensive support strategy that considers all possible complications should be prepared.

We have presented here a novel technique for acetabular reconstruction surgery in patients with massive bone loss secondary to failed THA. Although careful follow-up is needed, we obtained a good short-term outcome. Acetabular reconstruction surgery in patients with catastrophic destruction of the acetabulum is extremely difficult, and there are no standard treatment strategies. Originality and ingenuity in the surgical treatment of individual cases are very important in our quest to improve clinical outcomes.

Consent

The patient provided written informed consent for publication of this case report and accompanying images.

Conflicts of Interest

The authors declare that they have no conflicts of interest.

References

[1] J. Petrie, A. Sassoon, and G. J. Haidukewych, "Pelvic discontinuity: current solutions," *The Bone & Joint Journal*, vol. 95-B, no. 11, Supplement A, pp. 109–113, 2013.

[2] N. A. Beckmann, S. Weiss, M. C. M. Klotz, M. Gondan, S. Jaeger, and R. G. Bitsch, "Loosening after acetabular revision: comparison of trabecular metal and reinforcement rings. A systematic review," *The Journal of Arthroplasty*, vol. 29, no. 1, pp. 229–235, 2014.

[3] B. A. Rogers, P. M. Whittingham-Jones, P. A. Mitchell, O. A. Safir, M. D. Bircher, and A. E. Gross, "The reconstruction of periprosthetic pelvic discontinuity," *The Journal of Arthroplasty*, vol. 27, no. 8, pp. 1499–1506.e1, 2012.

[4] W. G. Paprosky, P. G. Perona, and J. M. Lawrence, "Acetabular defect classification and surgical reconstruction in revision arthroplasty. A 6-year follow-up evaluation," *The Journal of Arthroplasty*, vol. 9, no. 1, pp. 33–44, 1994.

[5] H. Akiyama, K. Yamamoto, M. Tsukanaka et al., "Revision total hip arthroplasty using a Kerboull-type acetabular reinforcement device with bone allograft: minimum 4.5-year follow-up results and mechanical analysis," *The Journal of Bone and Joint Surgery*, vol. 93-B, no. 9, pp. 1194–1200, 2011.

[6] J. Hori, Y. Yasunaga, T. Yamasaki et al., "Mid-term results of acetabular reconstruction using a Kerboull-type acetabular reinforcement device," *International Orthopaedics*, vol. 36, no. 1, pp. 23–26, 2012.

[7] D. Regis, A. Sandri, I. Bonetti, O. Bortolami, and P. Bartolozzi, "A minimum of 10-year follow-up of the Burch-Schneider cage and bulk allografts for the revision of pelvic discontinuity," *The Journal of Arthroplasty*, vol. 27, no. 6, pp. 1057–63.e1, 2012.

[8] T. Iwase, T. Ito, and D. Morita, "Massive bone defect compromises postoperative cup survivorship of acetabular revision hip arthroplasty with impaction bone grafting," *The Journal of Arthroplasty*, vol. 29, no. 12, pp. 2424–2429, 2014.

[9] M. A. Buttaro, F. Comba, R. Pusso, and F. Piccaluga, "Acetabular revision with metal mesh, impaction bone grafting, and a cemented cup," *Clinical Orthopaedics and Related Research*, vol. 466, no. 10, pp. 2482–2490, 2008.

[10] J. D. Bobyn, G. J. Stackpool, S. A. Hacking, M. Tanzer, and J. J. Krygier, "Characteristics of bone ingrowth and interface mechanics of a new porous tantalum biomaterial," *Journal of Bone and Joint Surgery*, vol. 81, no. 5, pp. 907–914, 1999.

21

Intra-Articular Entrapment of the Medial Epicondyle following a Traumatic Fracture Dislocation of the Elbow in an Adult

Hicham G. Abdel Nour ⓘ, George S. El Rassi ⓘ, Jack C. Daoud ⓘ, Youssef G. Hassan, Rami A. Ayoubi ⓘ, and Nabih I. Joukhadar

Department of Orthopedic Surgery and Traumatology, Saint Georges University Medical Center, Balamand University, P.O. Box 166378, Achrafieh, Beirut 1100 2807, Lebanon

Correspondence should be addressed to Hicham G. Abdel Nour; hicham.abdelnour.dr@gmail.com

Academic Editor: Johannes Mayr

Medial epicondyle entrapment after an acute fracture dislocation of the elbow is a common finding in the pediatric population, but a rare finding in adults. We present a case of an adult patient diagnosed with a traumatic fracture dislocation of the elbow joint with intra-articular entrapment of the medial epicondyle. After initial evaluation, closed reduction was done. Stability testing after reduction showed an unstable joint; thus, open reduction and internal fixation was decided.

1. Introduction

Medial epicondyle entrapment after an acute fracture dislocation of the elbow is a common finding in the pediatric population, but a rare finding in adults. The medial epicondyle is the last ossification center to fuse in the distal humerus, making the simple avulsion fracture very unlikely to occur after closure of the epiphyseal line [1]. The medial epicondyle fragment avulses due to a traction force by the medial collateral ligament typically by increased valgus stress or frequently an elbow dislocation [2]. A complex elbow instability posttraumatic elbow dislocation is a challenging entity to deal with and may have unsatisfactory results if not treated adequately [3]. We report here a case of an adult patient presenting with a traumatic posterolateral fracture dislocation of the left elbow with intra-articular entrapment of the medial epicondyle fragment.

2. Case

A 24-year-old male patient presented to our emergency department with severe left elbow pain and limited range of motion after falling from height on an outstretched hand 1 hour prior to his presentation. To note, the patient has no history of prior elbow dislocation or trauma during his childhood. On clinical examination, the patient was found to have posterolateral dislocation of his left elbow joint with severe tenderness over the medial aspect. There was minimal numbness over his left 4th and 5th fingers, but no other vascular involvement was noted. Anteroposterior and lateral radiographs of the left elbow were done that showed posterolateral dislocation of the left elbow joint with concomitant medial epicondyle avulsion fracture with intra-articular entrapment of that fragment (Figure 1).

Closed reduction was done under sedation, and after multiple failed attempts due to the entrapped medial epicondyle fragment, subsequent reduction of the medial epicondyle fragment was achieved (Figure 2).

After the reduction, and for proper postreduction evaluation, varus and valgus stress tests under fluoroscopy were done that showed grand instability of the elbow joint. A computed tomography scan with 3D reconstruction was then ordered to rule out any associated missed fracture on radiograph and for adequate preoperative planning. The CT scan showed a displaced medial epicondyle avulsion fracture but no other associated bony injuries (Figure 3).

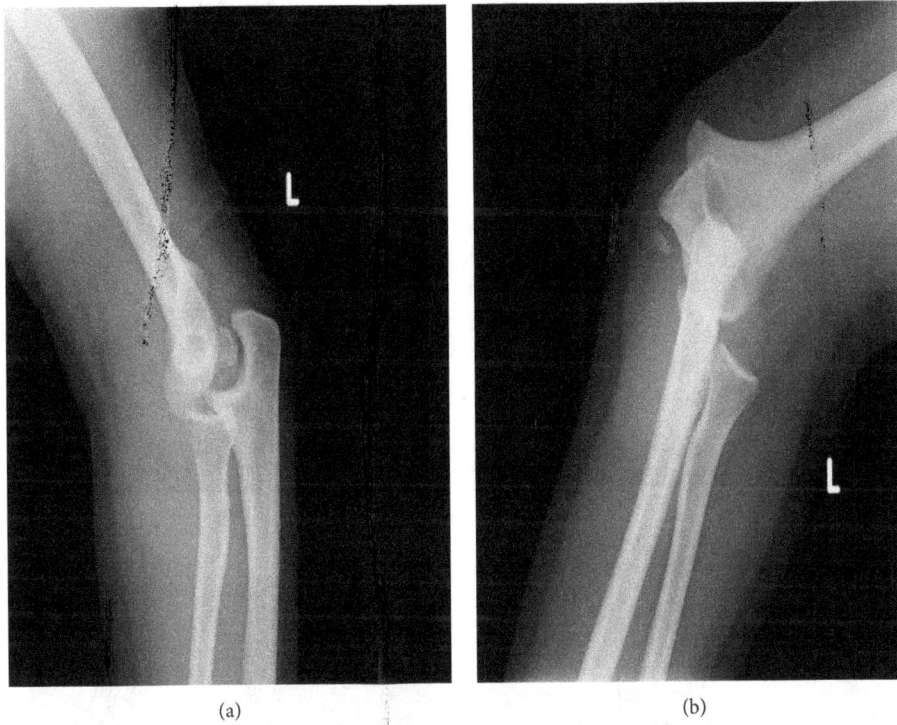

FIGURE 1: Lateral and anteroposterior radiographs of the left elbow joint showing posterolateral fracture dislocation with intra-articular entrapment of the avulsed medial epicondyle fragment. True lateral and anteroposterior radiographs could not be obtained due to the pain and the dislocation.

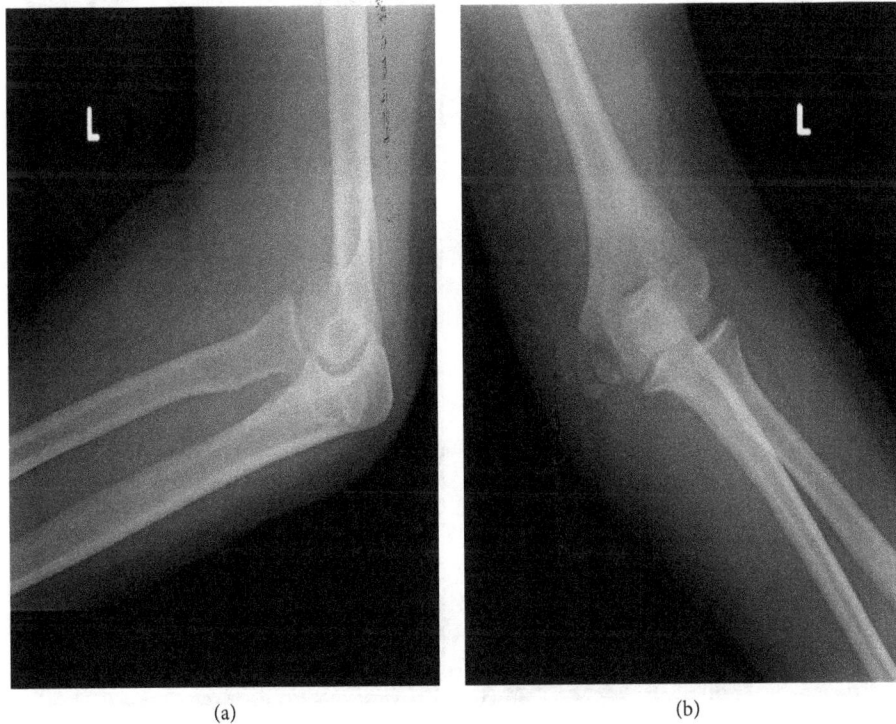

FIGURE 2: Anteroposterior and lateral radiographs of the left elbow joint after closed reduction showing a displaced medial epicondyle avulsion fracture.

The next day, the patient was transferred to the operating theater for open reduction and internal fixation. In the operating room, with the patient placed in the supine position, general anesthesia and prophylactic antibiotics were administered. With his left upper limb on a hand table, a medial approach to the left elbow joint was done with

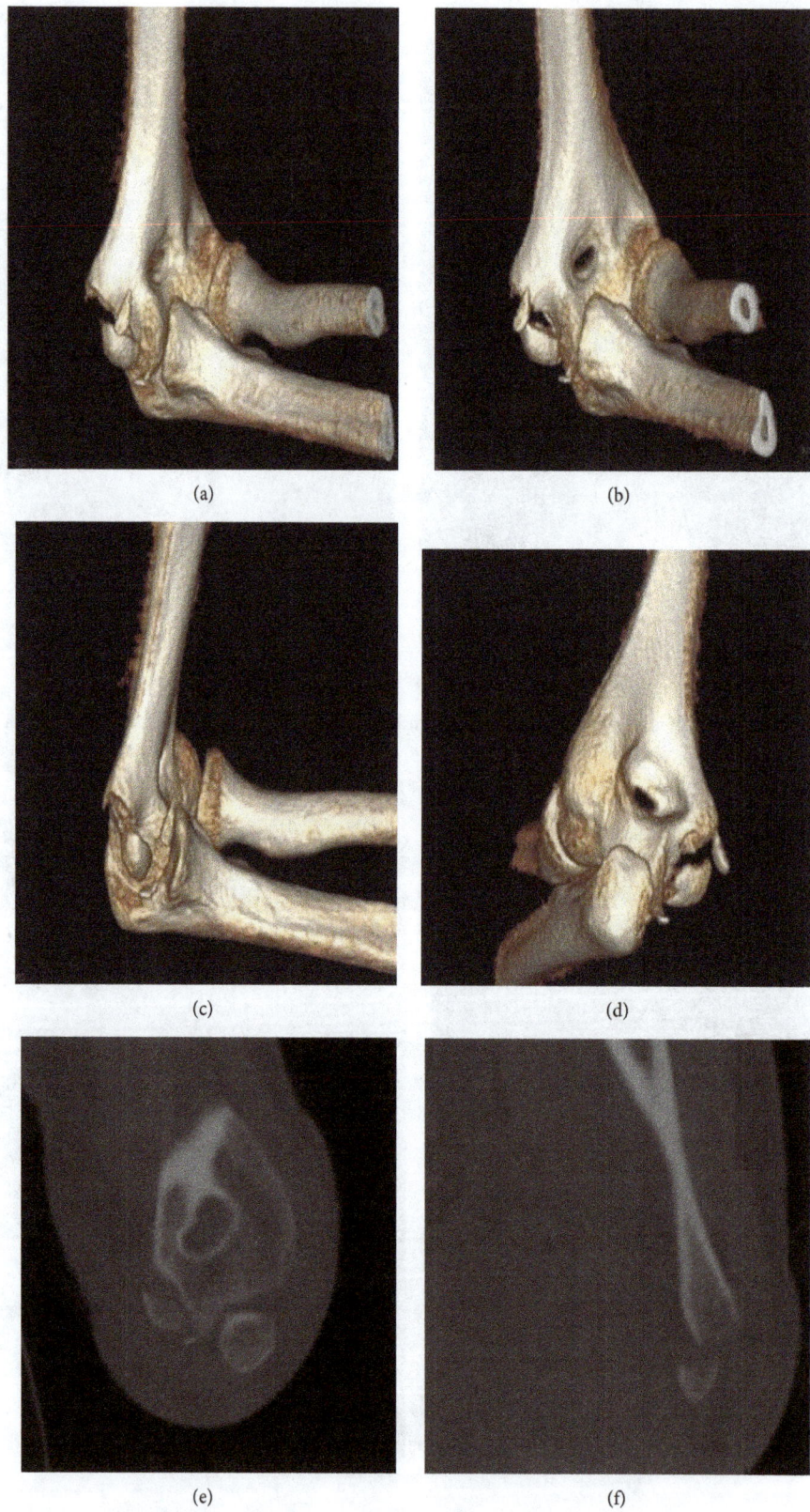

FIGURE 3: CT scan with 3D reconstruction after closed reduction showing a displaced medial epicondyle avulsion fracture with no other associated bony injury.

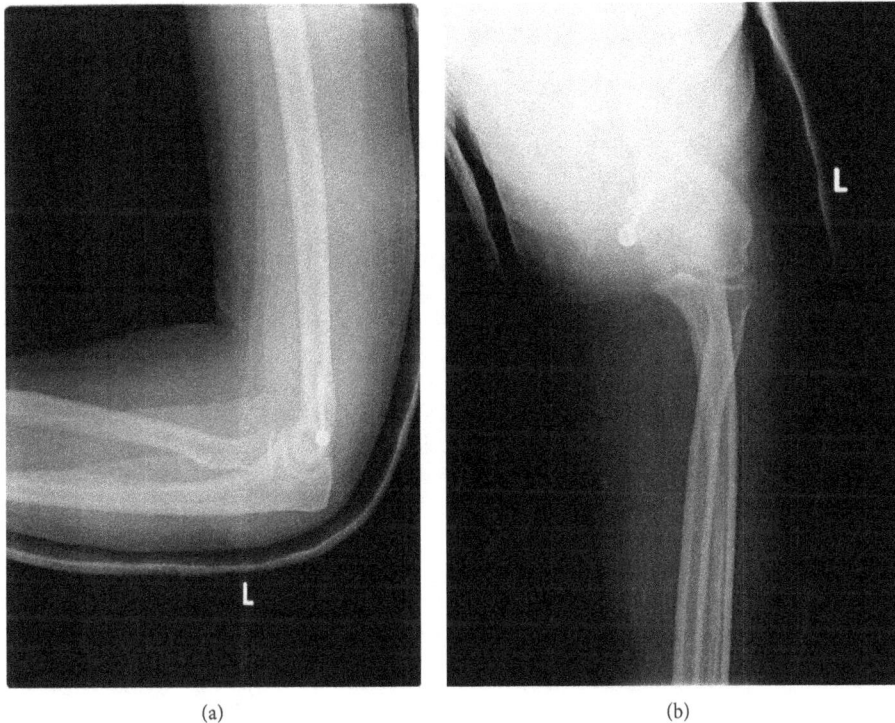

(a)   (b)

FIGURE 4: Postoperative control X-rays showing good reduction and compression of the medial epicondyle fragment. To note, the patient has an above-the-elbow posterior cast splint.

a longitudinal 5 cm incision over the medial epicondyle. After appropriate dissection, the medial epicondyle fragment was identified, still partially entrapped in the ulno-humeral joint line, with its unruptured intact medial collateral ligamentous complex. The fragment was reduced with 1 K wire and fixed with 1 cannulated half-threaded 40 mm × 4.5 mm screw and a washer (Figure 4).

A washer was used in order to optimize compression and not taking the risk of unintentional intrusion of the screw head through the cortical bone or fracturing the fragment. Careful inspection was done, leaving no entrapped soft tissue inside the fracture site during reduction. Postoperatively an above-the-elbow posterior splint was applied to the elbow joint in 90° of flexion with neutral forearm rotation. After 1 week, making sure that the swelling decreased and the 4th and 5th finger paresthesia has resolved, a full-circular above-the-elbow cast was applied in the same previous anatomic position. Control X-rays were done at 3 weeks postop that showed proper integrity of the reduction (Figure 5).

So the decision was taken to remove the cast and keep the right arm in an arm sling for 1 more week with minimal careful range of motion. After that, physiotherapy was started consisting only of passive progressive flexion/extension range of motion with no varus or valgus stress for the following 3 weeks. At 12 weeks postop, the patient had full range of motion of his elbow joint and adequate varus and valgus stability, and control X-rays done showed union of the avulsed medial epicondyle fragment (Figure 6). At this point, the patient was allowed to get back to normal daily activities and will be allowed to resume sports activities at 6 months

postoperatively. The future plan was removal of the screw at 6 months after the surgery.

3. Discussion

Medial epicondyle fractures are commonly described fractures in the pediatric age groups, as its epiphyseal line is the last ossification center to fuse in the distal humerus between ages 15 and 20 [1, 2]. Medial epicondyle fractures present most commonly posttraumatic pediatric elbow dislocation, and in 15% to 25% of these cases, the medial epicondyle becomes entrapped in the ulnohumeral joint. If the medial epicondyle fragment is seen at the level of the joint line after closed reduction of a traumatic elbow dislocation, partial entrapment should at least be considered [1]. This entity is rarely described throughout the literature in adults.

Purser mentioned two cases of adult fracture dislocation of the elbow with intra-articular inclusion of the medial epicondyle fragment. One of them was treated with open reduction but no fixation after multiple failed trials of closed reduction. The second case was a nonunion of a medial epicondyle fracture with recent posttraumatic intra-articular entrapment of that fragment. The latter patient was treated with closed reduction only. Purser concluded that in case the medial epicondyle fragment was really entrapped, then the affected joint would re-dislocate after full extension after closed reduction [4].

Khan and Zahid [2] reported two adult cases of fracture dislocation of the elbow with intra-articular inclusion of the medial epicondyle fragment. One case was treated with closed reduction, and the other required open reduction and

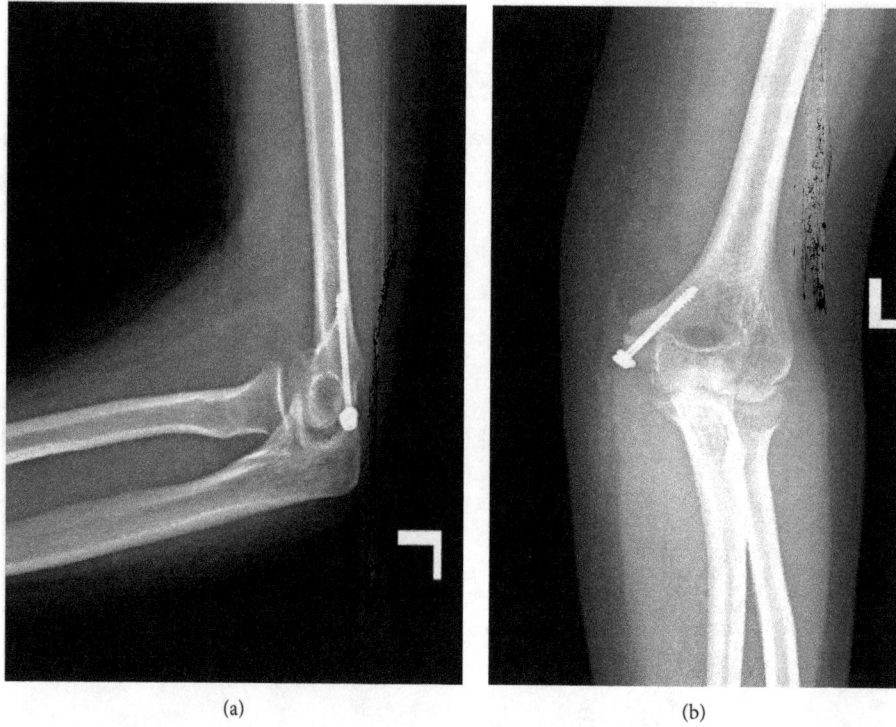

(a)   (b)

FIGURE 5: Left elbow control X-rays done at 3 weeks postop that showed proper integrity of the reduction.

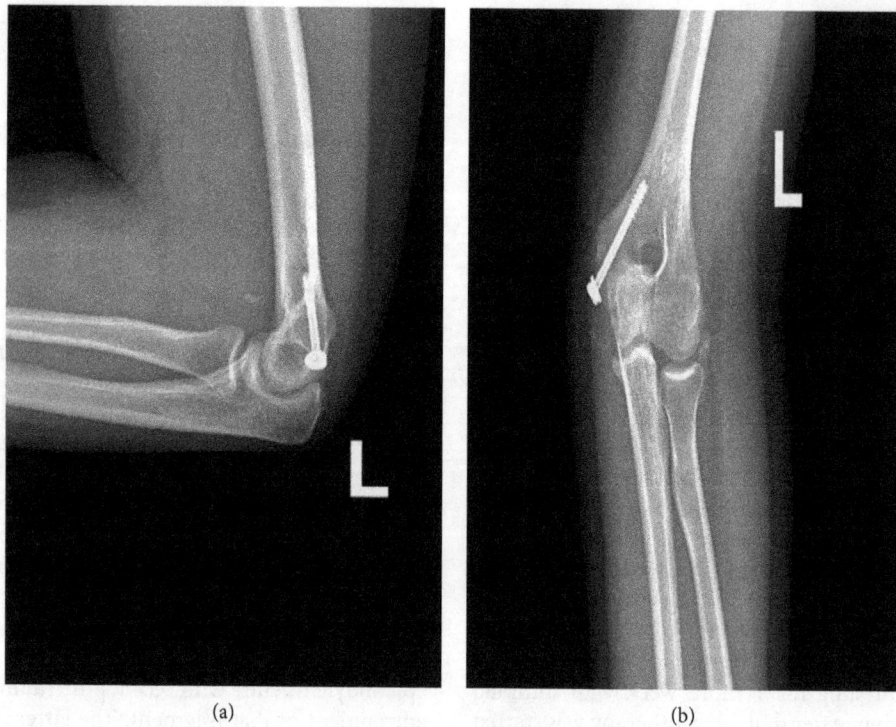

(a)   (b)

FIGURE 6: Lateral and anteroposterior radiographs of the left elbow joint 12 weeks postop showing union of the avulsed medial epicondyle fragment. Anterior and lateral ossifications seen indicate possible partial ligamentous injury that calcified with time and were not seen on previous radiographs.

fixation with 2 K wires. They noted one case with redislocation after full extension trial after closed reduction.

Rodriguez-Martin et al. [3] reported a case of a post-traumatic medial fracture dislocation of the elbow with a medial epicondyle displaced fracture but with an associated coronoid process fracture and severe soft tissue injury.

In a retrospective study done in a hospital in Montpellier, France, Louahem et al. [5] reported 130 pediatric cases with displaced medial epicondyle fractures. All cases were treated with open reduction and internal fixation with either K wires or compression screws. They concluded that operative fixation is a necessity in such fractures to ensure proper union and prevent valgus instability.

In our case, testing after closed reduction showed only valgus and varus instability, but no redislocation was noted in full extension. A preoperative CT scan for evaluating any associated missed fracture on radiograph is not always mandatory. An MRI in this case could have been helpful for evaluating any associated ligamentous injuries. Decision was taken to perform an open reduction and internal fixation with a compression screw and a washer to ensure proper reduction, subsequent union with minimal risk of un-intentional screw head intrusion into the fragment, and ensure early range of motion to prevent elbow stiffness. Keeping the cast for 4 weeks was not obligatory but was done to guarantee proper healing of the ligaments in order to obtain good elbow stability afterwards even if it could take few more physiotherapy sessions to regain full range of motion.

4. Conclusion

Fracture of the medial epicondyle is a rare entity in adults but frequent in the pediatric age group as traction of the medial collateral ligament can easily cause an avulsion of the nonfused medial epicondyle [2]. In addition, associated intra-articular entrapment of the medial epicondyle after elbow dislocation is rarely mentioned in the reported cases throughout the literature. Careful preoperative planning, operative treatment, and postoperative management are essential and if not managed properly can frequently result in unsatisfactory outcomes.

Conflicts of Interest

The authors declare no conflicts of interest regarding the publication of this article.

References

[1] S. D. Dodds, B. A. Flanagin, D. D. Bohl, P. A. DeLuca, and B. G. Smith, "Incarcerated medial epicondyle fracture following pediatric elbow dislocation: 11 cases," *Journal of Hand Surgery*, vol. 39, no. 9, pp. 1739–1745, 2014.

[2] S. A. Khan and M. Zahid, "Dislocation of the elbow with intra-articular entrapment of the medial epicondyle in adults. Report of two cases," *Acta Orthopaedica Belgica*, vol. 68, no. 1, pp. 83–86, 2002.

[3] J. Rodriguez-Martin, J. Pretell-Mazzini, D. Cecilia-Lopez, and C. Resines-Erasun, "Medial complex elbow dislocation: an unusual pattern of injury," *Journal of Orthopaedic Trauma*, vol. 24, no. 3, pp. e21–e24, 2010.

[4] D. W. Purser, "Dislocation of the elbow joint and inclusion of the medial epicondyle in the adult," *Journal of Band Joint Surgery*, vol. 36-B, no. 2, pp. 247–249, 1954.

[5] D. M. Louahem, S. Bourelle, F. Buscayret et al., "Displaced medial epicondyle fractures of the humerus: surgical treatment and results. A report of 139 cases," *Archives of Orthopaedic and Trauma Surgery*, vol. 130, no. 5, pp. 649–655, 2010.

22

Long-Term Follow-Up of Adamantinoma of the Tibia Complicated by Metastases and a Second Unrelated Primary Cancer

Brendan R. Southam ⓘ,[1] Alvin H. Crawford,[2] David A. Billmire,[3] James Geller,[4] Daniel Von Allmen,[5] Adam P. Schumaier ⓘ,[1] and Sara Szabo[6]

[1]Department of Orthopaedics and Sports Medicine, University of Cincinnati, Cincinnati, OH 45220, USA
[2]Department of Orthopaedics, Cincinnati Children's Hospital Medical Center, Cincinnati, OH 45229, USA
[3]Department of Plastic Surgery, Cincinnati Children's Hospital Medical Center, Cincinnati, OH 45229, USA
[4]Department of Oncology, Cincinnati Children's Hospital Medical Center, Cincinnati, OH 45229, USA
[5]Department of Surgery, Cincinnati Children's Hospital Medical Center, Cincinnati, OH 45229, USA
[6]Department of Pathology, Cincinnati Children's Hospital Medical Center, Cincinnati, OH 45229, USA

Correspondence should be addressed to Adam P. Schumaier; adam.schumaier@uc.edu

Academic Editor: Wan Ismail Faisham

Adamantinoma is a rare, low-grade malignant tumor of the bone which grows slowly and typically occurs in the diaphysis of long bones, particularly in the tibia. Adamantinomas have the potential for local recurrence and may metastasize to the lungs, lymph nodes, or bone. We report a case of a 14-year-old female with a tibial adamantinoma who underwent wide resection with limb salvage and has subsequently been followed up for 18 years. The patient went on to have both a local soft tissue recurrence 5 years after the resection and metastases to both an inguinal lymph node and the right lower lobe of the lung 8 years after that recurrence, all of which have been treated successfully with marginal resections. Unique to this case, the patient was also incidentally found to have chromophobe-type renal cell carcinoma when undergoing a partial nephrectomy to resect a presumed metastasis of her adamantinoma. Genetic testing has not revealed any known genetic predisposition to cancer.

1. Introduction

Adamantinomas are rare, accounting for less than 1% of primary malignancies of the bone [1–4]. Classically, adamantinomas occur in the long bones, particularly in the tibia in up to 80 to 90% of patients, and have a predilection for the mid-diaphyseal region [3, 5–7]. Involvement of a synchronous lesion in the ipsilateral fibula has been reported in approximately 10% of cases [5, 8, 9]. Adamantinomas occur most frequently in adolescents and young adults with a mean age of 25–35 years [2, 5, 9–11]. Previous series have identified a slight male predominance [8, 12]. Given the indolent nature of this malignancy, it typically has a long, progressive clinical course characterized by swelling, pain, and deformity prior to diagnosis [3, 5, 9].

Radiographically, the tumor tends to be eccentric, expansile, and osteolytic with a sharply or poorly defined sclerotic margin [5, 9, 13]. Not infrequently, multiple lytic foci are present with surrounding sclerosis giving the lesion a so-called "soap bubble appearance" [3, 5, 9, 13]. Significant anterior cortical disruption of the tibia is common and may be present with extension of the lesion into the medullary canal or the surrounding soft tissues resulting in anterior bowing [5, 9, 11]. MRI has proven crucial for determining the amount of intramedullary and soft tissue involvement of these tumors, assisting in preoperative planning [10, 14–17]. CT may also be useful for assessing cortical destruction and detecting subtle pathologic fractures, present in up to 23% of patients [10, 18].

Histologically, adamantinomas are low-grade biphasic malignant tumors, with a typically nesting or cord-like epithelial component in a bland osteofibrous stroma. Considerable variability in the relative amounts of these two components may be observed. In the well-differentiated variant, an osteofibrous dysplasia-like stromal component predominates, with small-to-inconspicuous epithelial nests and peripheral woven bone spicules that are rimmed by osteoblasts [3, 5, 7, 9]. This variant more commonly affects patients in the first two decades of life. The typical presentation of tumors in adults and metastatic lesions is the classic variant; in the classic variant, the epithelial component predominates, and its patterns may be described as spindle, squamous, basaloid, and tubular type [3, 5, 10, 19]. Another intermediate histological variant osteofibrous dysplasia- (OFD-) like adamantinoma has also been recognized in the literature. Similar to OFD, this subtype presents typically within the first two decades of life, producing an intracortical lesion of the tibia [9, 10, 20]. Histologically, it is characterized by a similar stroma to OFD with small scant nests of epithelial cells detectable with light microscopy [9, 20, 21]. The other top differential diagnoses to be considered based on histology and location are osteofibrous dysplasia and adamantinoma-like Ewing sarcoma.

Adamantinomas were historically thought to be localized malignancies with limited metastatic potential given their typically indolent course [22]. However, more recent literature has demonstrated relatively high rates of local recurrence and metastases, particularly following an incomplete resection. Given the relative rarity of these tumors, most of the literature has been limited to case series with inadequate long-term follow-up, making it challenging to determine definitive treatment guidelines for these patients. Chemotherapy and radiation have largely proven ineffective, and amputation was historically considered the mainstay of treatment [9, 10, 12, 23–26]. More recently, wide en bloc resection with subsequent reconstruction has proven highly effective for limb preservation with good functional outcomes and equivocal rates of recurrence, metastases, and survival [5, 12, 18, 23, 27, 28]. A variety of options for limb reconstruction exist including intercalary allografts, vascularized and nonvascularized fibular autografts, distraction osteogenesis, and segmental metallic implants [18, 27, 29–32]. Intercalary allografts, however, have emerged as the preferred form of reconstruction in the literature [3, 18].

We report a case of a tibial adamantinoma that was treated with a limb salvage procedure utilizing an intercalary tibial allograft and a free vascularized osteocutaneous graft of the fibula. The patient later had a local recurrence treated with a secondary salvage procedure and subsequent metastases to the lung and an inguinal lymph node treated with marginal resections. A second rare primary cancer, chromophobe-type renal cell carcinoma, was later discovered incidentally in this patient, despite no known genetic predisposition. A review of the literature is provided.

2. Case Study

A 14-year-old Caucasian female presented initially to an outside provider with a mass in the right midshin which had grown slowly in size over the course of two years causing increasing discomfort. Initial conservative management included observation and rest. Due to an acute exacerbation of pain, radiographs of the right tibia and fibula were obtained demonstrating a predominantly cortical-based lobulated lesion of the distal tibial diaphysis with overlying soft tissue irregularity (Figure 1). The patient underwent curettage and bone grafting of the lesion. Permanent pathology sections revealed an adamantinoma with epithelial cells in tubular and squamous patterns which had diffuse CD99 reactivity and cytokeratin-positive staining [3, 5, 10, 33]. This prompted referral to our institution for definitive treatment. The patient's past medical history was unremarkable, and family history of cancer was only notable for prostate cancer in a paternal grandfather.

A metastatic workup including a bone scan revealed increased uptake in the midtibia consistent with the previously diagnosed tumor. Additionally, a CT scan of the chest revealed several small nodules in the left upper lobe of the lung which were felt to be consistent with metastatic disease; however, an open biopsy demonstrated only evidence of chronic pleuritis with fibrosis (Figure 2).

After thorough preoperative counseling, the patient elected to undergo resection of the adamantinoma with limb salvage. A 19 cm section of the medial tibial shaft was resected along with a 20 × 5 cm section of the overlying skin and subcutaneous tissue down to the level of the anteromedial fascia, as this was assumed to have been contaminated from the original biopsy (Figure 3). The defect was then partially reconstructed laterally with an intercalary tibial allograft which was fixed both proximally and distally. Prior to placing the graft, the proximal metaphyseal tibia had been curetted for the bone graft which was placed into the intramedullary canal adjacent to the allograft. Simultaneously, plastic surgeons elevated an osteocutaneous fibular flap from the lateral aspect of the left leg. The free vascularized osteocutaneous graft of the fibula was placed to fill the remaining defect of the right medial tibia adjacent to the previously placed allograft (Figures 4 and 5). End-to-end and end-to-side anastomoses were performed with the microsurgical technique between the peroneal and posterior tibial veins and arteries, respectively. A tibialis anterior muscle flap was used for coverage of the allograft on the reconstructed right tibia. On the left donor-site side, a syndesmotic screw was placed to fix the distal fibula. Skin grafts from the left lateral thigh were obtained to provide coverage of the remaining skin defects on both legs. Frozen sections reviewed intraoperatively and permanent sections all confirmed negative margins. The patient was made non-weight-bearing after surgery to allow for graft consolidation.

The patient had an uneventful recovery, and serial radiographs demonstrated slow incorporation of the allograft. She later developed a stress fracture of the graft two and a half years postoperatively that subsequently healed. Four years after the initial resection, the patient began to experience recurrent pain and swelling of the right lower extremity. Radiographs demonstrated medial and pretibial soft tissue swelling over the previous tibial reconstruction, but a CT scan failed to demonstrate any lesion. Following conservative management with ibuprofen 800 mg and a compressive wrap with symptomatic control, nine months later, she elected for removal of hardware as this was thought to potentially be the source of her pain. The patient subsequently developed palpable masses on the right lower leg several months after the hardware was removed. MRI demonstrated

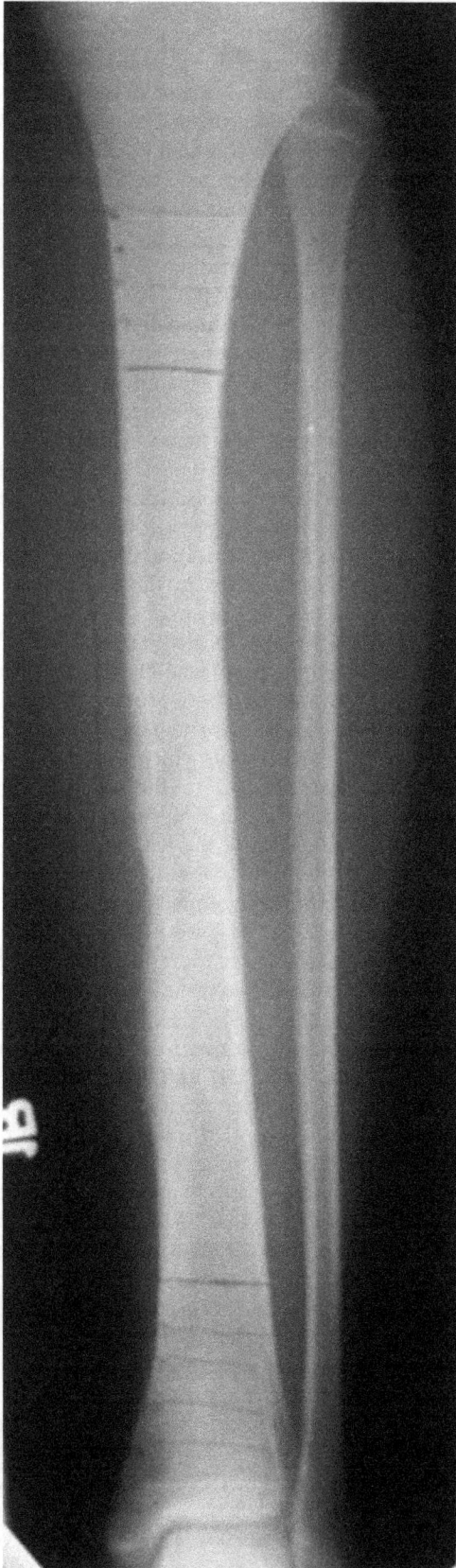

FIGURE 1: An anteroposterior radiograph of the right tibia and fibula obtained following curettage and bone grafting demonstrating a predominantly cortical-based expansile lesion involving the distal diaphysis consistent with adamantinoma.

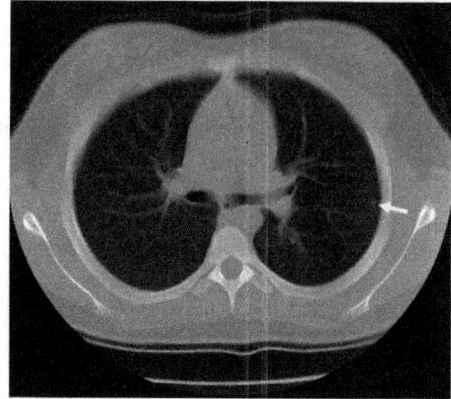

FIGURE 2: An axial computed tomography (CT) scan of the chest demonstrating a subpleural lesion (white arrow) identified at the time the adamantinoma was originally diagnosed. The lesion was biopsied due to concerns of metastasis, and the biopsy revealed benign fibrous lung tissue.

a dumbbell-shaped mass measuring $5.4 \times 1.7 \times 2.1$ cm in size arising in the soft tissues of the anterolateral aspect of the shin involving both the extensor hallucis longus and extensor digitorum longus muscles (Figure 6). A positron emission tomography (PET) scan, bone scan, and contrasted CT of the chest abdomen and pelvis were obtained and were unremarkable for metastatic disease. An open biopsy was performed and confirmed the diagnosis of recurrent adamantinoma.

After multiple discussions with the family regarding amputation versus a repeat limb salvage procedure, the patient elected to undergo local resection. The entirety of the anterior compartment was resected leaving a 10×25 cm soft tissue defect which plastic surgery reconstructed using a free-flap transfer of the entire left rectus muscle. The inferior epigastric vessels were anastomosed with the microsurgical technique to the anterior tibial vessels, and a skin graft was obtained from the previous donor site to cover the remaining skin defect from the resection. All margins of the soft tissue resection were negative. The patient was left with a residual drop foot following the procedure and 6 months later underwent a subtalar arthroereisis and peroneal tenodesis along with a posterior tibialis tendon transfer to anterior tibialis tendon transfer (Figure 7). Following this period, the patient returned every 6 months for regular surveillance including radiographs and an MRI of the right lower extremity.

At the age of 25, 11 years after initial presentation, the patient began to experience erythema and swelling of the skin graft on the right lower leg managed with oral antibiotics and subsequently by topical corticosteroids. The swelling resolved and was later assumed to be an allergic reaction from wearing compression stockings. At this time, she also noticed a mobile palpable mass in her right groin which bothered her only when she was exercising. This was felt to be an enlarged lymph node, and the decision was made to continue to follow the patient closely. Two years later, an MRI demonstrated a 2 cm round lesion in the right thigh with increased T2 signal and peripheral enhancement. A PET scan was also obtained which showed increased

(a)

(b)

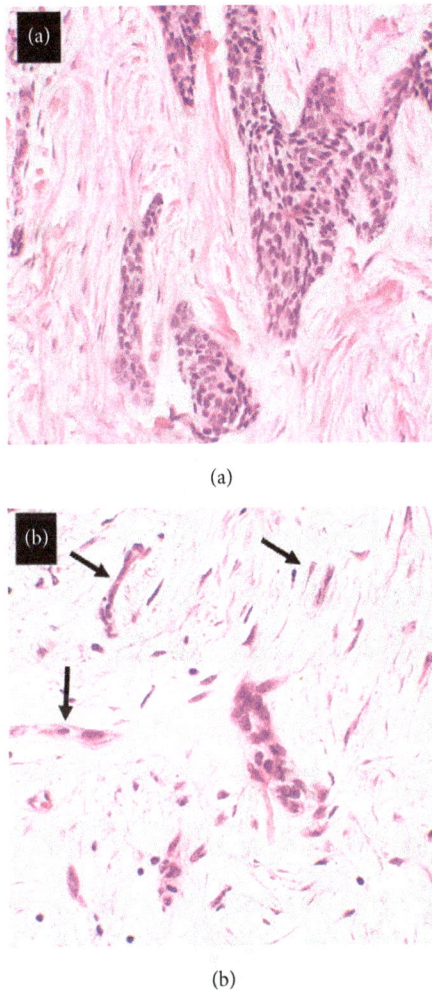

FIGURE 3: (a) Well-differentiated variants of adamantinoma including cords and islands of epithelial cells with a basaloid appearance, with some squamoid differentiation, were observed in this patient. (b) In other areas sampled, double rows of epithelial cells impart a tubular appearance or occur in single-cell cords (black arrows).

(a)

(b)

(c)

(d)

FIGURE 4: (a) A clinical image demonstrating the planned resection margins of the right lower extremity prior to the limb salvage procedure. The osteocutaneous flap from the contralateral extremity has also been marked out. (b) A postoperative image demonstrates that the medial osteocutaneous flap is well perfused. (c) Osteocutaneous free vascularized fibula flap. (d) The flap went on to incorporate well.

uptake in the right inguinal region. Thus, the patient underwent an excisional biopsy of the lymph node that revealed a metastasis of the adamantinoma (Figure 8). The patient subsequently had a CT of the chest, abdomen, and pelvis performed which revealed lesions in her bilateral kidneys and spleen and a large lesion in the right lower lobe of the lung (Figure 9).

General surgery performed a right lower lobectomy via thoracotomy which also revealed metastatic disease. Two months later, the patient underwent a robot-assisted laparoscopic splenectomy and partial nephrectomies of both kidneys. Pathology revealed that the right kidney and splenic lesions were both benign cysts, but the left kidney was stage T1A chromophobe-type renal cell carcinoma (chRCC), a second primary cancer, with microscopic positive margins (Figure 10). Given the improved prognosis with this subtype of RCC and a lower risk for metastasis, the decision was made to monitor the patient closely with serial imaging at

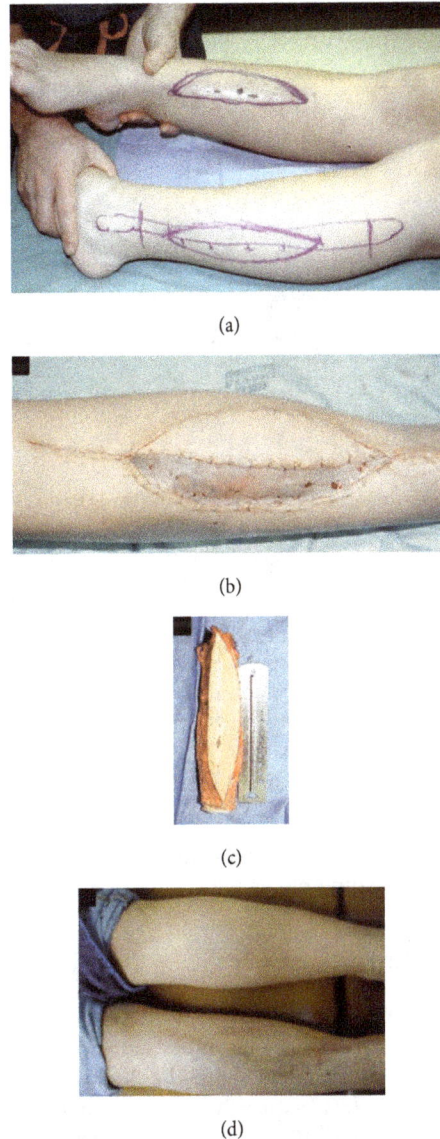

3-month intervals [34]. The patient developed a postsplenectomy thrombocytosis that has been monitored closely, and she completed two years of penicillin VK for sepsis prophylaxis. She has had no recurrence of either cancer on surveillance imaging. Given the history of two primary cancers, the patient later elected to undergo genetic testing involving an 18-gene panel of known renal cancer genes and was found to have no known genetic predisposition. Four years after the final resections, the patient developed a small mass at the base of her right neck just superior to the shoulder blade. An MRI was obtained which demonstrated the mass with a thin capsule and a fatty signal. She elected to

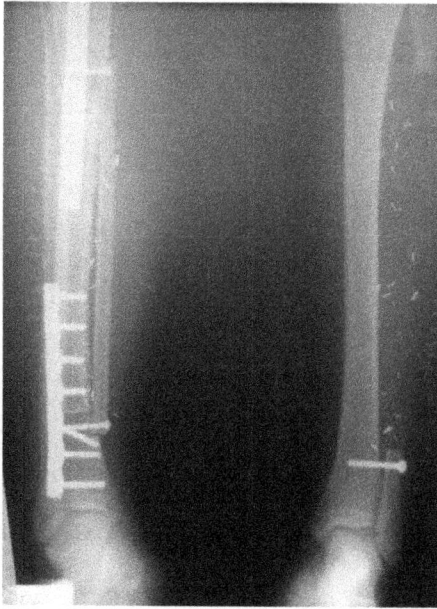

FIGURE 5: An anteroposterior radiograph of the bilateral lower legs following adamantinoma resection and limb reconstruction. On the right, the allograft is positioned laterally with the vascularized fibular graft placed overlying it medially. The grafts are fixed by plates and screws. On the left, the fibula has been resected and the ankle mortise has been stabilized proximally with a screw.

have the mass removed, and pathology revealed adipose tissue consistent with a lipoma.

3. Discussion

Although adamantinomas are low-grade malignancies, local recurrence and metastases are not uncommon. The most frequent sites of metastases are the lungs. Lymph node metastases occur less frequently, with rare metastases to the bone reported as well [8, 12, 14]. In the series by Moon and Mori, 21 patients had 29 sites of clinical metastases at the time of death: 16 of the sites were pulmonary and 5 were in the inguinal lymph nodes [12]. In a review by Keeney et al. of 85 cases of adamantinoma, 31% of patients had recurrent local disease, 15% developed lung metastases, and 7% developed lymph node metastases. Of those patients with lung metastases, 69% had a preceding local recurrence as was the case in this patient.

In a review of 28 patients with a diagnosed adamantinoma from the Netherlands Bone Tumor Registry, nine patients (32%) had a local recurrence after a mean 7-year follow-up. All of these patients had undergone an intralesional or marginal resection. Of these, three patients went on to have metastatic disease. An additional five patients without local recurrence also developed metastatic disease. However, no patients who had undergone an en bloc resection developed local recurrence or metastases. Thus, an overall rate of metastases of 29% was observed. Intralesional or marginal resection was found to be the most significant risk factor for a local recurrence or metastasis [23]. Other significant risk factors for recurrence included duration of

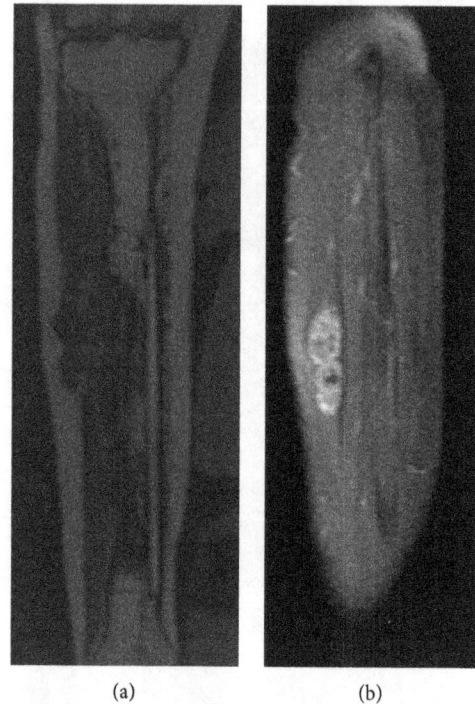

(a)   (b)

FIGURE 6: (a) A coronal T1-weighted magnetic resonance image showing a dumbbell-shaped mass in the anterolateral subcutaneous tissues involving the underlying extensor hallucis longus and extensor digitorum longus muscles. (b) The mass enhances diffusely after gadolinium administration, consistent with a soft tissue mass.

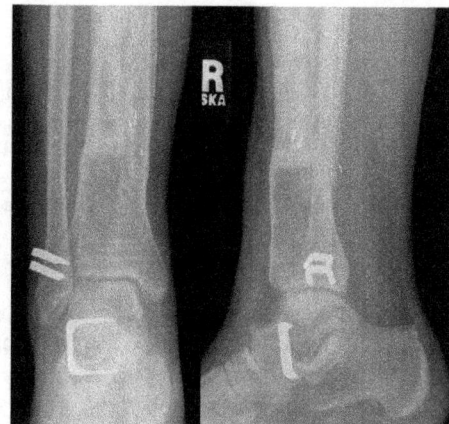

FIGURE 7: An AP and lateral view of the right ankle following a posterior-to-anterior tibialis tendon transfer, peroneal tenodesis, and subtalar fusion for an acquired foot drop resulting from resection of the soft tissue recurrence in the anterior compartment.

symptoms less than one year, pain at the time of presentation, and an age less than twenty years at the time of diagnosis.

In a recent international multicenter retrospective review of 70 cases of adamantinoma, 91% of patients had a limb salvage procedure performed with roughly half the patients receiving an intercalary allograft reconstruction. The limb preservation rate at a median follow-up of 7 years

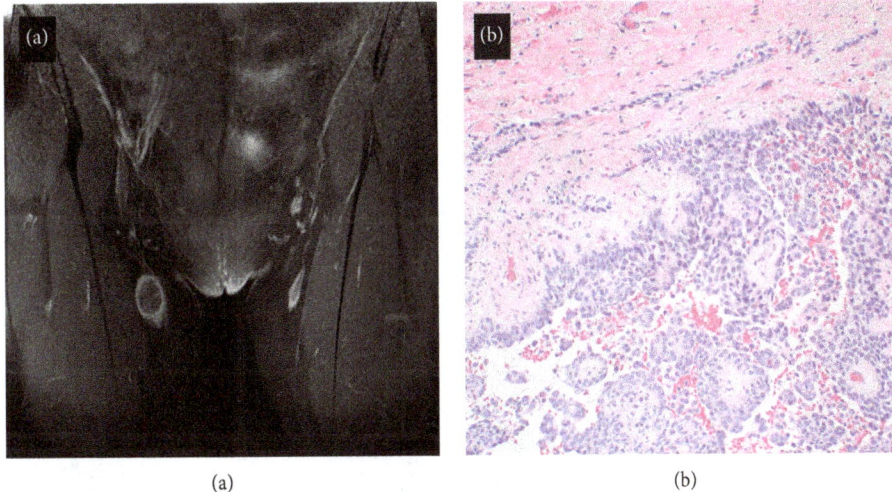

(a)

(b)

FIGURE 8: (a) A coronal fat-suppressed T1 image with gadolinium enhancement demonstrating a mass in the right groin with an irregular rim of peripheral enhancement. This mass was excised and found to be a metastasis of the adamantinoma to an inguinal lymph node. (b) The epithelial component of the metastasis regionally imparts a pseudopapillary appearance, with intervening hemorrhage.

was 84%. The rate of metastasis was 10%, and the rate of local recurrence at 10-year follow-up was 18.6%, with a 10-year survival rate of 87.2%. En bloc tumor resection with wide operative margins at the time of limb salvage was associated with a significantly lower risk of local recurrence. In patients who underwent reconstructions, nonunion and fracture were the most common complications, occurring in 24% and 23% of patients, respectively [18]. In this case, the patient experienced both delayed union and allograft fracture that subsequently healed.

Previously, the use of vascularized fibular grafts with massive allografts has been described in the literature [30, 35–37]. This well-established technique combines the mechanical strength of the allograft with the biologic potential of the fibular graft to revascularize and incorporate. This reduces the inherent risks associated with pure intercalary allograft reconstructions which include delayed unions, nonunions, and stress fractures as previously discussed, as well as an increased risk of infection [30, 35–38]. More recently, osteocutaneous fibular grafts used in combination with allografts have been described for the management of long bone defects. Halim et al. achieved favorable long-term outcomes in a series of 12 patients with a mean follow-up of 63 months who underwent this technique. They noted that osteocutaneous flaps provided soft tissue coverage at the time of reconstruction and allowed for a tensionless closure which did not compromise microvascular anastomoses. Three vascularized flaps in this series developed venous thrombosis recognized by the reduced Doppler signal and congestion of the skin paddle. This allowed for early detection and intervention leading to successful salvage of the flap in all cases [38].

Due to the slow-growing nature of adamantinomas, local recurrences and metastases have been documented in the literature up to 36 years after the original diagnosis

[8, 9, 39–43]. Therefore, long-term surveillance (>15 years) is warranted in these patients as was highlighted by the late metastases observed in the present case [14, 23, 41, 44]. Furthermore, imaging of the lungs and physical examination for lymphadenopathy may be considered on an annual basis or at the time of local recurrence to monitor for metastases [10]. Metastases and recurrences discovered through routine surveillance should be managed by surgical resection [10, 42, 44].

In this patient, routine surveillance resulted in the incidental detection of a second primary malignancy which may have otherwise been missed. It also resulted in additional morbidity with the patient undergoing a partial nephrectomy, splenectomy, and a prior open biopsy of the lung, all of which revealed benign tissue. However, in light of this patient, we feel that suspected metastases to unusual locations outside of the lungs, lymph nodes, or bone should be evaluated carefully as these may represent other malignancies.

To the best of our knowledge, this is the only reported case in the literature of a second primary malignancy in a patient with adamantinoma [45]. There are no known germline mutations associated with adamantinoma. Cytogenetic analyses of 9 cases of adamantinoma and osteofibrous dysplasia have identified several trisomies which have potentially been implicated with the histogenesis of these lesions, including trisomies 7, 8, 12, 19, and 22 [46]. Interestingly, chRCC is also a rare malignancy accounting for roughly 5–10% of cases of diagnosed RCC, which translates to projected 3200–6400 cases in the United States in 2016 [47, 48]. Although most cases of chRCC are sporadic, some are associated with a familial form known as Birt–Hogg–Dubé syndrome which is caused by an inactivating mutation of the *FLCN* gene [48, 49]. However, this patient was found not to be a carrier of this mutation. Given multiple metachronous primary cancers in one patient, it is possible that

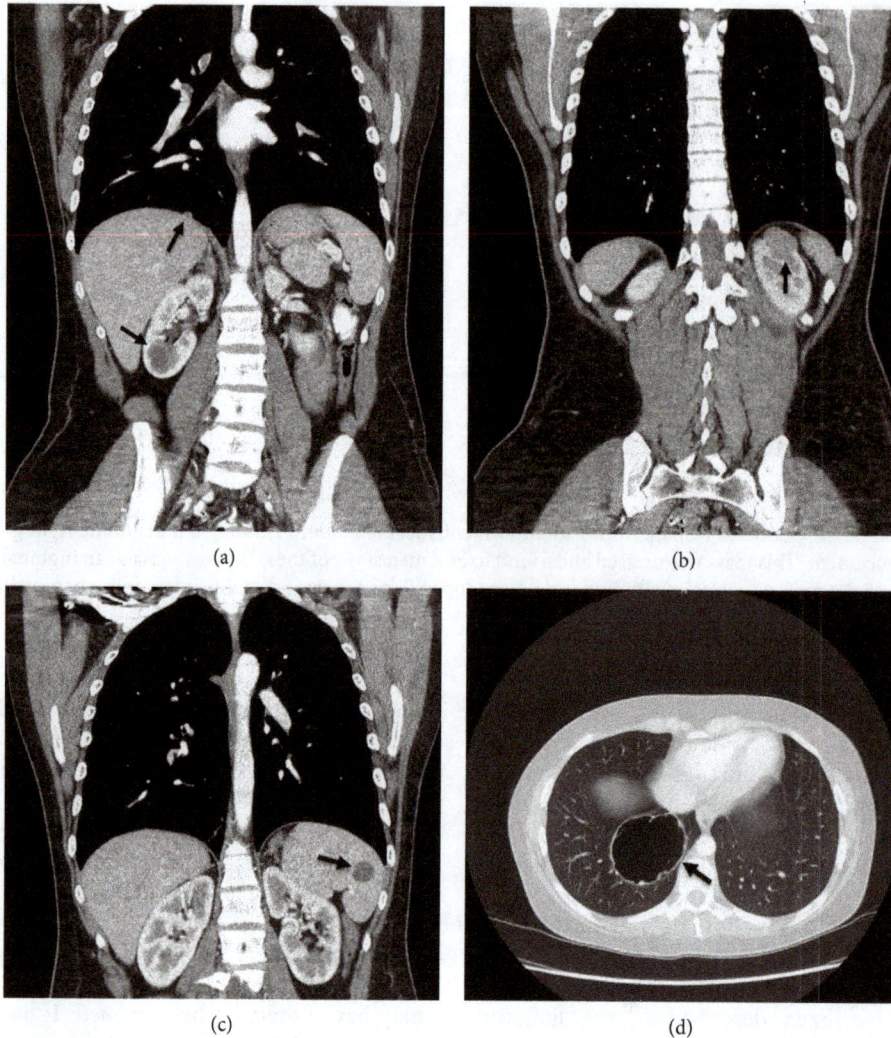

FIGURE 9: Computed tomography scans of the chest, abdomen, and pelvis demonstrating multiple lesions including a hypodense lesion of the spleen, bilateral kidney lesions, and a large cystic lesion with mural nodularity in the right lower lobe of the lung. The image on the top right demonstrates the lesion that was found to be chromophobe-type renal cell carcinoma in the upper pole of the left kidney, and the image on the bottom right shows the large metastatic adamantinoma lesion in the right lung.

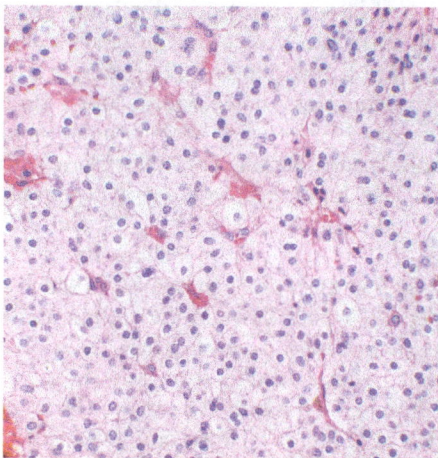

FIGURE 10: A hematoxylin and eosin stain demonstrating representative histomorphology of the incidentally diagnosed chromophobe-type renal cell carcinoma.

she is a carrier of a genetic mutation that has not yet been identified which predisposes her to malignancy [50].

4. Conclusion

Adamantinoma is a rare, low-grade malignant tumor of the bone associated with an indolent course due to its slow growth. However, high rates of late local recurrence and metastases have been reported in the literature. En bloc resection with wide operative margins followed by limb reconstruction has now become the standard of care, producing good functional outcomes along with high rates of limb preservation and overall survival. It is imperative to continue to follow these patients for greater than 15 years to allow for early detection of recurrent disease or metastases. In the case of presumed metastases, consideration of other malignancies is warranted, particularly when these lesions are identified in areas uncommon for adamantinoma metastases.

Conflicts of Interest

The authors declare that they have no conflicts of interest.

References

[1] J. M. Mirra, P. Picci, and R. H. Gold, *Bone Tumors: Clinical, Radiologic, and Pathologic Correlations*, Lea & Febiger, Philadelphia, PA, USA, 1989.

[2] K. K. Unni, D. C. Dahlin, J. W. Beabout, and J. C. Ivins, "Adamantinomas of long bones," *Cancer*, vol. 34, no. 5, pp. 1796–1805, 1974.

[3] P. J. Papagelopoulos, A. F. Mavrogenis, E. C. Galanis, O. D. Savvidou, C. Y. Inwards, and F. H. Sim, "Clinico-pathological features, diagnosis, and treatment of adamantinoma of the long bones," *Orthopedics*, vol. 30, no. 3, pp. 211–217, 2007.

[4] S. E. Puchner, R. Varga, G. M. Hobusch et al., "Long-term outcome following treatment of adamantinoma and osteofibrous dysplasia of long bones," *Orthopaedics & Traumatology: Surgery & Research*, vol. 102, no. 7, pp. 925–932, 2016.

[5] D. Jain, V. K. Jain, R. K. Vasishta, P. Ranjan, and Y. Kumar, "Adamantinoma: a clinicopathological review and update," *Diagnostic Pathology*, vol. 3, no. 1, p. 8, 2008.

[6] R. Van Rijn, J. Bras, G. Schaap, H. van den Berg, and M. Maas, "Adamantinoma in childhood: report of six cases and review of the literature," *Pediatric Radiology*, vol. 36, no. 10, pp. 1068–1074, 2006.

[7] K. K. Unni and C. Y. Inwards, *Dahlin's Bone Tumors: General Aspects and Data on 10,165 Cases*, Lippincott Williams & Wilkins, Philadelphia, PA, USA, 2010.

[8] G. L. Keeney, K. K. Unni, J. W. Beabout, and D. J. Pritchard, "Adamantinoma of long bones. A clinicopathologic study of 85 cases," *Cancer*, vol. 64, no. 3, pp. 730–737, 1989.

[9] L. B. Kahn, "Adamantinoma, osteofibrous dysplasia and differentiated adamantinoma," *Skeletal Radiology*, vol. 32, no. 5, pp. 245–258, 2003.

[10] M. J. Most, F. H. Sim, and C. Y. Inwards, "Osteofibrous dysplasia and adamantinoma," *Journal of American Academy of Orthopaedic Surgeon*, vol. 18, no. 6, pp. 358–366, 2010.

[11] S. S. Desai, N. Jambhekar, M. Agarwal, A. Puri, and N. Merchant, "Adamantinoma of tibia: a study of 12 cases," *Journal of Surgical Oncology*, vol. 93, no. 5, pp. 429–433, 2006.

[12] N. F. Moon and H. Mori, "Adamantinoma of the appendicular skeleton–updated," *Clinical Orthopaedics and Related Research*, vol. 204, pp. 215–237, 1986.

[13] S. M. Levine, R. E. Lambiase, and C. N. Petchprapa, "Cortical lesions of the tibia: characteristic appearances at conventional radiography," *RadioGraphics*, vol. 23, no. 1, pp. 157–177, 2003.

[14] D. M. Holden, M. J. Joyce, and M. Sundaram, "Adamantinoma," *Orthopedics*, vol. 37, no. 6, pp. 362–422, 2014.

[15] J. W. Young, S. C. Aisner, C. S. Resnik, A. M. Levine, H. D. Dorfman, and N. O. Whitley, "Case report 660: adamantinoma of tibia," *Skeletal Radiology*, vol. 20, no. 2, pp. 152–156, 1991.

[16] M. Camp, R. Tompkins, S. Spanier, J. Bridge, and C. Bush, "Adamantinoma of the tibia and fibula with cytogenetic analysis," *RadioGraphics*, vol. 28, no. 4, pp. 1215–1220, 2008.

[17] H.-J. Van der Woude, H.-M. Hazelbag, J. L. Bloem, A. H. M. Taminiau, and P. C. W. Hogendoorn, "MRI of adamantinoma of long bones in correlation with histopathology," *American Journal of Roentgenology*, vol. 183, no. 6, pp. 1737–1744, 2004.

[18] A. A. Qureshi, S. Shott, B. A. Mallin, and S. Gitelis, "Current trends in the management of adamantinoma of long bones," *Journal of Bone and Joint Surgery-American Volume*, vol. 82, no. 8, p. 1122, 2000.

[19] S. W. Weiss and H. D. Dorfman, "Adamantinoma of long bone. An analysis of nine new cases with emphasis on metastasizing lesions and fibrous dysplasia-like changes," *Human Pathology*, vol. 8, no. 2, pp. 141–153, 1977.

[20] B. Czerniak, R. R. Rojas-Corona, and H. D. Dorfman, "Morphologic diversity of long bone adamantinoma. The concept of differentiated (regressing) adamantinoma and its relationship to osteofibrous dysplasia," *Cancer*, vol. 64, no. 11, pp. 2319–2334, 1989.

[21] G. Kuruvilla and G. C. Steiner, "Osteofibrous dysplasia-like adamantinoma of bone: a report of five cases with immunohistochemical and ultrastructural studies," *Human Pathology*, vol. 29, no. 8, pp. 809–814, 1998.

[22] J. C. Mandard, Y. Le Gal, and M. Fievez, "Adamantinoma of the long bones," *Annales D'Anatomie Pathologique*, vol. 16, no. 4, pp. 483–497, 1971.

[23] H. M. Hazelbag, A. H. Taminiau, G. J. Fleuren, and P. C. Hogendoorn, "Adamantinoma of the long bones. A clinicopathological study of thirty-two patients with emphasis on histological subtype, precursor lesion, and biological behavior," *Journal of Bone & Joint Surgery*, vol. 76, no. 10, pp. 1482–1499, 1994.

[24] J. Lokich, "Metastatic adamantinoma of bone to lung. A case report of the natural history and the use of chemotherapy and radiation therapy," *American Journal of Clinical Oncology*, vol. 17, no. 2, pp. 157–159, 1994.

[25] A. D. Liman, A. K. Liman, J. Shields, B. Englert, and R. Shah, "A case of metastatic adamantinoma that responded well to sunitinib," *Case Reports in Oncological Medicine*, vol. 2016, Article ID 5982313, 5 pages, 2016.

[26] A. G. Huvos and R. C. Marcove, "Adamantinoma of long bones. A clinicopathological study of fourteen cases with vascular origin suggested," *Journal of Bone and Joint Surgery-American Volume*, vol. 57, no. 2, pp. 148–154, 1975.

[27] M. C. Gebhardt, F. C. Lord, A. E. Rosenberg, and H. J. Mankin, "The treatment of adamantinoma of the tibia by wide resection and allograft bone transplantation," *Journal of Bone and Joint Surgery-American Volume*, vol. 69, no. 8, pp. 1177–1188, 1987.

[28] A. Minami, K. Kutsumi, N. Takeda, and K. Kaneda, "Vascularized fibular graft for bone reconstruction of the extremities after tumor resection in limb-saving procedures," *Microsurgery*, vol. 16, no. 2, pp. 56–64, 1995.

[29] M. A. Bus, J. M. Bramer, G. R. Schaap et al., "Hemicortical resection and inlay allograft reconstruction for primary bone tumors: a retrospective evaluation in the Netherlands and review of the literature," *Journal of Bone and Joint Surgery-American Volume*, vol. 97, no. 9, pp. 738–750, 2015.

[30] K. Rabitsch, W. Maurer-Ertl, U. Pirker-Frühauf, C. Wibmer, and A. Leithner, "Intercalary reconstructions with vascularised fibula and allograft after tumour resection in the lower limb," *Sarcoma*, vol. 2013, Article ID 160295, 8 pages, 2013.

[31] S. P. Frey, J. Hardes, H. Ahrens, W. Winkelmann, and G. Gosheger, "Total tibia replacement using an allograft (in a patient with adamantinoma). Case report and review of literature," *Journal of Cancer Research and Clinical Oncology*, vol. 134, no. 4, pp. 427–431, 2008.

[32] A. F. Mavrogenis, V. I. Sakellariou, H. Tsibidakis, and P. J. Papagelopoulos, "Adamantinoma of the tibia treated with a new intramedullary diaphyseal segmental defect implant,"

Journal of International Medical Research, vol. 37, no. 4, pp. 1238–1245, 2009.

[33] G. M. Sherman, T. A. Damron, and Y. Yang, "CD99 positive adamantinoma of the ulna with ipsilateral discrete osteofibrous dysplasia," *Clinical Orthopaedics and Related Research*, vol. 408, pp. 256–261, 2003.

[34] M. A. Lopez-Costea, L. Fumadó, D. Lorente, L. Riera, and E. F. Miranda, "Positive margins after nephron-sparing surgery for renal cell carcinoma: long-term follow-up of patients on active surveillance," *BJU International*, vol. 106, no. 5, pp. 645–648, 2010.

[35] S. L. Moran, A. Y. Shin, and A. T. Bishop, "The use of massive bone allograft with intramedullary free fibular flap for limb salvage in a pediatric and adolescent population," *Plastic and Reconstructive Surgery*, vol. 118, no. 2, pp. 413–419, 2006.

[36] D. W. Chang and K. L. Weber, "Use of a vascularized fibula bone flap and intercalary allograft for diaphyseal reconstruction after resection of primary extremity bone sarcomas," *Plastic and Reconstructive Surgery*, vol. 116, no. 7, pp. 1918–1925, 2005.

[37] R. Capanna, D. A. Campanacci, N. Belot et al., "A new reconstructive technique for intercalary defects of long bones: the association of massive allograft with vascularized fibular autograft. Long-term results and comparison with alternative techniques," *Orthopedic Clinics of North America*, vol. 38, no. 1, pp. 51–60, 2007.

[38] A. S. Halim, S. C. Chai, W. F. Wan Ismail, W. S. Wan Azman, A. Z. Mat Saad, and Z. Wan, "Long-term outcome of free fibula osteocutaneous flap and massive allograft in the reconstruction of long bone defect," *Journal of Plastic, Reconstructive & Aesthetic Surgery*, vol. 68, no. 12, pp. 1755–1762, 2015.

[39] F. De Keyser, J. Vansteenkiste, P. Van Den Brande, M. Demedts, and K. P. Van de Woestijne, "Pulmonary metastases of a tibia adamantinoma. Case report and review of the literature," *Acta Clinica Belgica*, vol. 45, no. 1, pp. 31–33, 1990.

[40] J. X. Van Schoor, J. H. Vallaeys, G. F. Joos, H. J. Roels, R. A. Pauwels, and M. E. Van Der Straeten, "Adamantinoma of the tibia with pulmonary metastases and hypercalcemia," *Chest*, vol. 100, no. 1, pp. 279–281, 1991.

[41] D. K. Giannoulis, A. Gantsos, D. Giotis et al., "Multiple recurrences and late metastasis of adamantinoma in the tibia: a case report," *Journal of Orthopaedic Surgery*, vol. 22, no. 3, pp. 420–422, 2014.

[42] M. Szendroi, I. Antal, and G. Arató, "Adamantinoma of long bones: a long-term follow-up study of 11 cases," *Pathology & Oncology Research*, vol. 15, no. 2, pp. 209–216, 2009.

[43] D. K. Filippou, V. Papadopoulos, E. Kiparidou, and N. T. Demertzis, "Adamantinoma of tibia: a case of late local recurrence along with lung metastases," *Journal of Postgraduate Medicine*, vol. 49, no. 1, pp. 75–77, 2003.

[44] A. N. Van Geel, H. M. Hazelbag, R. Slingerland, and M. I. Vermeulen, "Disseminating adamantinoma of the tibia," *Sarcoma*, vol. 1, no. 2, pp. 109–111, 1997.

[45] V. Sharma, A. H. Crawford, J. Evans, and M. H. Collins, "Sequential Ewing's sarcoma and osteosarcoma," *Journal of Pediatric Orthopaedics B*, vol. 17, no. 6, pp. 333–337, 2008.

[46] H. M. Hazelbag, J. W. Wessels, P. Mollevangers, E. van den Berg, W. M. Molenaar, and P. C. Hogendoorn, "Cytogenetic analysis of adamantinoma of long bones: further indications for a common histogenesis with osteofibrous dysplasia," *Cancer Genetics and Cytogenetics*, vol. 97, no. 1, pp. 5–11, 1997.

[47] National Cancer Institute, *Common Cancer Types*, 2017, https://www.cancer.gov/types/common-cancers.

[48] F. E. Vera-Badillo, E. Conde, and I. Duran, "Chromophobe renal cell carcinoma: a review of an uncommon entity,"

International Journal of Urology, vol. 19, no. 10, pp. 894–900, 2012.

[49] M. J. Welsch, A. Krunic, and M. M. Medenica, "Birt-Hogg–Dubé syndrome," *International Journal of Dermatology*, vol. 44, no. 8, pp. 668–673, 2005.

[50] A. Luciani and L. Balducci, "Multiple primary malignancies," *Seminars in Oncology*, vol. 31, no. 2, pp. 264–273, 2004.

23

Successful Complete Response of Tumor Thrombus after Combined with Chemotherapy and Irradiation for Ewing Sarcoma

Yusuke Minami,[1] Seiichi Matsumoto ⓘ,[1] Keisuke Ae,[1] Taisuke Tanizawa,[1] Keiko Hayakawa,[1] Yuki Funauchi,[1] Sakae Okumura,[2] and Yutaka Takazawa[3]

[1]Department of Orthopedic Surgery, The Cancer Institute Hospital of the Japanese Foundation for Cancer Research, Tokyo, Japan
[2]Department of Thoracic Surgery, The Cancer Institute Hospital of the Japanese Foundation for Cancer Research, Tokyo, Japan
[3]Department of Pathology, The Cancer Institute Hospital of the Japanese Foundation for Cancer Research, Tokyo, Japan

Correspondence should be addressed to Seiichi Matsumoto; smatsumoto@jfcr.or.jp

Academic Editor: Elke R. Ahlmann

Pelvic Ewing sarcoma is associated with a worse prognosis. Thromboembolic events are relatively common in pediatric patients with cancers including sarcomas. We have presented a case of Ewing sarcoma arising from the left iliac bone with tumor thrombus of inferior vena cava (IVC) which was obtained complete response by both chemotherapy and irradiation. Magnetic resonance imaging (MRI) scan demonstrated that the tumor arising from the left iliac bone extended into the left side of sacral bone, suggesting the difficulty of surgical resection. Computed tomography (CT) revealed the existence of the tumor thrombus of IVC. We performed irradiation (31.2 Gy) and chemotherapy (combination of VCR, Act-D, IFM, and ADR). The tumor was controlled successfully, and the tumor thrombus of IVC has completely vanished. Four years after the treatment, coin lesion in the left upper lung appeared. Suspected of metastasis, segmental resection of the left upper lung was performed. Fourteen years after the surgery, the patient has been remained free of recurrence. It is clinically significant for surgeons to treat pelvic Ewing sarcoma with tumor thrombus.

1. Introduction

Ewing sarcoma family of tumors (ESFTs) are rare, but high-grade malignant tumors of unclear etiology which mainly occurs in childhood [1]. Particularly, pelvic Ewing sarcoma commonly resulted in a poor prognosis [2]. Cancer and thromboembolic events are strongly associated. Venous thromboembolic events are often occurred in pediatric patients with sarcomas [3]. A few papers have been reported so far in sarcomas with tumor thrombus: osteosarcomas [4], [5], chondrosarcomas [6], clear cell sarcomas [7–9], leiomyosarcomas [10–12], rhabdomyosarcomas [13], and liposarcomas [14]. As far as we investigated, no case report of tumor thrombus with Ewing sarcomas has been reported.

2. Case Presentation

A 14-year-old male with continuous left low back pain, suspected of malignancy, referred to our hospital. He had been aware of left low back pain for the last 3 months. A clinical examination revealed spontaneous pain of his left low back and the paresthesia of left S1, 2 lesion. Plain radiograph of the pelvic bone showed osteolytic changes of the left iliac bone (Figure 1). CT and MRI demonstrated that a $7.2 \times 9.5 \times 3.0$ cm tumor arising from the left iliac bone extended into the left side of sacral bone (Figures 2(a) and 2(b)). The large mass showed low intensity on T1-weighted images and high intensity on T2-weighted images and was enhanced by contrast agent (Figure 2(b)). A contrast-enhanced

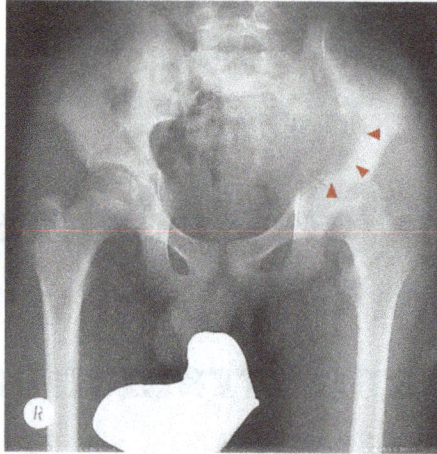

FIGURE 1: Plain radiograph showing osteolytic changes at the medial side of the left iliac bone.

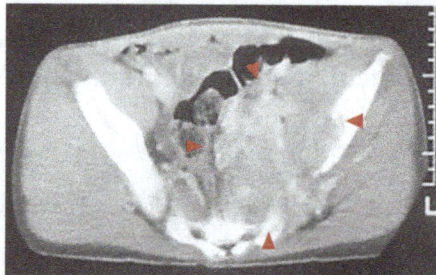

(a)

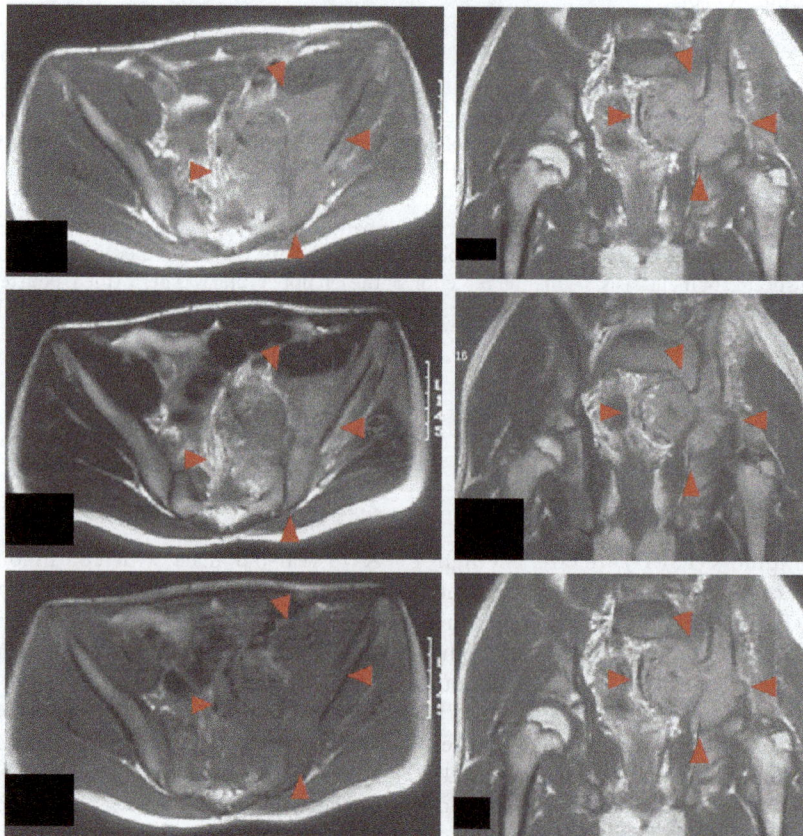

(b)

FIGURE 2: (a) $7.2 \times 9.5 \times 3.0$ cm mass arising from the left iliac bone and extended into the sacral bone. (b) The large mass showing low intensity on T1-weighted images and high intensity on T2-weighted images and sparsely enhanced by contrast agent.

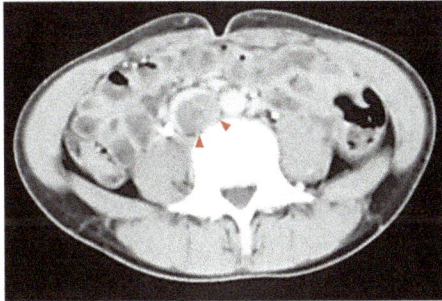

FIGURE 3: A contrast-enhanced CT suggesting the existence of the tumor thrombus of IVC.

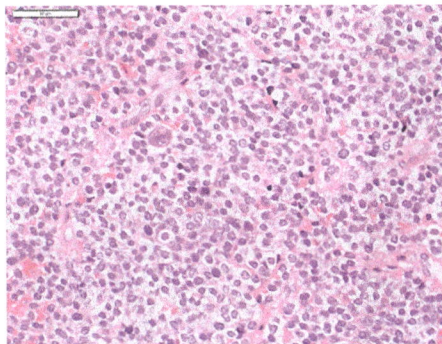

FIGURE 4: The tumor cells are small and round shaped and have abundant glycogen.

CT suggested the existence of the tumor thrombus of IVC (Figure 3). Open biopsy of the tumor was performed. Histopathologically, the tumor cells were small and round shaped and have abundant glycogen (Figure 4). Immuno-staining analysis showed MIC2 positive and NSE positive. The histopathological diagnosis was Ewing sarcoma. Before treatment, insertion of permanent IVC filter was performed to prevent fatal pulmonary embolism [15]. We performed irradiation (total 31.2 Gy) and total 4 cycles of chemotherapy (combination of VCR, Act-D, IFM, and ADR) because it was considered to be difficult to resect the mass surgically. After irradiation and a 1 cycle of chemotherapy, the tumor volume was reduced successfully and radiologically evaluated as partial response (PR) by both CT and MRI (Figures 5(a) and 5(b)). Moreover, the tumor thrombus of IVC has completely vanished (Figure 6). In addition, we performed 3 cycles of chemotherapy. 4 years after the treatment, coin lesion of the left upper lung appeared (Figure 7). Suspected of lung metastasis, segmental excision of the left upper lung was performed. The histopathological diagnosis was equally Ewing sarcoma. 14 years after the surgery, the patient has been remained free of any evidence of recurrence and tumor thrombus (Figures 8(a)–8(c)).

3. Discussion

The combination of surgery, chemotherapy, and irradiation for pelvic Ewing sarcoma has only resulted in about 40% five-year survival rate [16]. We have presented a case of Ewing sarcoma arising from the left iliac bone which caused

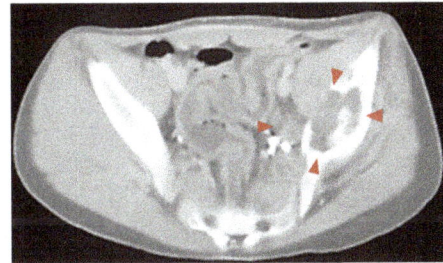

(a)

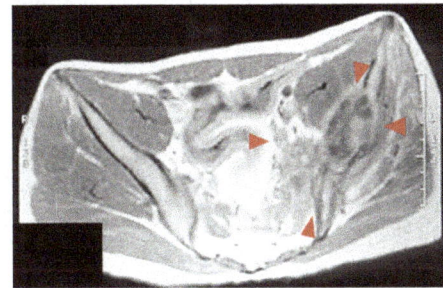

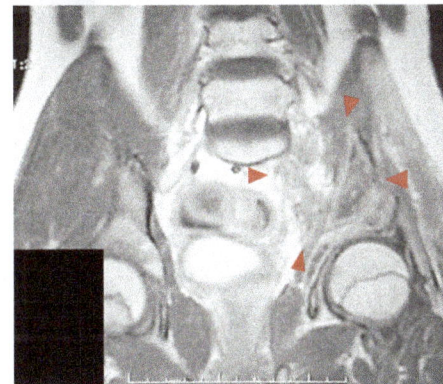

(b)

FIGURE 5: (a, b) The tumor volume was reduced successfully and judged as partial response (PR).

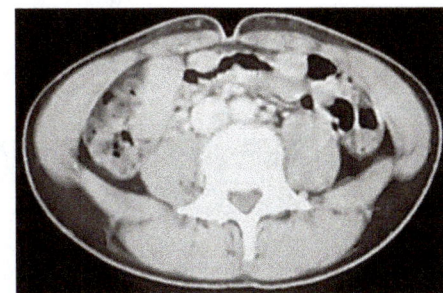

FIGURE 6: The tumor thrombus of IVC has completely vanished after irradiation and a 1 cycle of chemotherapy.

tumor thrombus of inferior vena cava (IVC). The tumor was obtained complete response by both chemotherapy and irradiation. The tumor thrombus of IVC has vanished without any anticoagulant therapy, which indicates that the content of IVC was not a venous thrombus but the tumor thrombus. We did not perform surgical procedures except

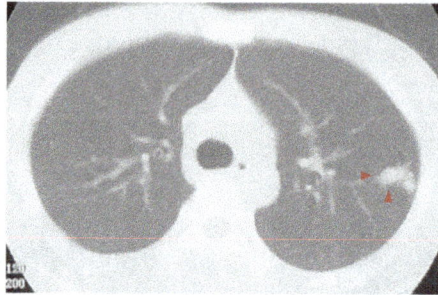

FIGURE 7: Four years after the treatment, coin lesion in the left upper lung appeared.

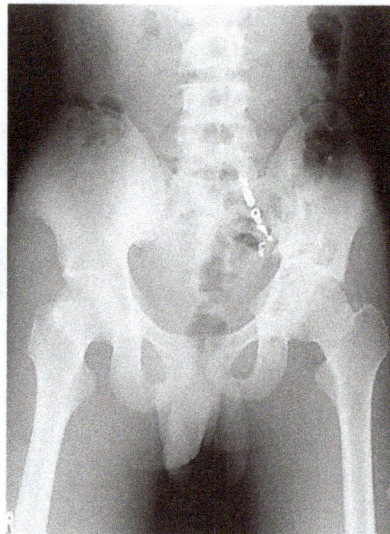

(a)

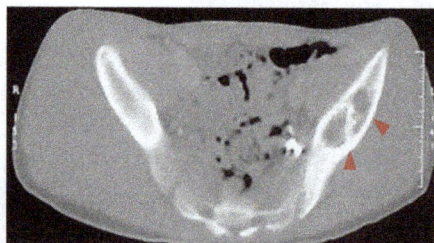

(b)

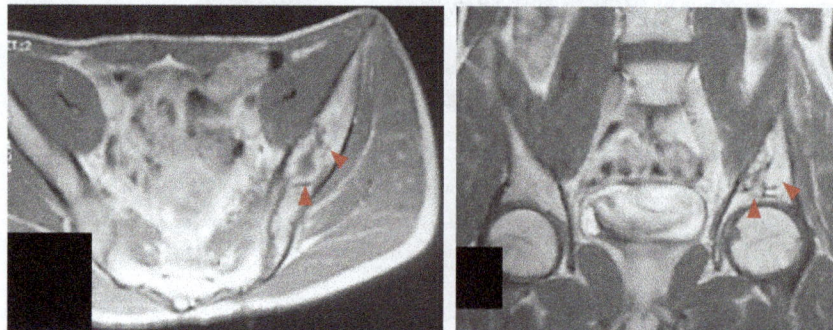

(c)

FIGURE 8: (a–c) 14 years after the surgery, the patient has remained with no evidence of recurrence.

for segmental excision of the left upper lung for lung metastasis. Previous papers showed that there was no significant difference in outcomes of patients with pelvic Ewing sarcoma treated with surgery and/or irradiation, although surgical resection was associated with superior outcomes for osteosarcoma and chondrosarcoma [17]. In this case, if we performed the curative surgery, both left hip amputation and tumor evacuation of IVC should be required. The surgical procedure itself might be very difficult and risky for the patient. Moreover, small round cell sarcomas such as Ewing sarcomas are known to be relatively sensitive to chemotherapy and irradiation [18]. On the other hand, spindle cell sarcomas require the curative surgery.

It is clinically very important that the pelvic Ewing sarcoma with the tumor thrombus of IVC could be controlled successfully by irradiation and chemotherapy without any surgical procedure. Our case report should be taken into consideration for surgeons to decide the treatment of pelvic Ewing sarcomas with tumor thrombus.

Consent

The patient and his family were informed that data from the case would be submitted for publication and gave their consent.

Conflicts of Interest

The authors declare that they have no conflicts of interest.

Acknowledgments

The authors thank Dr. Sakae Okumura for the performance of segmental excision of the left upper lung, Dr. Yutaka Takazawa for the histopathological diagnosis, and members of their department for helpful discussions.

References

[1] T. Ozaki, "Diagnosis and treatment of Ewing sarcoma of the bone: a review article," *Journal of Orthopaedic Science*, vol. 20, no. 2, pp. 250–263, 2015.

[2] C. Hoffmann, S. Ahrens, J. Dunst et al., "Pelvic Ewing sarcoma: a retrospective analysis of 241 cases," *Cancer*, vol. 85, no. 4, pp. 869–877, 1999.

[3] I. Paz-Priel, L. Long, L. J. Helman, C. L. Mackall, and A. S. Wayne, "Thromboembolic events in children and young adults with pediatric sarcoma," *Journal of Clinical Oncology*, vol. 25, no. 12, pp. 1519–1524, 2007.

[4] P. Navalkele, S. M. Jones, J. K. Jones et al., "Osteosarcoma tumor thrombus: a case report with a review of the literature," *Texas Heart Institute Journal*, vol. 40, no. 1, pp. 75–78, 2013.

[5] A. Kawai, A. G. Huvos, P. A. Meyers, and J. H. Healey, "Osteosarcoma of the pelvis. Oncologic results of 40 patients," *Clinical Orthopaedics and Related Research*, vol. 348, pp. 196–207, 1998.

[6] C. N. Hsu, H. Y. Chen, Y. C. Wu, C. F. Yang, and T. C. Hsieh, "Huge tumor thrombus of chondrosarcoma on FDG PET/CT," *Clinical Nuclear Medicine*, vol. 36, no. 10, pp. e142–145, 2011.

[7] S. B. Bhayani, H. Liapis, and A. S. Kibel, "Adult clear cell sarcoma of the kidney with atrial tumor thrombus," *Journal of Urology*, vol. 165, no. 3, pp. 896-897, 2001.

[8] N. Ohtake, A. Shiono, K. Okabe et al., "Clear cell sarcoma extending into the inferior vena cava," *Nihon Hinyokika Gakkai Zasshi*, vol. 86, no. 7, pp. 1298–1301, 1995.

[9] A. Zigman and I. Shen, "Clear cell sarcoma of the kidney with cavo-atrial tumor thrombus: complete resection in a child," *Journal of Pediatric Surgery*, vol. 41, no. 8, pp. 1464–1466, 2006.

[10] M. Cimino, C. Mussi, P. Colombo, F. Lutman, and V. Quagliuolo, "Leiomyosarcoma arising from the inferior mesenteric vein draining in the splenomesenteric angle with a tumour thrombus at the splenomesenteric confluence: a case report and review of the literature," *Updates in Surgery*, vol. 65, no. 4, pp. 313–316, 2013.

[11] T. Kato, Y. Nakai, Y. Miyagawa et al., "Leiomyosarcoma of the kidney with tumor thrombus to the inferior vena cava," *Hinyokika kiyo. Acta Urologica Japonica*, vol. 56, no. 12, pp. 687–690, 2010.

[12] K. Tomonori, T. Kato, S. Sakamoto et al., "Primary adrenal leiomyosarcoma with inferior vena cava thrombosis," *International Journal of Clinical Oncology*, vol. 9, no. 3, pp. 189–192, 2004.

[13] L. Garcia-Covarrubias, T. A. Salerno, P. G. Robinson, and G. Ciancio, "Right atrial and pulmonary tumor embolism from renal rhabdomyosarcoma," *Journal of Cardiac Surgery*, vol. 23, no. 6, pp. 778–780, 2008.

[14] Z. Vajtai, E. Korngold, J. E. Hooper, B. C. Sheppard, B. R. Foster, and F. V. Coakley, "Suprarenal retroperitoneal liposarcoma with intracaval tumor thrombus: an imaging mimic of adrenocortical carcinoma," *Clinical Imaging*, vol. 38, no. 1, pp. 75–77, 2014.

[15] B. Tuy, C. Bhate, K. Beebe, F. Patterson, and J. Benevenia, "IVC filters may prevent fatal pulmonary embolism in musculoskeletal tumor surgery," *Clinical Orthopaedics and Related Research*, vol. 467, no. 1, pp. 239–245, 2009.

[16] J. Zang, W. Guo, and H. Y. Qu, "Ewing's sarcoma of the pelvis: treatment results of 31 patients," *Zhonghua Wai Ke Za Zhi*, vol. 50, no. 6, pp. 524–528, 2012.

[17] M. U. Jawad, A. A. Haleem, and S. P. Scully, "Malignant sarcoma of the pelvic bones: treatment outcomes and prognostic factors vary by histopathology," *Cancer*, vol. 117, no. 7, pp. 1529–1541, 2011.

[18] S. L. Lessnick, A. P. Dei Tos, P. H. Sorensen et al., "Small round cell sarcomas," *Seminars in Oncology*, vol. 36, no. 4, pp. 338–346, 2009.

24

Resolution of Right Hemidiaphragm Paralysis following Cervical Foraminotomies

Neal Singleton ⓘ**, Matthew Bowman, and David Bartle**

Orthopaedic Department, Tauranga Hospital, Cameron Road, Tauranga, New Zealand

Correspondence should be addressed to Neal Singleton; nealsingleton@hotmail.com

Academic Editor: Koichi Sairyo

Introduction. Hemidiaphragm paralysis secondary to phrenic nerve palsy is a well-recognised medical condition. There are few case reports in the literature documenting resolution of hemidiaphragm paralysis following cervical spine surgery. This case report documents our experience with one such case. *Case Presentation.* A 64-year-old man was referred to the orthopaedic service with right hemidiaphragm paralysis. He had a previous history of asbestos exposure and polio and was initially seen and investigated by the respiratory physicians. He also reported intermittent neck pain and an MRI scan showed right-sided cervical foraminal stenosis. He underwent posterior right C3/4 and C4/5 foraminotomies, and by three months postoperatively, his hemidiaphragm paralysis had resolved and his shortness of breath had also improved. *Conclusion.* This report documents a unique case of resolution of hemidiaphragm paralysis following posterior unilateral cervical foraminotomies.

1. Introduction

The phrenic nerves (C3/4/5) supply motor function to the hemidiaphragms. The motor supply of each hemidiaphragm comes purely from the phrenic nerves, and so conditions affecting the phrenic nerve or its nerve roots cause hemidiaphragm paralysis. Hemidiaphragm paralysis secondary to phrenic nerve palsy is a well-recognised medical condition with multiple causes. However, there are few case reports in the literature documenting resolution of hemidiaphragm paralysis following the cervical spine surgery. The cases that have previously been described involve patients with concomitant tetraparesis treated with spinal cord decompression with or without foraminotomies. This case report documents resolution of hemidiaphragm paralysis and improved respiratory function with unilateral cervical nerve root decompression alone, a finding that has not previously been described.

2. Case Report

A 64-year-old man was referred to the orthopaedic service with right hemidiaphragm paralysis. He had initially presented to his general practitioner reporting subjective shortness of breath after stand-up paddleboarding. His past medical history was significant for asbestos exposure and polio. Chest radiograph revealed an elevated right hemidiaphragm (Figures 1 and 2). A previous chest radiograph taken five years before showed normal diaphragmatic contours. He was subsequently referred to the respiratory physicians where workup included a chest CT scan (which revealed no intrathoracic abnormality) and dynamic fluoroscopic sniffing test (which confirmed complete right hemidiaphragm paralysis). He reported innocuous injuries to his neck in the past and intermittent neck pain for which he had previously consulted both a chiropractor and an osteopath. An MRI scan was undertaken which showed right-sided cervical foraminal stenosis (with uncovertebral and facet joint osteophytic changes at C3/4 and C4/5) (Figure 3). He was therefore referred to the orthopaedic service. On examination, he had no focal cervical spine tenderness with a well-preserved range of motion. He did have some generalized right shoulder girdle and upper limb wasting and weakness compared to the left (presumed to be secondary to his postpolio syndrome). His upper limb reflexes were intact and symmetrical with the contralateral side.

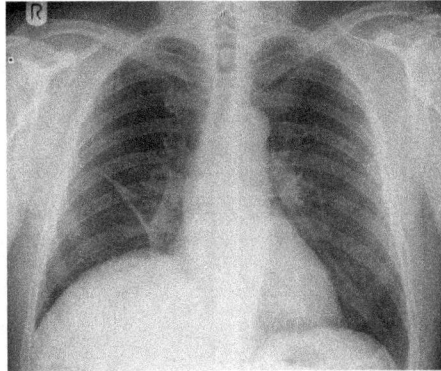

FIGURE 1: Preoperative chest radiograph in a 64-year-old man with right-sided stenosis at C3/4 and C4/5 demonstrating an elevated right hemidiaphragm.

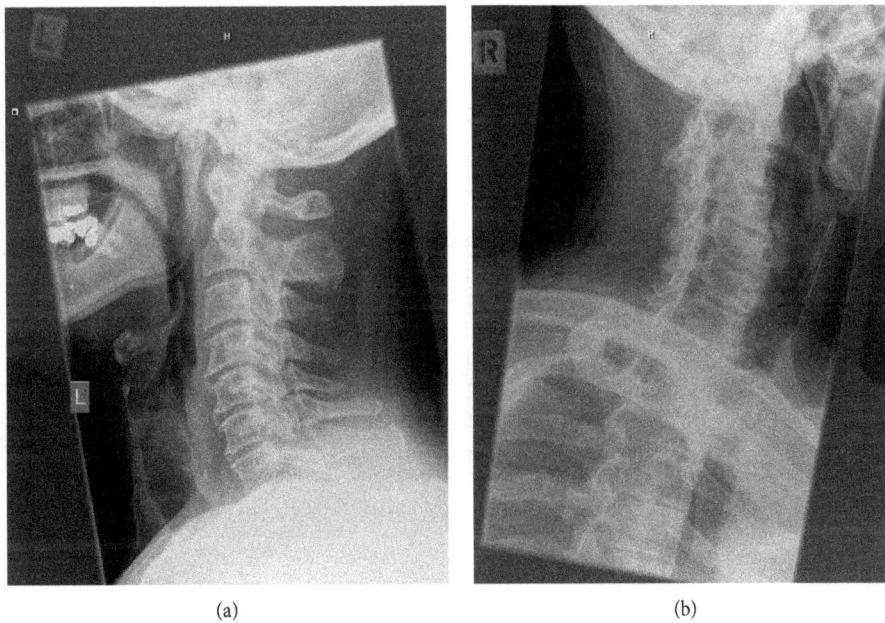

(a)

(b)

FIGURE 2: Preoperative AP and oblique cervical spine radiographs showing degenerative spondylosis.

The underlying cause for his hemidiaphragm paralysis, whether it was related to his cervical foraminal stenosis or postpolio syndrome, was indeterminant (Figure 4).

After obtaining multiple subspecialist opinions, a decision was made to proceed with posterior right C3/4 and C4/5 foraminotomies accepting that this may not have any effect on his shortness of breath. Surgery proceeded uneventfully as did postoperative recovery. By three months postoperatively, his hemidiaphragm paralysis had completely resolved on chest radiograph, and his shortness of breath had also improved (Figure 5). Comparison of preoperative and postoperative spirometry lung function showed significant improvements in all parameters tested: increases in FVC from 3.88L to 4.86L, FEV1 from 2.44L to 3.13L, TLC from 5.11L to 7.65L, FRCpl from 2.61 to 3.63, and RV from 1.23L to 2.58L. A graphic representation of these findings is shown in Figure 6. A satisfactory outcome was thus achieved.

3. Discussion

The phrenic nerve originates from cervical nerve roots C3–5 with the dominant supply coming from C4. The phrenic nerves are the sole motor supply to the hemidiaphragms and also provide proprioceptive fibres to the central part of each hemidiaphragm. Common causes of phrenic nerve palsy include idiopathic, malignancy (primary lung tumour or metastatic disease), trauma (penetrating injury and postsurgical, following central venous catheterisation and cervical manipulation), neuromuscular disease (polio or multiple sclerosis), inflammation (pneumonia or HSV), brachial plexus palsies, and direct compression (aortic aneurysm). However, the aetiology of diaphragmatic paralysis remains unidentified in more than two-thirds of patients [1].

It is possible that these idiopathic cases are caused by unidentified nerve root compression in the cervical spine.

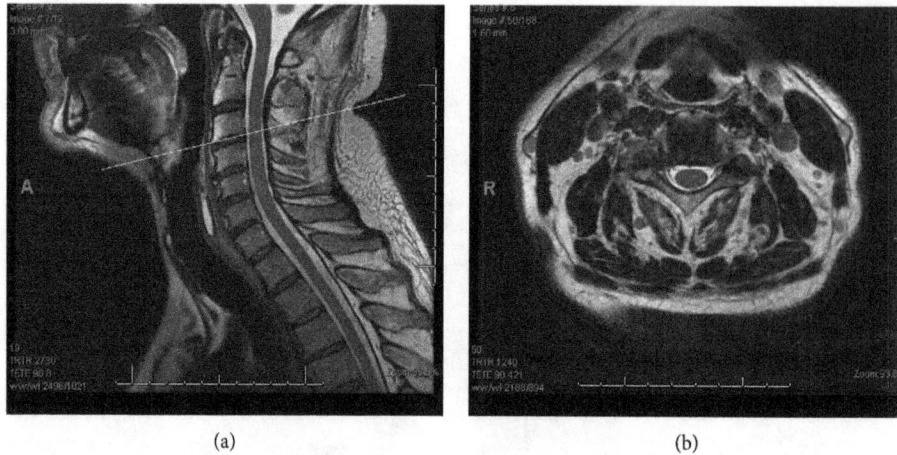

(a)

(b)

FIGURE 3: Preoperative T2-weighted sagittal MRI scan at the C3/4 level with corresponding axial sequence illustrating right-sided foraminal stenosis due to a combination of disc bulge, uncovertebral osteophyte, and facet joint hypertrophy.

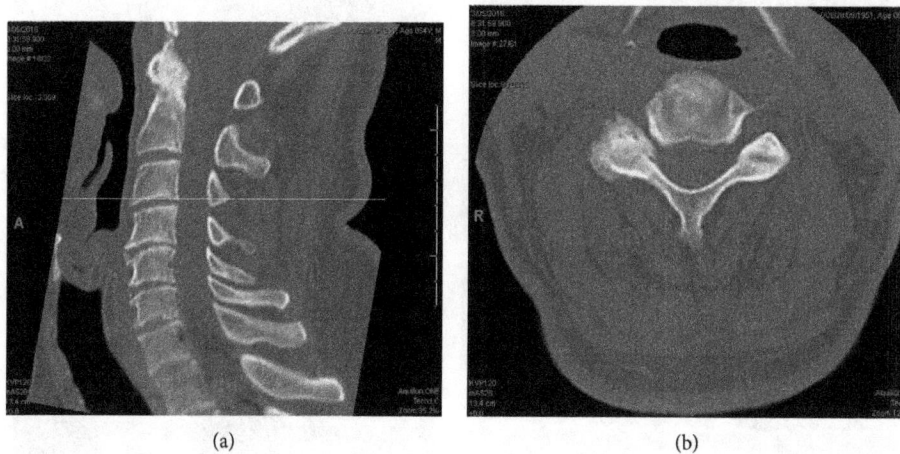

(a)

(b)

FIGURE 4: Preoperative CT scan of the cervical spine with sagittal slice and corresponding axial slice at the C3/4 level illustrating right-sided foraminal stenosis.

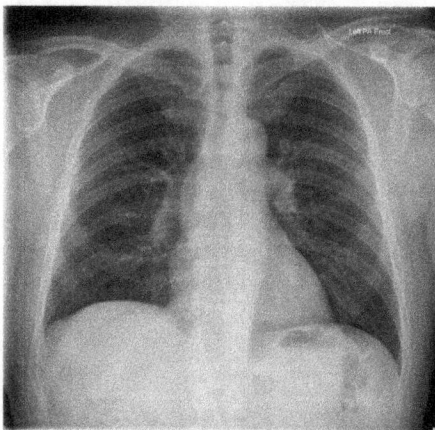

FIGURE 5: Chest radiograph three months postoperatively showing resolution of right hemidiaphragm paralysis.

Poliomyelitis can result in the degeneration of the anterior horn cells, innervating both hemidiaphragms and the accessory respiratory muscles. Additional damage to the axons of the surviving anterior horn cells as a result of nerve root compression may result in clinically significant respiratory dysfunction as was evident in this patient.

Acute dyspnoea secondary to diaphragmatic paralysis can also occur following minor cervical trauma. Parke and Whalen described two patients with severe cervical myelopathy who developed respiratory insufficiency related to phrenic nerve palsy after cervical manipulation [2]. Merino-Ramirez et al. also reported on two patients who developed hemidiaphragm paralysis, one after chiropractic cervical manipulation and the other following a motorcycle accident [3].

Respiratory compromise is a known complication of acute cervical spinal cord injury but rarely is it considered in less acute settings such as in cases of degenerative cervical spondylosis.

There are few case reports in the literature documenting resolution of diaphragmatic paralysis due to cervical nerve root compression following cervical spine surgery. Hayashi et al. reported on a 64-year-old man with dyspnoea who had bilateral hemidiaphragm paralysis secondary to cervical spondylosis [4]. Following cervical laminoplasty, his diaphragm

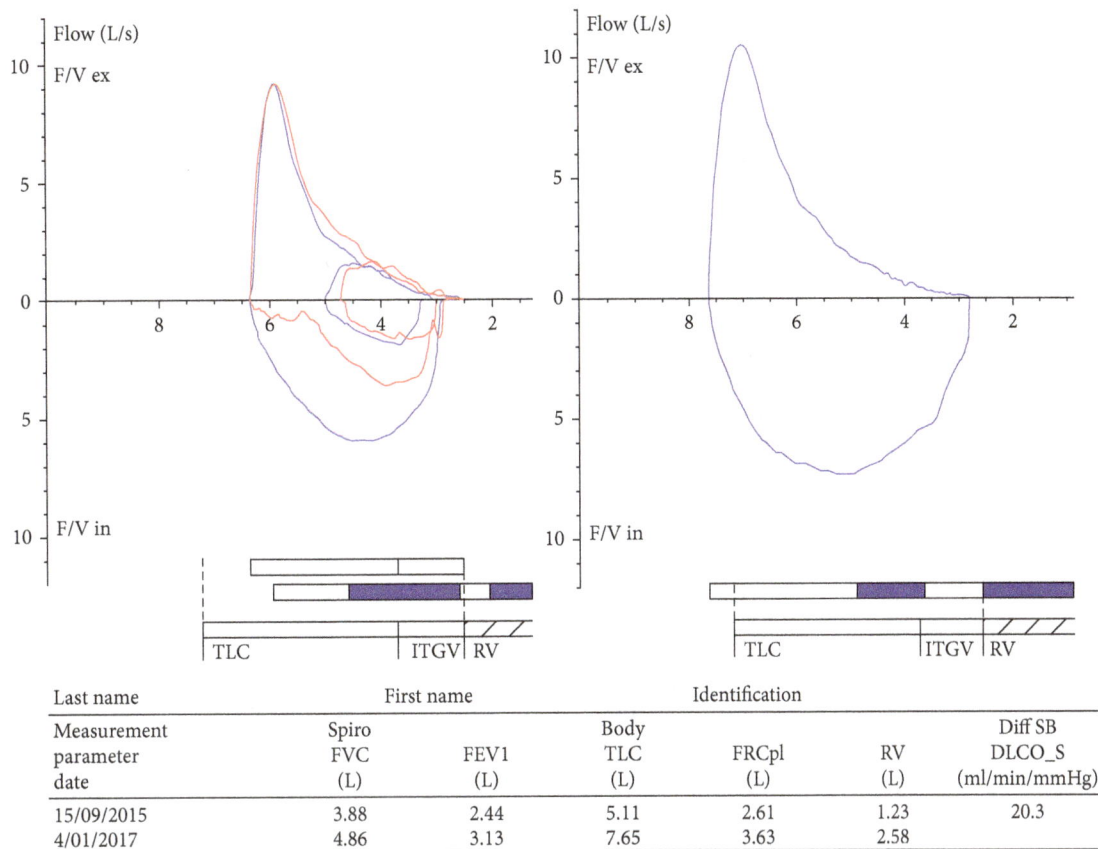

Last name		First name		Identification		
Measurement parameter date	Spiro FVC (L)	FEV1 (L)	Body TLC (L)	FRCpl (L)	RV (L)	Diff SB DLCO_S (ml/min/mmHg)
15/09/2015	3.88	2.44	5.11	2.61	1.23	20.3
4/01/2017	4.86	3.13	7.65	3.63	2.58	

FIGURE 6: Comparison of preoperative and postoperative spirometry results showing marked improvement in respiratory function.

paralysis completely resolved, and his respiratory symptoms and spirometry also improved. Fregni et al. reported a case of phrenic nerve palsy in a 53-year-old with cervical spondylotic myelopathy [5]. Buszek et al. reported on a case of left hemidiaphragm paralysis with shortness of breath secondary to C3/4 neural foramen compression which resolved completely after laminectomy [6]. Rudrappa and Kokatnur reported on a 64-year-old man with acute shortness of breath and dyspnoea and an elevated left hemidiaphragm with severe cervical spondylosis on MRI [7]. Following cord decompression, his respiratory symptoms resolved. Yu et al. reported the case of an 82-year-old man who presented with respiratory symptoms [8]. He went on to have cardiac angiography and ultimately triple coronary artery bypass grafting which failed to improve his symptoms. He then developed generalised weakness, and an MRI showed C2–7 central canal stenosis and myelomalacia. Following laminectomy and instrumented fusion, his respiratory symptoms completely resolved. To our knowledge, this is the first case that shows resolution of hemidiaphragm paralysis and improved subjective and objective respiratory function after cervical foraminotomies alone.

There are numerous studies in the literature that show impaired respiratory function in patients presenting with cervical pathology. Ishibe and Takahashi compared 84 patients with cervical pathology with an age-matched control group of patients without cervical pathology and found that those in the cervical group had significantly lower respiratory function (vital capacity and percent forced vital capacity) [9]. Within the cervical group those with more cephalad pathology (C4 and cephalad) had more severe respiratory dysfunction. Postoperatively, those in the cephalad cervical group were shown to have significantly improved respiratory function. Similarly, Yanaka et al. reported on 12 patients with cervical myelopathy treated with laminoplasty [10]. Pre- and postoperative spirometry was performed, and it was found that tidal volume increased significantly.

4. Conclusion

Similar to other case reports in the literature, this report documents a case of resolution of right hemidiaphragm paralysis following C4 and C5 nerve root decompression via posterior cervical foraminotomies (C3/4 and C4/5 levels), a finding not previously described. Although rare, cervical nerve root compression as a cause of phrenic nerve palsy should be considered in patients presenting with hemidiaphragm paralysis and respiratory symptoms as surgical management can result in resolution of paralysis and potential improvement in respiratory symptoms.

Conflicts of Interest

The authors declare that they have no conflicts of interest.

References

[1] G. J. Gibson, "Diaphragmatic paresis: pathophysiology, clinical features, and investigation," *Thorax*, vol. 44, no. 11, pp. 960–970, 1989.

[2] W. Parke and J. Whalen, "Phrenic paresis—a possible additional spinal cord dysfunction induced by neck manipulation in cervical spondylotic myelopathy: a report of two cases with anatomical and clinical considerations," *Clinical Anatomy*, vol. 14, no. 3, pp. 173–178, 2001.

[3] M. Merino-Ramirez, G. Juan, M. Ramon, J. Cortijo, and E. Morcillo, "Diaphragmatic paralysis following minor cervical trauma," *Muscle and Nerve*, vol. 36, no. 2, p. 267, 2007.

[4] H. Hayashi, S. Kihara, M. Hoshimaru, and N. Hashimoto, "Diaphragmatic paralysis caused by cervical spondylosis. Case report," *Journal of Neurosurgery: Spine*, vol. 2, no. 5, pp. 604–607, 2005.

[5] F. Fregni, S. Conceicao, G. Souza, M. Taricco, and E. Mutarelli, "Phrenic paresis and respiratory insufficiency associated with cervical spondylotic myelopathy," *Acta Neurochirurgica*, vol. 146, no. 3, pp. 309–312, 2004.

[6] M. Buszek, T. Szymke, J. Honet, J. Raikes, W. Leuchter, and S. Bendix, "Hemidiaphragmatic paralysis: an unusual complication of cervical spondylosis," *Archives of Physical Medicine and Rehabilitation*, vol. 64, no. 12, pp. 601–603, 1983.

[7] M. Rudrappa and L. Kokatnur, "Dyspnea due to osteoarthritis. Diaphragmatic palsy caused by cervical spondylosis," *World Journal of Pharmaceutical and Medical Research*, vol. 2, no. 5, pp. 214–216, 2016.

[8] E. Yu, N. Romero, T. Miles, S. Hsu, and D. Kondrashov, "Dyspnea as the presenting symptom of cervical spondylotic myelopathy," *Surgery Journal*, vol. 2, no. 4, pp. e147–e150, 2016.

[9] T. Ishibe and S. Takahashi, "Respiratory dysfunction in patients with chronic-onset cervical myelopathy," *Spine*, vol. 27, no. 20, pp. 2234–2239, 2002.

[10] K. Yanaka, S. Noguchi, H. Asakawa, and T. Nose, "Laminoplasty improves respiratory function in elderly patients with cervical spondylotic myelopathy," *Neurologia Medico-Chirurgica*, vol. 41, no. 10, pp. 488–492, 2001.

25

Bilateral Greater Trochanteric Avulsion Fractures after Bilateral Simultaneous Total Hip Arthroplasty

Hiroaki Tagomori, Nobuhiro Kaku ⓘ, Tomonori Tabata, and Hiroshi Tsumura

Department of Orthopaedic Surgery, Oita University, Oita, Japan

Correspondence should be addressed to Nobuhiro Kaku; nobuhiro@oita-u.ac.jp

Academic Editor: Elke R. Ahlmann

We report a case of bilateral spontaneous greater trochanteric fracture after bilateral simultaneous total hip arthroplasty (THA) performed via the posterolateral approach during the early postoperative phase. A 75-year-old woman underwent bilateral simultaneous THA (BS-THA) for severe osteoarthritis with developmental dysplasia of the hip; she also presented a limited range of adduction. BS-THA was successful without any intraoperative complications. Rehabilitation with full weight-bearing exercises was initiated the day after the surgery. On the 14th postoperative day, she experienced a spontaneous left greater trochanteric fracture during a walking exercise without any trauma. Osteosynthesis was performed for the fracture on the 18th postoperative day. On the 20th postoperative day, a right spontaneous greater trochanteric avulsion fracture occurred during a transfer exercise without any trauma; this was treated on the 27th postoperative day. In the 18th postoperative month, although the right fragment showed slight upper migration, the patient had no complaints of coxalgia and both hip joints showed an excellent range of motion.

1. Introduction

Bilateral simultaneous total hip arthroplasty (BS-THA) yields clinical results comparable to those of two-staged procedures. BS-THA has several advantages such as a decrease in patient anxiety, total treatment cost, and hospitalization period; the use of a single, short anesthetic exposure; and achievement of a postoperative hip flexion angle [1]. Greater trochanteric fractures are one of the rare complications of THA, with an incidence of about 5%. Because greater trochanteric fractures occur due to intraoperative manipulations, they are frequently reported after THA that is performed via an anterior approach [2]. We present a rare case of bilateral greater trochanteric fracture after BS-THA that was performed via a posterolateral approach.

2. Case Presentation

A 75-year-old woman presented to our institution after 10 years of conservative treatment for hip osteoarthritis secondary to developmental dysplasia. The patient characteristics were as follows: height, 165 cm; body weight, 50.6 kg; and body mass index, 18 kg/m^2. Physical examination revealed an antalgic gait while ambulating with a cane. Tenderness was observed in both Scarpa triangles, and the Patrick test was positive for both legs. Her range of motion was moderately restricted, with hip flexion of 110°, extension of 5°, abduction of 30°, adduction of 10°, internal rotation of 10°, and external rotation of 30°. The Harris Hip Score was 52/51 (right/left (Rt/Lt)) points. The bone mineral density (BMD) of the femoral neck was 0.758/0.690 (Rt/Lt) g/cm^2 and of the lumbar spine was 0.857 g/cm^2. Although the BMD of the femoral neck (Rt/Lt) and the lumbar vertebra was more than 80% of the mean values in young adults, the patient's T-score was low.

Plain radiography indicated osteoarthritic changes, represented by hip joint narrowing, osteosclerotic changes in the subchondral bone, and osteophyte formation (Figure 1). However, preoperative magnetic resonance imaging did not

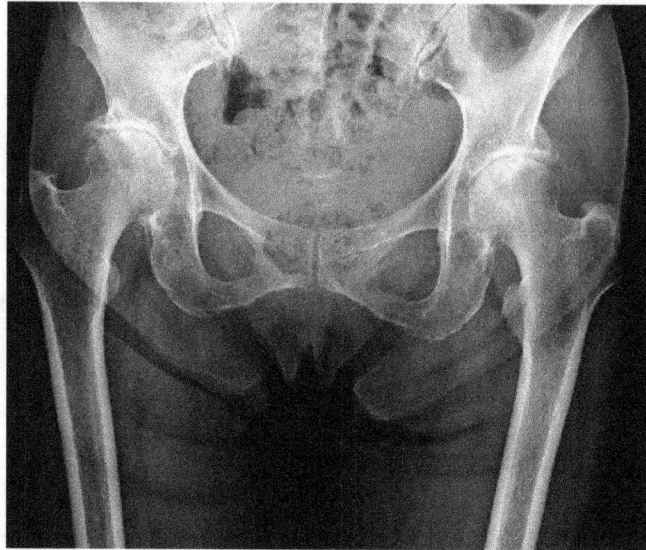

FIGURE 1: Preoperative radiograph showing osteoarthritis secondary to developmental dysplasia of the hips.

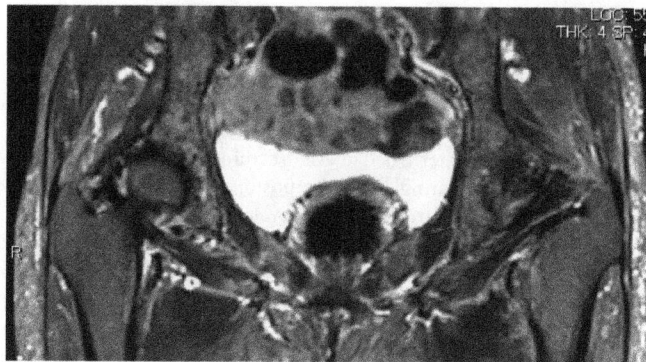

FIGURE 2: Preoperative magnetic resonance imaging. No abnormal findings are observed.

show any abnormal findings of the gluteus medius muscle (Figure 2).

The patient underwent BS-THA via a posterolateral approach, which was successful without intraoperative complications. We implanted acetabular cups with a computed tomography-based navigation system (VectorVision Compact Hip CT version 3.5.2; BrainLab, Munich, Germany). The implants included cementless hydroxyapatite-coated acetabular SQRUM cups (Kyocera Medical Co. Ltd., Osaka, Japan), polyethylene acetabular Aquala liners (Kyocera Medical Co. Ltd., Osaka, Japan), and tapered-wedge cementless hydroxyapatite-coated femoral J-Taper stems (Kyocera Medical Co. Ltd., Osaka, Japan). We detached the piriformis, short rotator muscles, and joint capsule from the femur during the posterolateral approach, created a few holes vertically in the intertrochanteric posterior crest before closing the surgical wound, and then attached the piriformis, short rotator muscles, and joint capsule to the intertrochanteric crest with sutures. The total operation time was 5 hours and 57 minutes with an estimated blood loss of 530 mL.

Postoperative radiographic evaluation demonstrated that the patient's right and left limbs were extended by 14 and

8 mm, respectively, when compared with the preoperative length (Figure 3). We measured the preoperative and postoperative distance from the anterior superior iliac spine to the greater trochanter tip using the ZedHip system (ZedHip Lexi Co. Ltd., Tokyo, Japan) (Figure 4).

Rehabilitation and full weight-bearing exercises were initiated soon after the surgery. The patient was able to perform exercises for walking, muscle strengthening, and range of motion without severe pain. However, on the 14th postoperative day, she complained of left coxalgia during a walking exercise without any falls. Plain radiographs revealed a left greater trochanteric avulsion fracture (Figure 5). This fracture was fixed using tension band wiring on the 18th postoperative day (Figure 6). She was allowed to ambulate but weight bearing of the left leg was prohibited. On the 20th postoperative day, right coxalgia occurred during a transfer exercise, and a greater trochanteric avulsion fracture on the right side was detected on plain radiographs (Figure 7). On the 27th postoperative day, her right fracture was treated with small plate and wiring (Figure 8). The patient was discharged home about a month after the last surgery.

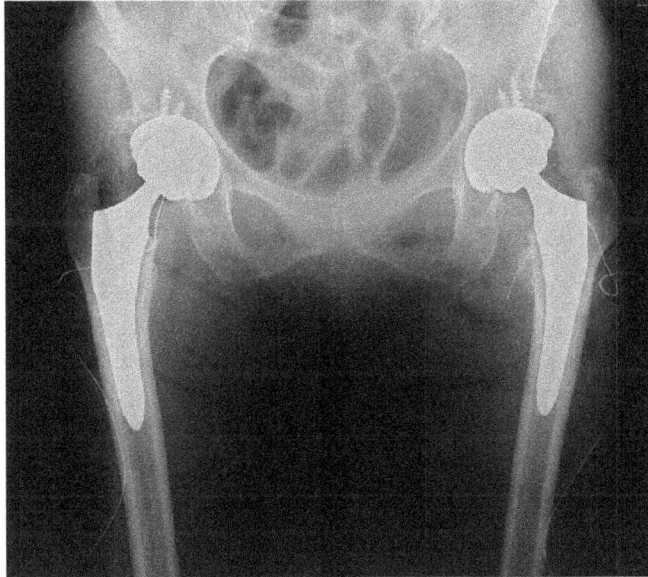

FIGURE 3: The patient underwent BS-THA via a posterolateral approach, which was successful without intraoperative complications.

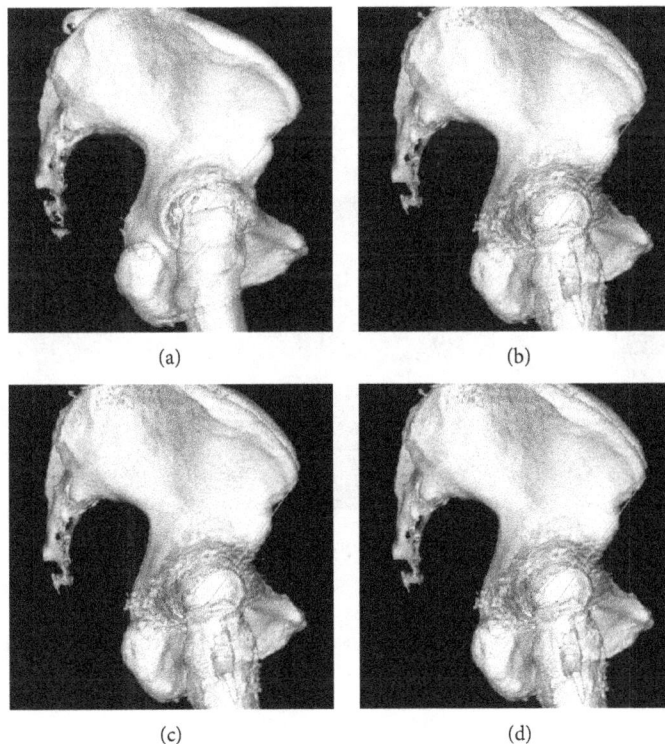

(a)

(b)

(c)

(d)

FIGURE 4: Measurement of the preoperative and postoperative distance from the anterior superior iliac spine to the greater trochanter tip by using the ZedHip system. (a) Preoperative, right. (b) Postoperative, right. (c) Preoperative, left. (d) Postoperative, left.

In the 18th postoperative month, although the right fragment showed slight upper migration, the patient had no complaints of coxalgia and both hip joints showed excellent range of motion. The Harris Hip Score was 89/89 (Rt/Lt) points with range of motion of 10° bilateral adduction (Figure 9). Informed consent was obtained from the patient to publish this case report. All surgical procedures were conducted in accordance with the Declaration of Helsinki

(1964). The report has been approved by the Ethical Committee/Institutional Review Board.

3. Discussion

BS-THA was first reported by Jaffe and Charnley in 1971 [8]. Previous reports have showed no difference in systemic complications between 1-stage bilateral THA and 2-stage

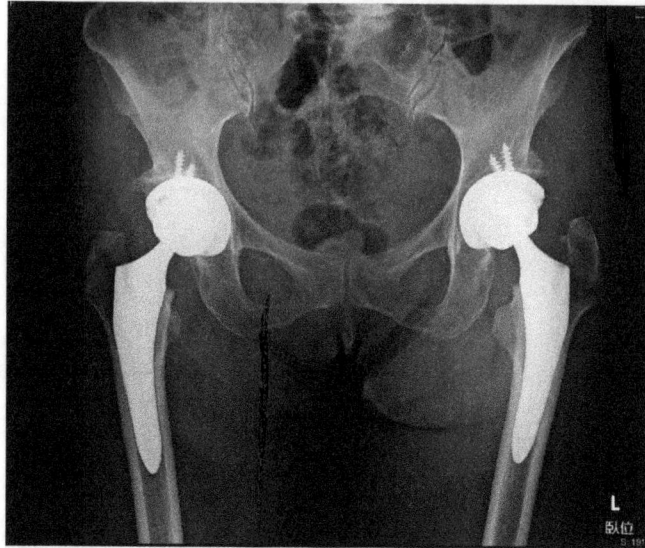

FIGURE 5: On the 14th postoperative day, the patient complained of left coxalgia during a walking exercise without any falls. Plain radiographs revealed a left greater trochanteric avulsion fracture.

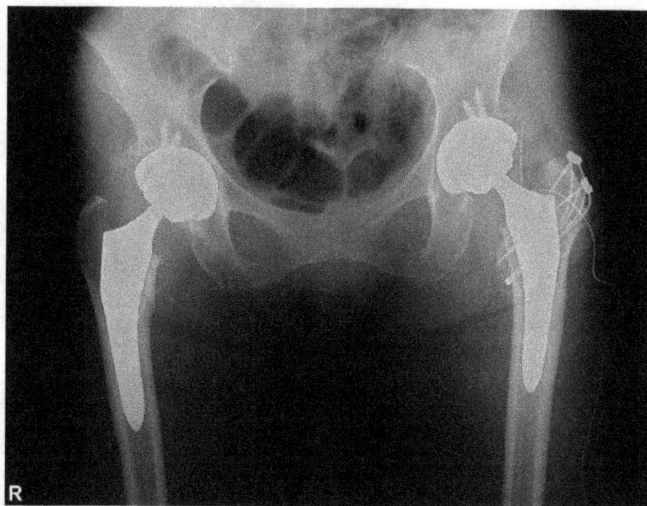

FIGURE 6: The fracture was fixed using tension band wiring on the 18th postoperative day.

unilateral THA, and no differences were observed in intraoperative fractures [3–7]. BS-THA was mostly performed either via the direct anterior approach or the posterior approach in previous reports. Greater trochanteric fractures after THA performed via direct anterior approach are not rare and have an incidence of about 12% because the greater trochanter is sometimes subject to excessive load stress due to the surgical procedure of lifting the femur for preparing the stem installation during surgery [1]. Our patient underwent BS-THA via a posterolateral approach and experienced spontaneous bilateral greater trochanteric fractures within the 20th postoperative day but not immediately after the surgery. Among the reports on fractures after BS-THA in the early postoperative phase, although there is a report of a fracture around the femoral stem occurring after BS-THA was performed using an anterior approach, no case of bilateral postoperative

femoral large trochanter avulsion fractures after BS-THA with a posterior approach has been reported. Thus, to the best of our knowledge, this case is the first to report such fractures.

Fractures are considered to be associated with multiple factors, such as osteopenia, contracture of the gluteus medius, the height and shape of the femoral neck osteotomy due to the stem design, repairing of the posterior soft tissue, increasing tension of the gluteus medius after operation, and the load of muscular strength training.

With regard to osteopenia, preoperative examination revealed that slight osteopenia was observed in the present case. To date, no reports have demonstrated the relationship between the decrease in BMD and fracture at the greater trochanter and showed frequent fractures at the greater trochanter after THA for elderly people with femoral neck

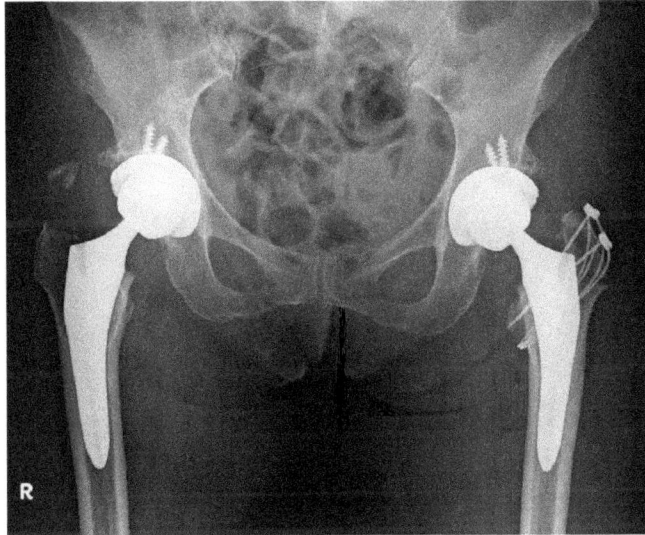

FIGURE 7: On the 20th postoperative day, right coxalgia emerged during a transfer exercise. The greater trochanteric avulsion fracture on the right side was detected on plain radiographs.

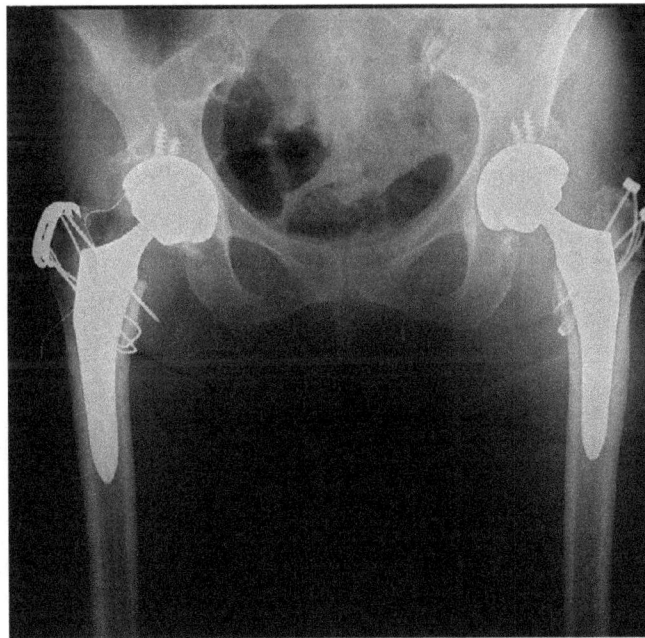

FIGURE 8: On the 27th postoperative day, the right fracture was treated with small plate and wiring.

fractures. Moreover, osteopenia is not considered a primary factor for greater trochanter fractures after THA. Osteopenia may have been a minor contributor to the fracture in this case.

Although severe multidirective preoperative hip joint contractures were not found clearly on medical examination, our patient's preoperative abduction was decreased, suggesting the reduction of gluteus medius extensibility.

The femoral stem design used to be one of the causes of greater trochanter fractures. The design of the Charnley cement stem does not usually require the removal of the cancellous bone in the great trochanter area. On the other hand,

with the condition wherein the shoulder of the cementless stem is larger and in the valgus femur, the remaining cancellous bone of the greater trochanter becomes very thin and brittle. The remaining bone width of the greater trochanter part in this case was not significantly thinner compared to that after THA using other stems. This is because a tapered wedge-type stem with a design that does not overhand the greater trochanter was used, and the height of femoral neck osteotomy was not too far from the top of the great trochanter, which usually occurs. Moreover, it is difficult to conclude based on the almost horizontal fracture line of our patient that the bone holes that were created vertically in the

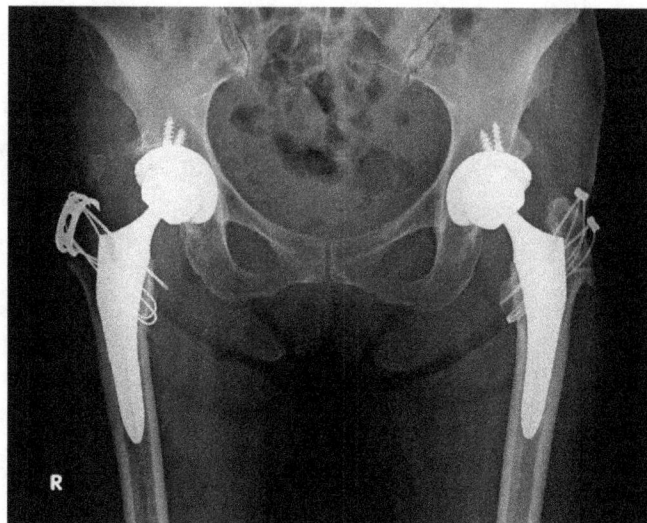

FIGURE 9: At the 18th postoperative month, the right fragment showed slight upper migration.

intertrochanteric posterior crest for the repair of the posterior soft tissue were the main cause. Thus, the kind of stem, osteotomy of the femoral neck fracture, and bone holes are unlikely to be important factors influencing the occurrence of fractures.

It was considered that the spontaneous pelvic coronal tilt toward the surgical side for alleviating the tension of the gluteus muscle, which was often found after unilateral surgery, was difficult to achieve in cases of BS-THA because the pelvis was pulled bilaterally due to the tension of the gluteus muscle, in a manner different from that in unilateral THA. Thus, the tension of the gluteus muscle after BS-THA would be relatively increased when the leg length and offset distance between the pelvis and femur would be longer than those before surgery. Although excessive tension of the affected medial gluteus muscle can be compensated for by abduction of the affected side in unilateral THA, BS-THA cannot prevent the gluteus medius muscle tension at the time of loading. Because the three-dimensional offset of the greater trochanter after operation was longer compared to that before the operation, the tensile strength was more likely to be applied to the attachment part of the greater trochanter gluteus medius muscle, causing fracture at the same part. Because there is no report of a similar case with BS-THA, bilateral great trochanteric fractures after BS-THA in this case are considered to occur due to a complex interaction among several factors.

This report has a limitation in that the cause of the fracture in the present case was not proven with clear evidence. However, to prevent the greater trochanter fracture after BS-THA, surgeons must carefully identify indications in cases with contracture of abduction, small range of motion to adduction, and severe osteoporosis. Additionally, it is necessary to correct the offset such that it is not longer than the preoperative offset.

Disclosure

Before the submission to *Case Reports in Orthopedics*, the manuscript then entitled as "A Case of Greater Trochanteric

Avulsion Fractures after Bilateral Simultaneous Total Hip Arthroplasty" was presented at the "Effort's 2017 Annual Meeting" by Dr. Hiroaki Tagomori in 2017.

Conflicts of Interest

The authors declare that they have no conflict of interest.

Acknowledgments

The authors would like to thank Editage for the English language editing.

References

[1] T. Alexandrov, E. R. Ahlmann, and L. R. Menendez, "Early clinical and radiographic results of minimally invasive anterior approach hip arthroplasty," *Advances in Orthopedics*, vol. 2014, Article ID 954208, 7 pages, 2014.

[2] S. L. Barnett, D. J. Peters, W. G. Hamilton, N. M. Ziran, R. S. Gorab, and J. M. Matta, "Is the anterior approach safe? Early complication rate associated with 5090 consecutive primary total hip arthroplasty procedures performed using the anterior approach," *The Journal of Arthroplasty*, vol. 31, no. 10, pp. 2291–2294, 2016.

[3] A. I. Stavrakis, N. F. SooHoo, and J. R. Lieberman, "Bilateral total hip arthroplasty has similar complication rates to unilateral total hip arthroplasty," *The Journal of Arthroplasty*, vol. 30, no. 7, pp. 1211–1214, 2015.

[4] E. Tsiridis, G. Pavlou, J. Charity, E. Tsiridis, G. Gie, and R. West, "The safety and efficacy of bilateral simultaneous total hip replacement: an analysis of 2063 cases," *The Journal of Bone and Joint Surgery: British Volume*, vol. 90-B, no. 8, pp. 1005–1012, 2008.

[5] J. Parvizi, A. E. Pour, E. L. Peak, P. F. Sharkey, W. J. Hozack, and R. H. Rothman, "One-stage bilateral total hip arthroplasty compared with unilateral total hip arthroplasty," *The Journal of Arthroplasty*, vol. 21, no. 6, pp. 26–31, 2006.

[6] S. Bhan, A. Pankaj, and R. Malhotra, "One- or two-stage bilateral total hip arthroplasty: a prospective, randomised, controlled study in an Asian population," *The Journal of*

Bone and Joint Surgery: British Volume, vol. 88-B, no. 3, pp. 298–303, 2006.

[7] M. E. Berend, M. A. Ritter, L. D. Harty et al., "Simultaneous bilateral versus unilateral total hip arthroplasty: an outcomes analysis," *The Journal of Arthroplasty*, vol. 20, no. 4, pp. 421–426, 2005.

[8] W. L. Jaffe and J. Charnley, "Bilateral Charnley low-friction arthroplasty as a single operative procedure. A report of fifty cases," *Bulletin of the Hospital for Joint Diseases*, vol. 32, no. 2, pp. 198–214, 1971.

26

Klippel–Feil Syndrome with Sprengel Deformity and Extensive Upper Extremity Deformity

John W. Stelzer ⓘ,[1] **Miguel A. Flores,**[2] **Waleed Mohammad,**[3] **Nathan Esplin ⓘ,**[3] **Jonathan J. Mayl,**[3] **and Christopher Wasyliw**[2]

[1]*Department of Orthopaedic Surgery, Massachusetts General Hospital, Harvard Medical School, Boston, MA, USA*
[2]*Department of Diagnostic Radiology, Florida Hospital, Orlando, FL, USA*
[3]*University of Central Florida College of Medicine, Orlando, FL, USA*

Correspondence should be addressed to John W. Stelzer; jwstelzer@gmail.com

Academic Editor: Koichi Sairyo

Introduction. Klippel–Feil syndrome (KFS) is a congenital anomaly resulting from fusion of cervical vertebral bodies secondary to the dysregulation of signaling pathways during somite development. It is commonly associated with scoliosis and Sprengel deformity. We present a case of KFS with commonly associated abnormalities as well as deformities that have not yet been reported in the literature. *Case Presentation.* A 3-year-old girl presented for further evaluation of a left upper extremity deformity following a negative genetic workup. Upon physical exam and radiographic imaging, the patient was diagnosed with KFS and associated abnormalities including cervical scoliosis, Sprengel deformity, and congenital deformity of the left upper extremity. Deformities of the left upper extremity include radioulnar synostosis, a four-rayed hand, and absent thenar musculature. The Sprengel deformity was corrected surgically with a Woodward procedure. *Discussion.* Congenital musculoskeletal deformities can be differentiated based upon spinal and limb embryology. The presence of extraspinal abnormalities not originating from somite differentiation may suggest a severe form of KFS. Important considerations in the workup of the KFS patient include looking for deformities of the shoulder girdle and upper extremities to identify abnormalities for intervention at a young age.

1. Introduction

Klippel–Feil syndrome (KFS) is a congenital anomaly resulting from fusion of cervical vertebral bodies, characterized by the triad of cervical vertebral body fusion, low posterior hairline, and short neck with limited range of motion [1–3]. KFS is a rare condition, seen in approximately 1 in 40,000–42,000 live births with approximately equal distribution in males and females [4–6]. Pathogenesis of the disorder likely involves various dominant and recessive genetic mutations including *GDF6*, *GDF3*, *MEOX1*, and *RIPPLY2* which are responsible for transcription regulation and signaling pathways involved in somite development during embryogenesis [7–12]. KFS may be associated with other deformities, including Sprengel deformity (a congenitally high scapula), scoliosis, hearing impairment, congenital heart disease, lung defects, and genitourinary malformation [13, 14].

2. Case Presentation

The patient is a 3-year-old girl from China who initially presented with an ongoing diagnosis of left upper extremity deformity. Previous radiographs showed a deformity within the left forearm and hand, but left radial aplasia was excluded. Holt–Oram syndrome was previously excluded due to the lack of cardiac malformations and, more definitively, the lack of mutations within the *TBX5* gene. Klippel–Trenaunay syndrome was previously excluded due to the lack of a port-wine stain or other vascular malformations and the absence of limb or tissue overgrowth. Previous genetic testing revealed no mutations within the *PIK3CA* gene, making Klippel–Trenaunay syndrome unlikely.

Physical examination demonstrated a left hand with only four digits, likely from congenital fusion of the first and second digits which functioned as a thumb, opposing to the fifth digit with very good strength. The patient's left forearm measured 2 centimeters shorter than the right with apparent synostosis of the left proximal radioulnar joint. Additionally, the left humerus measured 3 centimeters shorter than the right. The patient was unable to undergo passive pronation or supination of the hand with preserved flexion and extension at the elbow joint. Examination of the patient's back demonstrated a symmetrically higher left scapula with a hard prominence palpable at the cervicothoracic junction.

Initial outside radiographs of the cervical, thoracic, and lumbar spine demonstrated mild scoliosis of the cervical spine. Further imaging revealed partial fusion of the left cervicothoracic spine from C4 to T1 (Figure 1). Elevation of the left scapula with an associated omovertebral bone was also noted (Figures 2 and 3). These findings are consistent with Klippel–Feil syndrome with an associated Sprengel deformity. Additional imaging of the left upper extremity confirmed a proximal radioulnar synostosis (Figure 4). Incidental findings included a left cervical rib and tracheal bronchus. The patient suffered no hearing impairment and no congenital cardiac or genitourinary defects upon further workup. Although genetic testing to further support a diagnosis of KFS was offered, the parents of the patient declined, since the immediate treatment plans would remain unchanged regardless of the results. Additional conditions considered in the patient's differential diagnosis included Poland syndrome and MURCS (müllerian duct aplasia-renal aplasia-cervicothoracic somite dysplasia) association; however, these were unlikely due to the lack of symptomology classically associated with the musculoskeletal deformities seen in each condition.

3. Discussion

Klippel–Feil syndrome was described over 100 years ago by Maurice Klippel and André Feil. However, opinions regarding associated abnormalities and treatment options are still evolving [2, 3]. The classic cervical vertebral abnormalities of KFS are well known and associated with derangements within the signaling pathways during paraxial mesoderm differentiation and somite development [12]. The literature also reports occurrences of KFS with common associated anomalies. Our case is unique due to the multiple extraspinal manifestations identified in a single patient, including Sprengel deformity and significant left upper extremity deformities such as proximal radioulnar synostosis and a four-rayed hand without thenar musculature. To the best of the author's knowledge, oligodactyly with absence of thenar musculature has not yet been reported with KFS.

Cervical scoliosis, which is the most common associated abnormality with KFS, was seen in the case presented. The patient also demonstrated partial fusion of the left cervicothoracic spine from C4 to T1 (Figure 1). Vertebral anomalies at the cervicothoracic junction are secondary only to the C2-C3 junction in prevalence of fusion anomalies [15]. The classification system recently proposed by Samartzis et al. defines the cervical spine fusion patterns for patients with KFS. The classification is determined radiographically such that Type I patients are defined as having a single congenitally fused cervical segment. Type II patients have

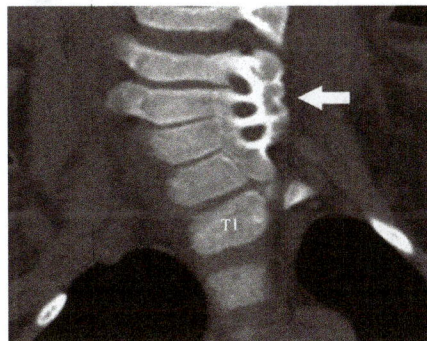

FIGURE 1: CT, coronal reformatted image demonstrates partial fusion involving the left cervicothoracic spine from C4 through T1 in a patient with Klippel–Feil syndrome (arrow). (*Courtesy of Miguel Flores, MD, Orlando, FL.*)

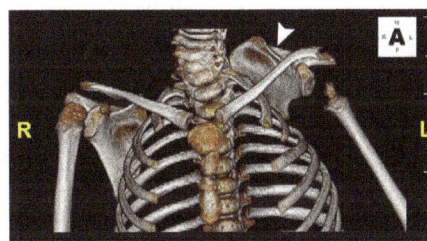

(a)

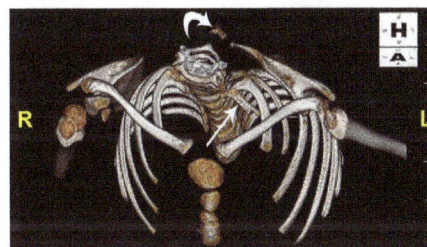

(b)

FIGURE 2: CT, 3D reconstructed images demonstrate Sprengel deformity in a patient with Klippel–Feil syndrome with abnormal elevation of the left scapula (a, arrowhead) and associated omovertebral bone (b, curved arrow). Incidental left cervical rib was also identified (b, arrow). (*Courtesy of Miguel Flores, MD, Orlando, FL.*)

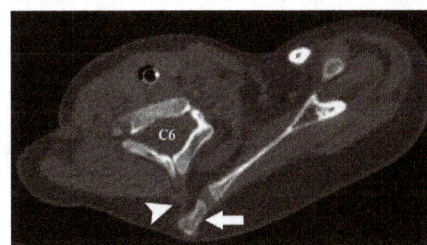

FIGURE 3: CT, axial image demonstrates Sprengel deformity with associated omovertebral bone (arrow) and fibrocartilaginous band (arrowhead). (*Courtesy of Miguel Flores, MD, Orlando, FL.*)

multiple, noncontiguous congenitally fused segments, and Type III patients have multiple contiguous, congenitally fused cervical segments [16]. Under this proposed classification, our patient would be classified as a Type III KFS.

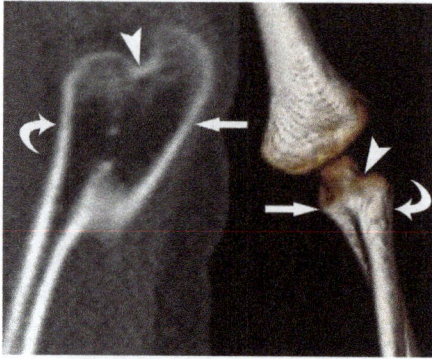

FIGURE 4: CT, sagittal reformatted (*left*) and 3D reconstructed (*right*) images demonstrate left radioulnar (radius = curved arrows, ulna = arrows) synostosis (arrowheads) in a patient with Klippel–Feil syndrome. (*Courtesy of Miguel Flores, MD, Orlando, FL.*)

No surgical intervention, such as disc arthroplasty or fusion of unstable adjacent cervical spine levels, was indicated for our patient, since neurologic symptoms to suggest radiculopathy or myelopathy were not evident. However, Type III KFS patients do have increased risk of developing radiculopathic or myelopathic symptoms when compared to Type I and II patients [16]. Typical age of onset of spine-related neurologic symptoms is between 10 and 11 years of age for KFS patients when the disorder is identified in childhood. However, patients with milder forms of KFS not detected in childhood can present with neurologic symptoms into their 40s [16–18]. For this reason, the patient was encouraged to continue routine follow-up to evaluate for future development of neurological deficit.

In addition to cervical scoliosis, the presence of a Sprengel deformity was identified. This deformity, the second most common deformity associated with KFS, was first described by Eulenberg in 1863 [13, 19]. Years later, others described cases of the congenitally elevated scapula, but it was Otto Sprengel who described the pathology and proposed a theory of its existence in 1891 [20, 21]. The accepted cosmetic classification of Sprengel deformity, the Cavendish classification, was proposed in 1972 [22].

The Cavendish classification system proposed grades based on the deformity. Grade 1 is described as a very mild deformity that is not noticeable when the patient is dressed. Grade 2 is described as a mild deformity that is visible as a lump in the web of the neck when the patient is dressed. Grade 3 is a moderate deformity described as an easily visible deformity with the shoulder joint elevated 2–5 centimeters. Grade 4 is a severe deformity with shoulder joint elevation greater than 5 centimeters or evidence of the superior angle of the scapula near the occiput with or without webbing. Grading can be difficult because of the variation in appearance within a single grade. Although this classification does not consider function, it is utilized in the management of the deformity for objective differentiation when surgical intervention is necessitated to correct both appearance and function.

In the case of our patient, the left shoulder was elevated with scapular elevation to the level of C4-5 on CT imaging (Figure 2), translating clinically to a Grade 3 Sprengel

deformity according to the Cavendish classification. The undescended scapula seen in Sprengel deformity is at times fixed in place to the adjacent vertebra by a pathognomonic omovertebral bone or fibrocartilaginous bridge preventing necessary scapular rotation during arm abduction past 90° (Figure 3) [23]. The arm is often unable to abduct and continue over the head due to the downward-facing glenoid cavity which may develop in the setting of a severely malrotated scapula.

The treatment for Sprengel deformity depends on the severity of the abnormality. For mild deformities classified as Cavendish Grades 1 and 2, nonsurgical options including physical therapy, stretching, and continued observation are most beneficial for the prevention of torticollis and decreased range of motion. Moderate and severe deformities that fall into the higher Cavendish classification grades are candidates for surgical intervention. Many surgical procedures for Sprengel deformity correction have been discussed in the literature, but the hallmark techniques involve resection of the omovertebral bone, if present, with caudal relocation of the scapula. Two of the most popular procedures are the Green's and Woodward procedures.

Green's procedure entails detaching muscles from their scapular insertion, elevating the trapezius muscle, and detaching the supraspinatus from the scapula followed by excision of the omovertebral bone. The supraspinous fossa of the scapula is resected, while being cautious not to injure the suprascapular neurovasculature, and the latissimus dorsi and serratus anterior are detached from the scapula as well. Once the scapula is descended to the corrected position, the muscles are reattached to it. Modifications have been made to the initial Green's procedure including a clavicular osteotomy to reduce the risk of brachial plexus injury, dissection of the insertion of the serratus anterior, and suturing of the inferior pole of the scapula to the thoracic cage into a pocket of the latissimus dorsi muscle [24].

The Woodward procedure was described in 1961 and is often the operation of choice for deformity correction. The procedure involves detaching the trapezius, rhomboid, and levator scapulae muscles at the midline origin followed by removing the omovertebral bone. Next, prominent bony portions of the scapula are removed as well, as the scapula is pulled downward and the muscle attachments are reattached distally to help secure the lowered scapula [25].

Surgical correction is recommended at a young age, usually between 3 and 8 years. However, a few studies have suggested that age does not influence outcomes [26, 27]. Since a higher-grade Sprengel deformity limits the patient's function by impeding necessary rotation of the scapula and shoulder girdle, surgical correction of the Sprengel deformity was indicated in our patient. Surgical correction would improve both function and aesthetics.

Limitations and complications specific to the surgical procedures for Sprengel deformity correction include hypertrophic scarring, regrowth of the resected bone, neurologic injury to the brachial plexus, and scapular winging [28–32]. Although cosmetic and functional improvements are not always optimally restored to normal, the improvements seen in the aesthetics and function of the scapula can be very significant. The mean arm abduction improvements in studies with correctional surgery for Sprengel deformity have been reported between 49° and 77°. Additionally, the mean improvement of Cavendish grading has been reported from 1.5 to 2.0 grades lower in follow-up studies after surgical correction [28, 33–38].

The Sprengel deformity was not the only musculoskeletal abnormality resulting in physical limitation. The patient's left upper extremity syndactyly and proximal radioulnar synostosis (Figure 4) only allowed for flexion and extension at the elbow joint. Pronation and supination were not possible secondary to the proximal radioulnar synostosis that kept the left arm fixed in 10 degrees of pronation. Surgical correction to restore pronation and supination, however, was not advised. Surgical correction for congenital radioulnar synostosis is rarely indicated except in cases of severe deformity (i.e., ≥60° of pronation) due to high recurrence rates and therefore was not performed [39–41].

4. Conclusion

Congenital musculoskeletal deformities can be differentiated based on mechanisms of spinal and limb embryology. The presence of extraspinal manifestations, not originating from somite differentiation, may be indicative of a more severe form of Klippel–Feil syndrome. Important considerations in the workup of the KFS patient include looking for deformities of the shoulder girdle and upper extremities. Identifying these associated abnormalities early is paramount to assess for potential surgical intervention at a young age.

Conflicts of Interest

The authors declare that they have no conflicts of interest.

References

[1] D. Samartzis, P. Kalluri, J. Herman, J. P. Lubicky, and F. H. Shen, ""Clinical triad" findings in pediatric Klippel-Feil patients," *Scoliosis and Spinal Disorders*, vol. 11, p. 15, 2016.

[2] M. Klippel and A. Feil, "Un cas d'absence des vertebres cerivales. Avec cage thoacique remontant jusqu'a la base lu crane (cage thoracique cervicale)," *Nouvelle Iconographie de la Salpêtrière*, vol. 25, pp. 223–250, 1912.

[3] A. Feil, *L'absence et la diminuation des vertebres cervicales (etude cliniqueet pathogenique); le syndrome dereduction numerique cervicales*, Ph.D. thesis, Université de Paris, Paris, France, 1919.

[4] E. O. Da Silva, "Autosomal recessive Klippel-Feil syndrome," *Journal of Medical Genetics*, vol. 19, no. 2, pp. 130–134, 1982.

[5] C. H. Gunderson, R. H. Greenspan, G. H. Glaser, and H. A. Lubs, "The Klippel-Feil syndrome: genetic and clinical reevaluation of cervical fusion," *Medicine*, vol. 46, no. 6, pp. 491–512, 1967.

[6] R. C. Juberg and J. J. Gershanik, "Cervical vertebral fusion (Klippel-Feil) syndrome with consanguineous parents," *Journal of Medical Genetics*, vol. 13, no. 3, pp. 246–249, 1976.

[7] M. Tassabehji, Z. M. Fang, E. N. Hilton et al., "Mutations in GDF6 are associated with vertebral segmentation defects in Klippel-Feil syndrome," *Human Mutation*, vol. 29, no. 8, pp. 1017–1027, 2008.

[8] M. Ye, K. M. Berry-Wynne, M. Asai-Coakwell et al., "Mutation of the bone morphogenetic protein GDF3 causes ocular and skeletal anomalies," *Human Molecular Genetics*, vol. 19, no. 2, pp. 287–298, 2010.

[9] F. Bayrakli, B. Guclu, C. Yakicier et al., "Mutation in MEOX1 gene causes a recessive Klippel-Feil syndrome subtype," *BMC Genetics*, vol. 14, p. 95, 2013.

[10] J. Y. Mohamed, E. Faqeih, A. Alsiddiky, M. J. Alshammari, N. A. Ibrahim, and F. S. Alkuraya, "Mutations in MEOX1, encoding mesenchyme homeobox 1, cause Klippel-Feil anomaly," *American Journal of Human Genetics*, vol. 92, no. 1, pp. 157–161, 2013.

[11] E. Karaca, O. O. Yuregir, S. T. Bozdogan et al., "Rare variants in the notch signaling pathway describe a novel type of autosomal recessive Klippel-Feil syndrome," *American Journal of Medical Genetics Part A*, vol. 167a, no. 11, pp. 2795–2799, 2015.

[12] K. M. Kaplan, J. M. Spivak, and J. A. Bendo, "Embryology of the spine and associated congenital abnormalities," *Spine Journal*, vol. 5, no. 5, pp. 564–576, 2005.

[13] R. N. Hensinger, J. E. Lang, and G. D. MacEwen, "Klippel-Feil syndrome; a constellation of associated anomalies," *Journal of Bone and Joint Surgery, American Volume*, vol. 56, no. 6, pp. 1246–1253, 1974.

[14] W. B. Moore, T. J. Matthews, and R. Rabinowitz, "Genitourinary anomalies associated with Klippel-Feil syndrome," *Journal of Bone and Joint Surgery, American Volume*, vol. 57, no. 3, pp. 355–357, 1975.

[15] D. Samartzis, J. Herman, J. P. Lubicky, and F. H. Shen, "Sprengel's deformity in Klippel-Feil syndrome," *Spine*, vol. 32, no. 18, pp. E512–E516, 2007.

[16] D. D. Samartzis, J. Herman, J. P. Lubicky, and F. H. Shen, "Classification of congenitally fused cervical patterns in Klippel-Feil patients: epidemiology and role in the development of cervical spine-related symptoms," *Spine*, vol. 31, no. 21, pp. E798–E804, 2006.

[17] A. Reyes-Sanchez, B. Zarate-Kalfopulos, and L. M. Rosales-Olivares, "Adjacent segment disease in a patient with Klippel-Feil syndrome and radiculopathy: surgical treatment with two-level disc replacement," *SAS Journal*, vol. 1, no. 4, pp. 131–134, 2007.

[18] S. A. Mirhosseini, S. M. M. Mirhosseini, R. Bidaki, and A. P. Boshrabadi, "Sprengel deformity and Klippel-Feil syndrome leading to cervical myelopathy presentation in old age," *Journal of Research in Medical Sciences*, vol. 18, no. 6, pp. 526–528, 2013.

[19] M. Eulenberg, "Casuistische Mittelheilungen aus dem Gembeite der Orthopadie," *Archiv fuer Klinische Chirurgie*, vol. 4, pp. 301–311, 1863.

[20] T. Kolliker, "Mittheilungen aus der chirurgischen Casuistik und Kleinere Mittheilungen. Bemerkungen zum Aufsatze von Dr. Sprengel. Die angeborene Verschiebung des Schulterblattes nach oben," *Archiv für Klinische Chirurgie*, vol. 42, p. 925, 1891.

[21] O. Sprengel, "Die angeborene Verschiebung des Schulterblattes nach oben," *Archiv für Klinische Chirurgie*, vol. 42, pp. 545–549, 1891.

[22] M. E. Cavendish, "Congenital elevation of the scapula," *Journal of Bone and Joint Surgery, British Volume*, vol. 54, no. 3, pp. 395–408, 1972.

[23] Y. Mikawa, R. Watanabe, and Y. Yamano, "Omoclavicular bar in congenital elevation of the scapula. A new finding," *Spine*, vol. 16, no. 3, pp. 376-377, 1991.

[24] G. Andrault, F. Salmeron, and J. M. Laville, "Green's surgical procedure in Sprengel's deformity: cosmetic and functional results," *Orthopaedics & Traumatology: Surgery & Research*, vol. 95, no. 5, pp. 330–335, 2009.

[25] D. P. Grogan, E. A. Stanley, and W. P. Bobechko, "The congenital undescended scapula. Surgical correction by the Woodward procedure," *Journal of Bone and Joint Surgery, British Volume*, vol. 65, no. 5, pp. 598–605, 1983.

[26] B. Greitemann, J. J. Rondhuis, and A. Karbowski, "Treatment of congenital elevation of the scapula. 10 (2–18) year follow-up of 37 cases of Sprengel's deformity," *Acta Orthopaedica Scandinavica*, vol. 64, no. 3, pp. 365–368, 1993.

[27] A. Khairouni, H. Bensahel, Z. Csukonyi, Y. Desgrippes, and G. F. Pennecot, "Congenital high scapula," *Journal of Pediatric Orthopaedics B*, vol. 11, no. 1, pp. 85–88, 2002.

[28] A. A. Ahmad, "Surgical correction of severe Sprengel deformity to allow greater postoperative range of shoulder abduction," *Journal of Pediatric Orthopaedics*, vol. 30, no. 6, pp. 575–581, 2010.

[29] J. L. Borges, A. Shah, B. C. Torres, and J. R. Bowen, "Modified Woodward procedure for Sprengel deformity of the shoulder: long-term results," *Journal of Pediatric Orthopaedics*, vol. 16, no. 4, pp. 508–513, 1996.

[30] P. Farsetti, S. L. Weinstein, R. Caterini, F. De Maio, and E. Ippolito, "Sprengel's deformity: long-term follow-up study of 22 cases," *Journal of Pediatric Orthopaedics B*, vol. 12, no. 3, pp. 202–210, 2003.

[31] W. G. Carson, W. W. Lovell, and T. E. Whitesides Jr., "Congenital elevation of the scapula. Surgical correction by the Woodward procedure," *Journal of Bone and Joint Surgery, American Volume*, vol. 63, no. 8, pp. 1199–1207, 1981.

[32] D. M. Ross and R. L. Cruess, "The surgical correction of congenital elevation of the scapula. A review of seventy-seven cases," *Clinical Orthopaedics and Related Research*, no. 125, pp. 17–23, 1977.

[33] S. J. Leibovic, M. G. Ehrlich, and D. J. Zaleske, "Sprengel deformity," *Journal of Bone and Joint Surgery, American Volume*, vol. 72, no. 2, pp. 192–197, 1990.

[34] M. Bellemans and J. Lamoureux, "Results of surgical treatment of Sprengel deformity by a modified Green's procedure," *Journal of Pediatric Orthopaedics B*, vol. 8, no. 3, pp. 194–196, 1999.

[35] I. McMurtry, G. C. Bennet, and C. Bradish, "Osteotomy for congenital elevation of the scapula (Sprengel's deformity)," *Journal of Bone and Joint Surgery, British Volume*, vol. 87, no. 7, pp. 986–989, 2005.

[36] D. C. Mears, "Partial resection of the scapula and a release of the long head of triceps for the management of Sprengel's deformity," *Journal of Pediatric Orthopaedics*, vol. 21, no. 2, pp. 242–245, 2001.

[37] J. J. Masquijo, O. Bassini, F. Paganini, R. Goyeneche, and H. Miscione, "Congenital elevation of the scapula: surgical treatment with Mears technique," *Journal of Pediatric Orthopaedics*, vol. 29, no. 3, pp. 269–274, 2009.

[38] Z. M. Zhang, J. Zhang, M. L. Lu, G. L. Cao, and L. Y. Dai, "Partial scapulectomy for congenital elevation of the scapula," *Clinical Orthopaedics and Related Research*, vol. 457, pp. 171–175, 2007.

[39] J. E. Cleary and G. E. Omer Jr., "Congenital proximal radio-ulnar synostosis. Natural history and functional assessment," *Journal of Bone and Joint Surgery, American Volume*, vol. 67, no. 4, pp. 539–545, 1985.

[40] D. L. Fernandez and E. Joneschild, ""Wrap around" pedicled muscle flaps for the treatment of recurrent forearm synostosis," *Techniques in Hand and Upper Extremity Surgery*, vol. 8, no. 2, pp. 102–109, 2004.

[41] J. M. Failla, P. C. Amadio, and B. F. Morrey, "Post-traumatic proximal radio-ulnar synostosis. Results of surgical treatment," *Journal of Bone and Joint Surgery, American Volume*, vol. 71, no. 8, pp. 1208–1213, 1989.

27

Reconstruction of Acute Patellar Tendon Rupture after Patellectomy

Kenjiro Fujimura [D],[1,2] **Koji Sakuraba,**[1,2] **Satoshi Kamura,**[1,2] **Kiyoshi Miyazaki,**[1,2] **Nobuo Kobara,**[1,2] **Kazumasa Terada,**[1,2] **and Hisaaki Miyahara**[1,2]

[1]*Clinical Research Institute, National Hospital Organization, Kyushu Medical Center, Fukuoka, Japan*
[2]*Department of Orthopaedic Surgery, National Hospital Organization, Kyushu Medical Center, Fukuoka, Japan*

Correspondence should be addressed to Kenjiro Fujimura; ksytfuji@gmail.com

Academic Editor: Georg Singer

Acute rupture of the knee extensor mechanism after patellectomy is extremely rare. We present the case of a patient with acute patellar tendon rupture who had undergone patellectomy 53 years before. Twelve days after the injury, the ruptured patellar tendon was repaired with end-to-end suture. Postoperatively, we splinted the knee for 6 weeks but permitted the patient to walk without limiting weight bearing at 1 week postoperatively. At one-year follow-up, the patient is able to move his knee almost full range of motion and the Lysholm knee score is 81. The patient is satisfied with the outcome. This is the first report to treat acute rupture of the patellar tendon in a patient who had undergone patellectomy. Although careful rehabilitation is required, end-to-end suture might be an adequate surgical procedure for acute rupture of the knee extensor mechanism after patellectomy.

1. Introduction

The most frequent cause of failure of the knee extensor mechanism is patellar fracture, while ruptures of the patellar tendon or quadriceps tendon are comparatively rare. Patellar tendon ruptures are reportedly the least frequent cause of knee extension failure [1–4]. Moreover, as patellectomy is only performed when there are no other methods for reconstructing the patella [3, 5], this procedure is currently rarely performed. Thus, acute rupture of the knee extensor mechanism after patellectomy is extremely rare. In fact, there is only one case report on acute quadriceps tendon rupture after patellectomy [6], while acute patellar tendon rupture after patellectomy has not yet been reported in the English literature.

The present report describes the case of a 73-year-old male patient who ruptured his left patellar tendon 53 years following patellectomy. The treatment modality and the outcome are presented.

2. Case Report

A 73-year-old male had a traffic accident while riding his bicycle and hit his left knee on the ground. He presented at our hospital 4 days after the accident. He could walk without crutches but could not extend his knee against gravity. We palpated a subcutaneous depression in the left knee.

The patient was 165.5 cm tall, weighed 63.8 kg, and had a BMI of $23.3 \, \text{kg/m}^2$. He had previously experienced a comminuted left patellar fracture and underwent a total patellectomy when he was 20 years old. After the patellectomy, he had no complaints and had a full range of movement in the left knee. The preinjury Lysholm knee score was 90 [7]. At 57 years of age, the patient had received mitral valve replacement for regurgitation at another hospital and had been on anticoagulant therapy since then.

Plain radiographic examination did not show any fracture of the left knee but detected the absence of the

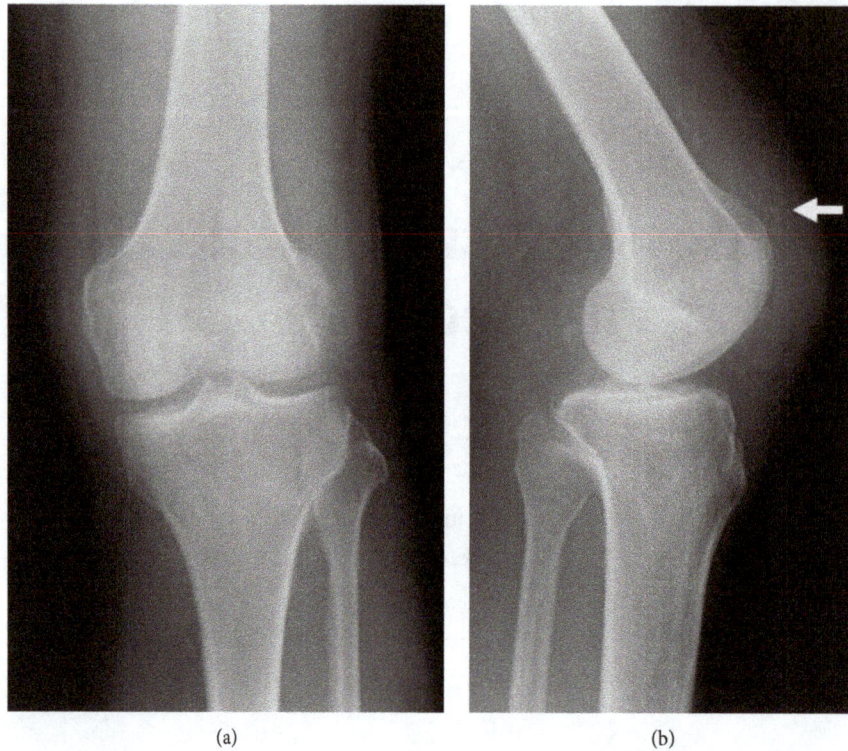

FIGURE 1: Plain radiographic anteroposterior view (a) and lateral view (b) of the left knee showing the absence of a patella and the presence of a small heterotopic calcification (white arrow) at the distal side of the quadriceps tendon.

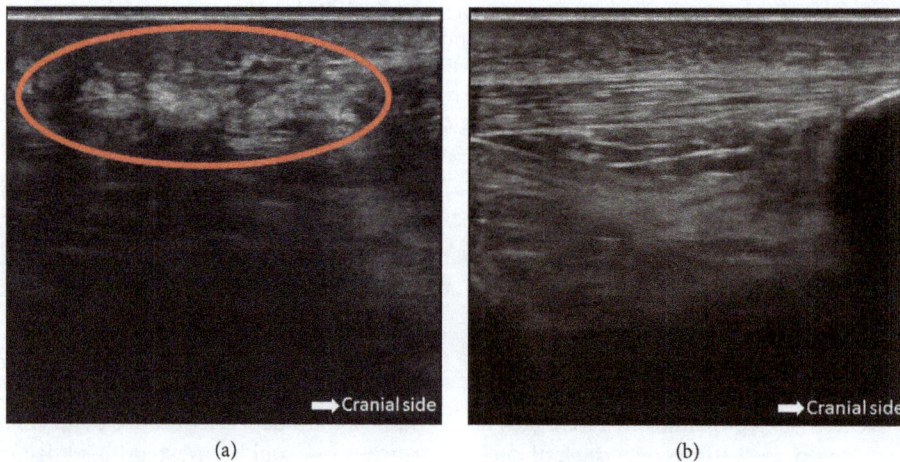

FIGURE 2: Ultrasound examination showed a loose patellar tendon (within red circle) (a) compared with the contralateral side (b). The right is the cranial side, and the patella can be seen on the far right in (b).

patella and a small heterotopic calcification at the distal side of the quadriceps tendon (Figure 1). Ultrasound examination showed a loose left patellar tendon compared with the contralateral side (Figure 2), although it could not identify the rupture site. Magnetic resonance imaging (MRI) revealed subcutaneous edema and tendon disruption at the proximal side of the left patellar tendon, which indicated patellar tendon rupture (Figure 3). We immediately immobilized the left knee with a splint and changed his anticoagulant therapy from warfarin to intravenous heparin.

Surgery to reconstruct the ruptured left patellar tendon was performed 12 days after the accident. We made a midline incision instead of an oblique incision along the previous scar and found a complete patellar tendon rupture with both medial and lateral patellar retinaculum rupture with about a 2.0 cm gap filled with a hematoma (Figure 4(a)). These ruptures were at the proximal side of the patellar tendon. We first washed and removed the hematoma and refreshed the ruptured tendon edge with scissors. The length of remained patellar tendon was about 5 cm. We then

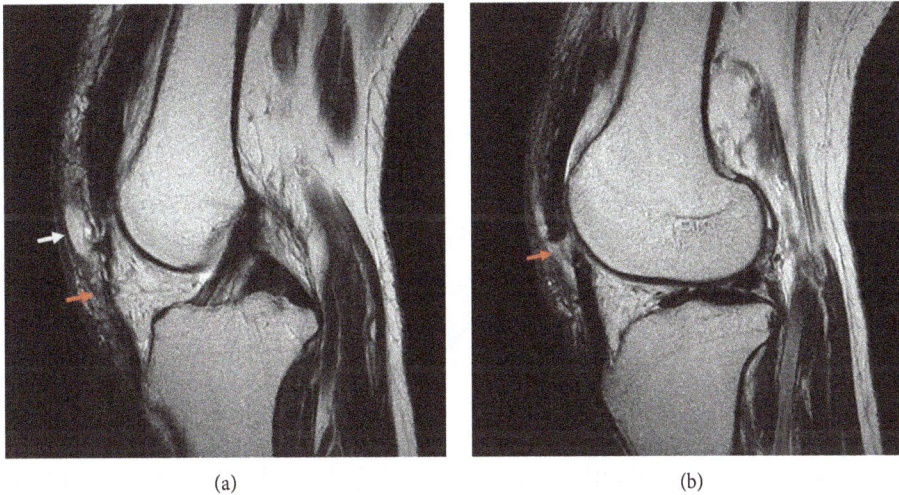

(a)   (b)

FIGURE 3: T2-weighted magnetic resonance imaging showed a loose patellar tendon (red arrow) and subcutaneous edema (white arrow) (a) and tendon disruption (red arrow) (b) at the proximal side of the patellar tendon.

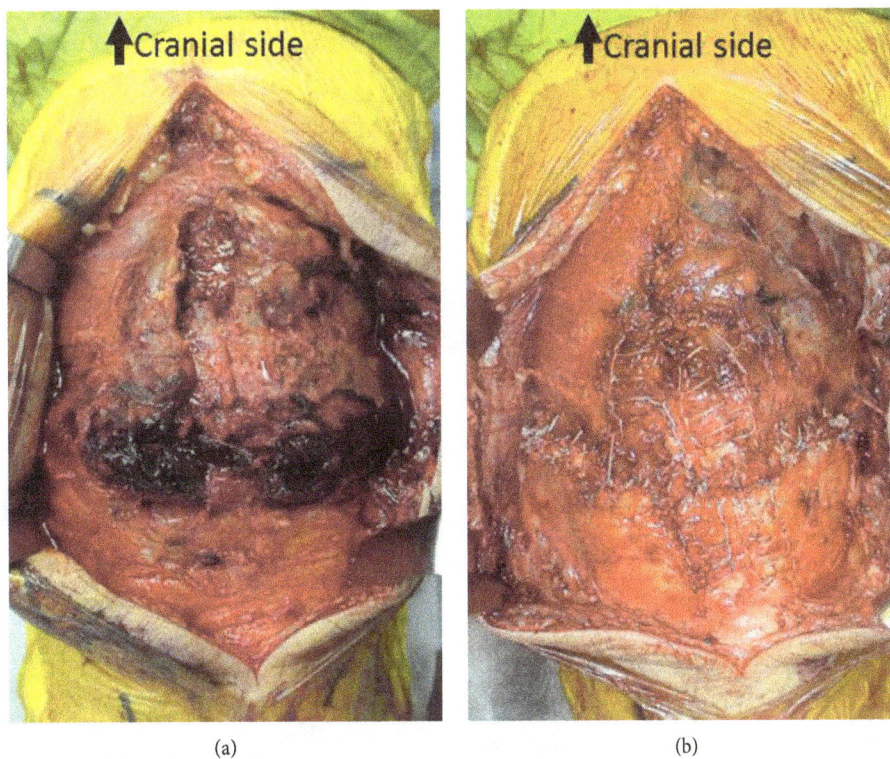

(a)   (b)

FIGURE 4: Intraoperative photographs. The top is cranial and the bottom is caudal. The patellar tendon and patellar retinaculum were completely ruptured. Hematoma filled the rupture site (a). We performed end-to-end suture with two Krackow locking stitches and figure-of-eight sutures (b).

performed end-to-end suturing with two Krackow locking stitches with #2 Hifi high-strength suture (CONMED, NY, USA) and added approximately twenty figure-of-eight sutures with #0 Hifi high-strength suture (Figure 4(b)).

Postoperatively, the left knee was protected with a splint for 6 weeks. The patient was permitted to walk without limiting weight bearing at 1 week postoperatively. After 6 weeks, knee flexion exercise was started, but the knee was protected in extension with a knee brace during walking for another 6 weeks. At postoperative 3 months, the patient could walk without any difficulty and could almost fully flex his left knee but had an extensor lag of 20° and left quadriceps muscle atrophy. Currently (at 1 year postoperatively), the patient can extend his knee with almost no extension lag and can flex fully but has persistent quadriceps muscle atrophy. The Lysholm knee score at 1 year postoperatively is 81. The patient is satisfied with the outcome.

Written consent was obtained from the patient for publication of the study.

3. Discussion

The knee extensor mechanism is comprised of the patella, quadriceps tendon, and patellar tendon. Loss of the knee extensor mechanism is most commonly caused by patellar fracture. Patellar tendon rupture is the rarest cause of knee extensor failure, and this mainly occurs due to indirect trauma in patients under 40 years of age [1–4]. Ruptures usually occur in weakened tendons that have degenerative changes caused by iterative microtrauma, local corticosteroid injections, or systemic diseases such as diabetes, thyroid disorders, renal disease, hyperlipidemia, and systemic inflammatory diseases [1–3]. Traumatic patellar tendon rupture is also reported [2], as seen in the present case. Currently, total patellectomy is considered the final method for treating severe osteomyelitis, severe comminuted fractures, or open fracture with bone loss, as clinical outcomes are unsatisfactory [3, 5]. Hence, it is extremely rare to encounter rupture of the knee extensor mechanism after patellectomy, and only few cases have been reported [6, 8–10]. Shanmugam and Maffulli reported the first case of acute quadriceps tendon rupture in a patient with patellectomy [6]. There are three other reports on rupture of the patellar tendon after patellectomy [8–10]; all of these ruptures occurred at the site of the tibial tubercle and were successfully treated at the chronic phase with either an Achilles tendon allograft [8], the iliotibial band from the contralateral side [9], or the gracilis and semitendinosus tendons [10]. This is the first report of treatment of an acute rupture of the patellar tendon in a patient who had previously undergone patellectomy. The present patient incurred this rupture by direct trauma, similarly to the patient in the report by Shanmugam and Maffulli [6].

Ultrasound and MRI examinations are reportedly better at diagnosing chronic patellar tendon ruptures compared with acute cases [3]. In the present case, ultrasound examination could not reveal the rupture site but detected only the loose patellar tendon; however, MRI examination was useful to detect the existence of a rupture at the patellar tendon side. Although loss of the knee extensor mechanism can be diagnosed relatively easily by palpation of a subcutaneous depression and failure of active knee extension [3], it might be difficult to determine the location of the rupture site in patients without a patella. The present case findings suggest that imaging examinations are also effective to clarify the details of the extensor mechanism of the knee.

Surgical treatment is required for patellar tendon rupture. In particular, end-to-end suture is selected for full-body rupture. Although reinforcement frames are often added to support the suture and avoid rerupture [2, 3], we selected end-to-end suture without reinforcement frames in the present case, as Shanmugam and Maffulli reported the successful use of this method [6]. They performed continuous

locked suture with heavy absorbable sutures [6]; however, we selected two Krackow locking stitches with approximately twenty figure-of-eight sutures with nonabsorbable suture material, as we considered that this would provide adequate strength. Shanmugam and Maffulli examined the teared tendon margins histopathologically and found chronic hypoxic tendon degeneration [6]. Although we did not perform such an analysis, we considered that the present case would likely have had the same findings. Hence, we also resected and refreshed the tendon margin to prevent failure of the suture site.

In terms of the timing of surgery, Siwek and Rao reported that the result of delayed repair (more than 2 weeks after injury) was worse than that of immediate repair [11]. Another report recommended that the repair should be performed within 1 week of injury to achieve satisfactory results, and they performed surgery within 24 hours of the injury [6]. However, there are cases in which surgery cannot be performed immediately because of comorbidities or anticoagulant therapy, such as in the present case. Although some studies report that early mobilization results in a favorable outcome [12–14], strict immobilization with a walking cast is generally recommended to avoid suture failure. Previous reports have recommended a duration of immobilization of at least 1 month [3] and at least 6 weeks [2]. Moreover, Langenhan et al. found no significant differences between limited versus early functional rehabilitation protocol after surgical repair of quadriceps tendon rupture [15]. Our patient could have started knee flexion exercise earlier, but we immobilized his knee with a splint for 6 weeks because we selected elective surgery.

This is the first report of treatment of acute rupture of the patellar tendon in a patient who had undergone patellectomy, and the outcome was satisfactory. From our patient's favorable result and as reported previously [6], end-to-end suture without reinforcement frames is adequate for treating acute phase rupture of the extensor mechanism of the knee, even in patients who have undergone patellectomy.

Conflicts of Interest

The authors declare that they have no conflicts of interest.

Acknowledgments

The authors thank Kelly Zammit, BSc, BVSc, from the Edanz Group (www.edanzediting.com/ac) for editing a draft of this manuscript.

References

[1] M. R. Garner, E. Gausden, M. B. Berkes, J. T. Nguyen, and D. G. Lorich, "Extensor mechanism injuries of the knee: demographic characteristics and comorbidities from a review of 726 patient records," *Journal of Bone and Joint Surgery-American Volume*, vol. 97, no. 19, pp. 1592–1596, 2015.

[2] A. Roudet, M. Boudissa, C. Chaussard, B. Rubens-Duval, and D. Saragaglia, "Acute traumatic patellar tendon rupture: early and late results of surgical treatment of 38 cases,"

Orthopaedics & Traumatology: Surgery & Research, vol. 101, no. 3, pp. 307–311, 2015.

[3] D. Saragaglia, A. Pison, and B. Rubens-Duval, "Acute and old ruptures of the extensor apparatus of the knee in adults (excluding knee replacement)," *Orthopaedics & Traumatology: Surgery & Research*, vol. 99, no. 1, pp. S67–S76, 2013.

[4] R. A. E. Clayton and C. M. Court-Brown, "The epidemiology of musculoskeletal tendinous and ligamentous injuries," *Injury*, vol. 39, no. 12, pp. 1338–1344, 2008.

[5] C. Gwinner, S. Märdian, P. Schwabe, K. D. Schaser, B. D. Krapohl, and T. M. Jung, "Current concepts review: fractures of the patella," *GMS Interdisciplinary Plastic and Reconstructive Surgery DGPW*, vol. 5, 2016.

[6] C. Shanmugam and N. Maffulli, "Traumatic quadriceps rupture in a patient with patellectomy: a case report," *Journal of Medical Case Reports*, vol. 1, p. 146, 2007.

[7] J. Lysholm and J. Gillquist, "Evaluation of knee ligament surgery results with special emphasis on use of a scoring scale," *American Journal of Sports Medicine*, vol. 10, no. 3, pp. 150–154, 1982.

[8] D. C. Wascher and C. D. Summa, "Reconstruction of chronic rupture of the extensor mechanism after patellectomy," *Clinical Orthopaedics and Related Research*, vol. 357, pp. 135–140, 1998.

[9] P. M. Poonnoose, R. J. Korula, and A. T. Oommen, "Chronic rupture of the extensor apparatus of the knee joint," *Medical Journal of Malaysia*, vol. 60, no. 4, pp. 511–513, 2005.

[10] C. C. Donken, J. J. Caron, and M. H. Verhofstad, "Functional reconstruction of a chronically ruptured extensor apparatus after patellectomy," *Journal of Knee Surgery*, vol. 22, no. 4, pp. 378–381, 2009.

[11] C. W. Siwek and J. P. Rao, "Ruptures of the extensor mechanism of the knee joint," *Journal of Bone & Joint Surgery*, vol. 63, no. 6, pp. 932–937, 1981.

[12] J. G. Enad and L. L. Loomis, "Primary patellar tendon repair and early mobilization: results in an active-duty population," *Journal of the Southern Orthopaedic Association*, vol. 10, no. 1, pp. 17–23, 2001.

[13] R. A. Marder and L. A. Timmerman, "Primary repair of patellar tendon rupture without augmentation," *American Journal of Sports Medicine*, vol. 27, no. 3, pp. 304–307, 1999.

[14] J. L. West, J. S. Keene, and L. D. Kaplan, "Early motion after quadriceps and patellar tendon repairs: outcomes with single-suture augmentation," *American Journal of Sports Medicine*, vol. 36, no. 2, pp. 316–323, 2008.

[15] R. Langenhan, M. Baumann, P. Ricart et al., "Postoperative functional rehabilitation after repair of quadriceps tendon ruptures: a comparison of two different protocols," *Knee Surgery, Sports Traumatology, Arthroscopy*, vol. 20, no. 11, pp. 2275–2278, 2012.

28

A Novel Minimally Invasive Reduction Technique by Balloon and Distractor for Intra-Articular Calcaneal Fractures

M. Prod'homme ⓘ, **S. Pour Jafar, P. Zogakis, and P. Stutz**

Orthopedic Surgery Department, Riviera-Chablais Hospital, Montreux, Switzerland

Correspondence should be addressed to M. Prod'homme; marcprod86@gmail.com

Academic Editor: Stamatios A. Papadakis

Treatment of displaced intra-articular fractures of the calcaneus remains a challenge for the orthopaedic surgeon. Conservative therapy is known to produce functional impairment. Surgical approach is plagued by soft-tissue complications and insufficient fracture reduction. We describe a minimally invasive technique that will hopefully improve these issues. We want to present our first experience through two cases. The first was a 46-year-old man who presented with a Sanders type IIBC calcaneal fracture, and the second was a 86-year-old woman with a type IIIBC calcaneal fracture. We introduced 2 Schanz screws in the talus and the calcaneus. After distraction, we introduced an inflatable balloon inside the calcaneus. By inflating the balloon, the articular surface was reduced by lifting it up. Then bone cement was injected in order to maintain the reduction. Additional screw fixation was used in the young patient. Postoperative imaging showed good congruence of the subtalar joint without leakage of cement, for the two cases. After 2 months, the patients had no pain and were without soft-tissue complications. We advocate this technique to perform a minimally invasive reduction and fixation of intra-articular calcaneal fractures because it preserves soft-tissues and provides good clinical results with early weight-bearing.

1. Introduction

Calcaneal fractures account for approximately 2% of all fractures, with displaced intra-articular fractures between 60 and 75% of these injuries [1].

Several treatment options are suggested: conservative, including cast immobilisation and/or Harris' traction; surgical, including percutaneous pinning, open reduction and internal fixation, primary arthrodesis and external fixation [2]. The question of surgical versus nonoperative treatment in calcaneal fractures is still controversial with no obvious benefit for some authors [3]. The main surgical difficulties are the reduction of the fracture and the approach. Especially with open approaches, soft-tissue damage is a well-known issue [4].

The calcaneus is continuously subjected to compressive forces with the articular facets of the midfoot and the subtalar joint. Fractures in this area lead to limitation in everyday activities and work [2, 4]. The fees for accident insurance,

such as the Suva (Schweizerische Unfallversicherungsanstalt) in Switzerland [5], are substantial: the treatment fees in Swiss Franc were a mean of 19,210 (range 581–49,843). The insurance costs were a mean of 60,656 (range 1759–159,539). The Suva indemnified a mean of 182 days off.

Many authors recommend minimally invasive procedure with good results, supported by studies comparing open fixation and minimally invasive treatment [6] with excellent American Orthopaedic Foot and Ankle Society (AOFAS) scale results [7, 8]. Using Schanz pins and Kirschner wires, cannulated screws, arthroscopically guided percutaneous fixation, and application of bone substitute, with lower complication rates found, the procedures were considered as promising [9].

We present two cases of intra-articular calcaneal fractures, treated by an innovative minimally invasive technique using the combination of a talocalcaneal distractor and a balloon to perform the reduction of the fracture.

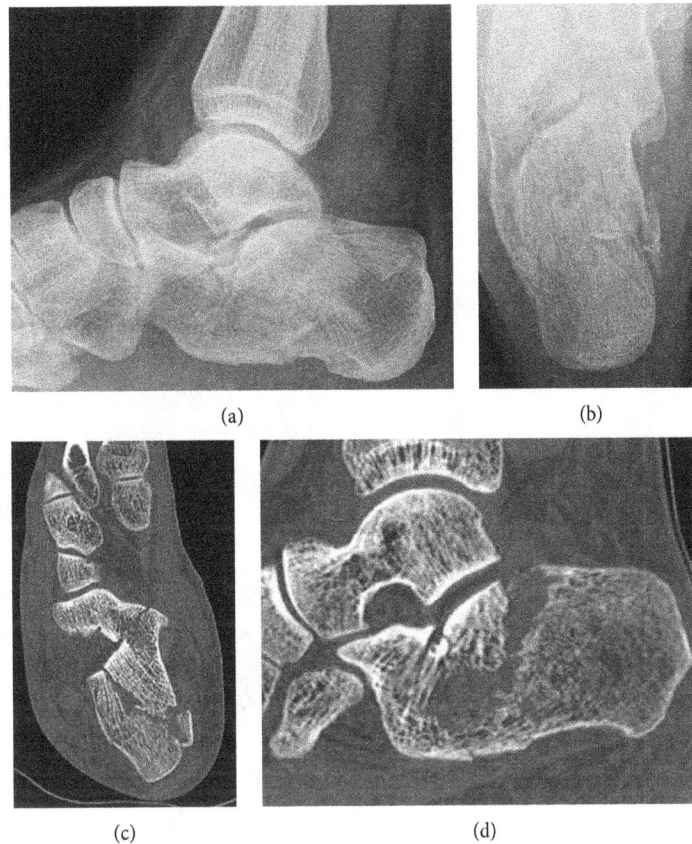

FIGURE 1: Preoperative imaging of the left foot. The upper part revealed a multifragmentary fracture of the calcaneus, with a Boehler's angle of 5 degrees. The CT scan permitted to classify the fracture as a Sanders type IIBC.

2. Cases Presentation

2.1. Case 1. A 46-year-old man fell from a stepladder corresponding to a height of 1.5 meters hitting his right heel. There was no torsion of his ankle. He presented with heel pain, increased by motion. We hospitalized him in our Orthopedic Surgery Department in order to investigate his lesions and perform the surgical procedure.

Clinically, he presented with a total functional impotence of his right foot. There was a lateral ankle oedema but no trophic complication. Passive mobilization of his ankle was painful, same as the palpation on the external collateral ligament and the Chopart joint. The Lisfranc joint was painless, and there was no laxity. There was no neurologic or vascular impairment.

The X-ray of the foot showed an intra-articular calcaneal fracture with a Boehler's angle of 5 degrees, as we can see in Figure 1. The contralateral Boehler's angle was measured as 26 degrees on another X-ray. The CT scan (Figure 1) revealed a multifragmentary fracture of the calcaneus, with a depression of the articular surface. There was also an impingement of the articular surface, on the internal and posterior part. There was no injury of the cuboidocalcaneal articular surface. According to Sanders [4], we classified the fracture as a type IIBC.

2.1.1. Surgical Technique. After few days of bed rest, surgery was performed in a ventral position and under general anesthesia. Cefazolin was used for antibiotic prophylaxis. No tourniquet was applied. Under control by image intensifier and by way of stab incisions, we introduced two 4 mm Schanz screws from the posterior side into the talus and the calcaneus. The center of the achilles tendon was longitudinally split before introducing the Schanz screw. Using the distraction device of an external fixator (Hoffmann, Stryker®), we distracted the subtalar joint by counterbalancing the forces of the sural triceps. This also produces a rotation in extension of the posterior fragment and thus a preliminary reduction. By way of a third stab incision, the tip of a Jamshidi needle (Medtronic®) was placed beneath the impacted anterior aspect of the posterior talar joint surface. The needle was replaced by a trocar whose end has the form of a halfpipe. A balloon (Inflate FX™ Gen II Kit, Medtronic) was then introduced into the trocar. By inflating the balloon with Iopamiro® until 400 psi, the depressed joint surface was lifted up and thus disimpacted, respectively, and anatomically reduced. The balloon was then deflated and removed. The cavity which was produced by the balloon was filled with about 4 to 7 cc absorbable phosphocalcic cement (injectable bone void filler; Kyphon®, Medtronic Spine LLC®) in the younger patient or PMMA in the older lady. In the young patient, a screw (diameter 4.0 mm, Synthes®) was introduced such as pointing the cuboidocalcaneal joint. Skin closure was performed by using standard suture. Both patients were operated by the senior author. The main steps are represented in Figure 2.

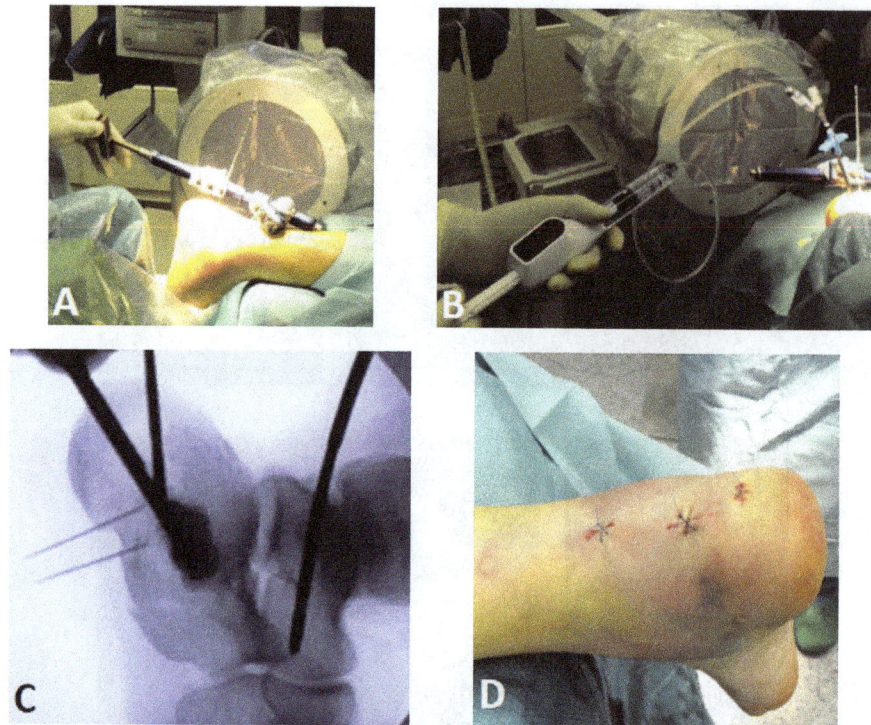

FIGURE 2: Operative procedure steps: (a) distractor use, (b) balloon reduction, (c) fluoroscopic control, and (d) skin incisions at the end of surgery.

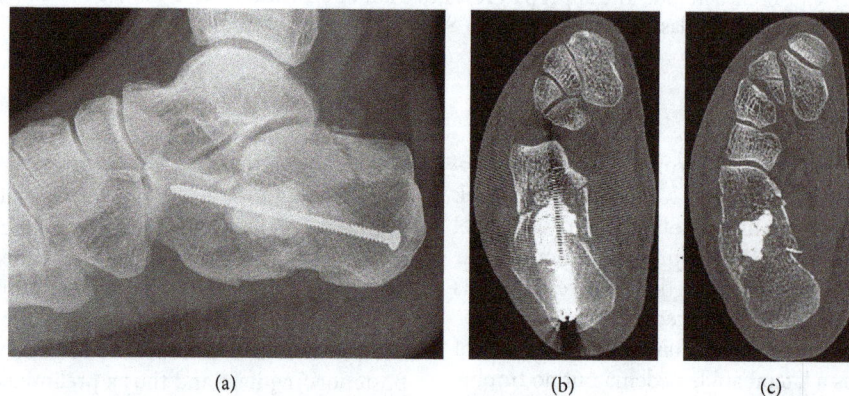

FIGURE 3: Postoperative imaging, showing a good reduction of the subtalar joint, with a Boehler's angle of 24 degrees, satisfying axis of the calcaneus, and no leakage of cement.

2.1.2. Follow-Up. We reported no intraoperative nor postoperative complication. The postoperative evolution was uneventful without any soft-tissue problem and with optimal pain control. 15 kg of weight-bearing was recommended since the first postoperative day. For prophylaxis of thromboembolism, Dalteparin natrium was administered daily (5000 IU sc) for the first 10 days and then switched to rivaroxaban (10 mg po per day) for 2 months.

The postoperative imaging of his right foot was in order (Figure 3).

The patient was discharged from the hospital at postoperative day 3.

We reassessed the patient at 2 months. Clinically, he had no pain. The tibiotalar motion was normal, but the talocalcaneal one was 70% of the opposite side. The X-ray revealed a Boehler's angle of 18 degrees versus 24 degrees postoperatively. The CT scan confirmed a partial (25%) lack of the initial reduction (Figure 4).

To prevent from a secondary displacement, we advocated the patient to keep 15 kg weight-bearing on his right foot, during the next two weeks. And after that time, normal weight-bearing was allowed.

After two years, the patient had an AOFAS score of 83/100 which means a good result.

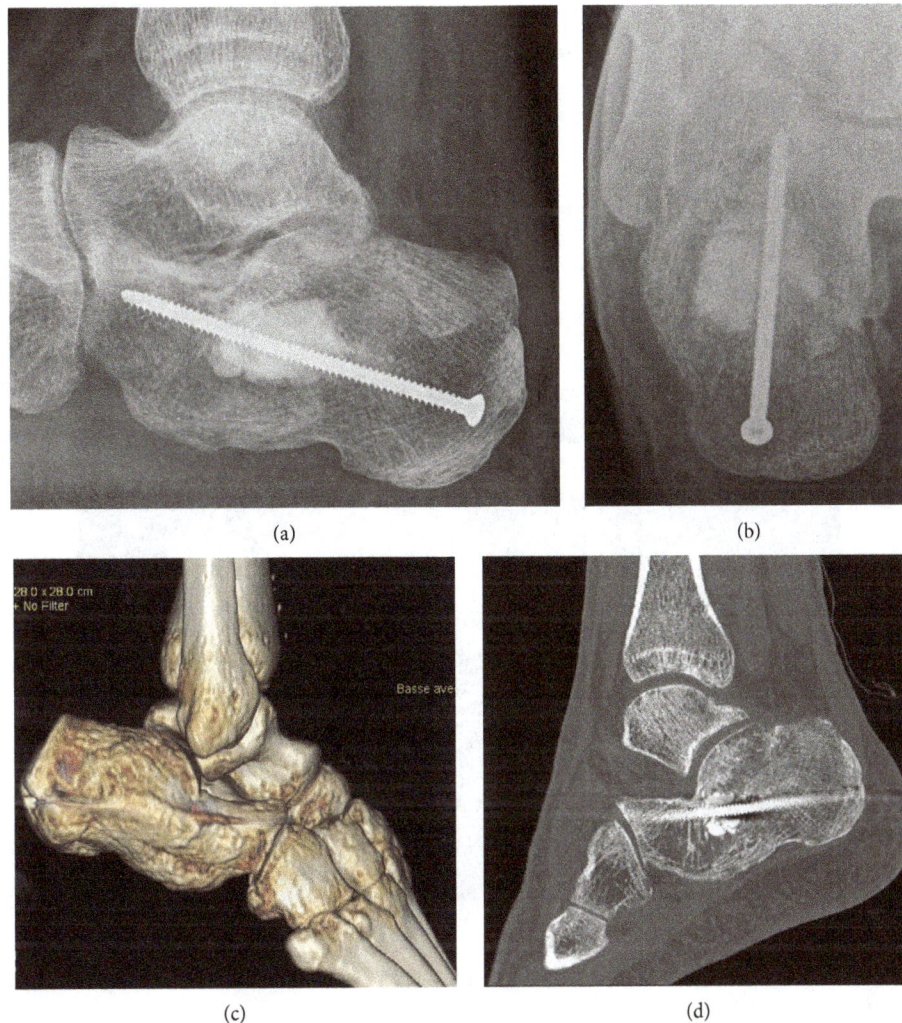

(a)

(b)

(c)

(d)

FIGURE 4: Imaging after 2 months, revealed a partial lack of fracture reduction, but good signs of bone healing.

2.2. Case 2. Our second patient was an 86-year-old woman with comorbidities, such as active tobacco abuse and osteoporosis, treated by clopidogrel. She fell from her height, describing torsion of her right ankle after walking on a stone. She presented with ankle hematoma and limping with functional impotence of her foot. There was severe pain at the palpation of the lateral malleolus and of the lateral collateral ligament. Ankle and foot motions were limited in all directions. The skin was not impaired.

The radiographs of the foot showed a Boehler's angle evaluated less than 5 degrees (Figure 5) and a comminuted fracture of the median and anterior parts of the calcaneus, especially with an intra-articular fracture at the level of the posterior subtalar joint, matching with severe osteoporosis.

The CT scan revealed an osteoporotic bony destructive fracture, more precisely of the average and anterior part of the calcaneus bone. There was a fracture regarding the posterior subtalar joint. We classified it as a Sanders type IIIBC [4].

The surgical approach and the procedure were the same as previously described, except that no screw was inserted

and we introduced PMMA cement inside the bone defect, because of severe osteoporosis.

Postoperative imagings (Figure 6) revealed a satisfying alignment of the bone fragments, with a Boehler's angle at 33 degrees (contralateral side was measured at 36 degrees) and a regular subtalar surface.

The stab incisions presented no complication. The patient could bear full weight-bearing on her right foot with the protection of a simple ankle and foot splint for a 2-month duration. The patient was discharged at postoperative day 10 to enter a rehabilitation center.

We assessed the patient at 2 months postoperative. The injured foot showed a good alignment. The tibiotalar joint motion was about 30 to 40% of the contralateral side. She had no pain. Nevertheless, the X-rays showed a Boehler's angle fall from 32 degrees postoperative to 13 degrees (69%). Unfortunately, after two years of follow-up, the patient was not achievable by phone and deceased.

None of the patients required any reoperation. None of them had pain at follow-up, and no joint subsidence nor arthritis was observed.

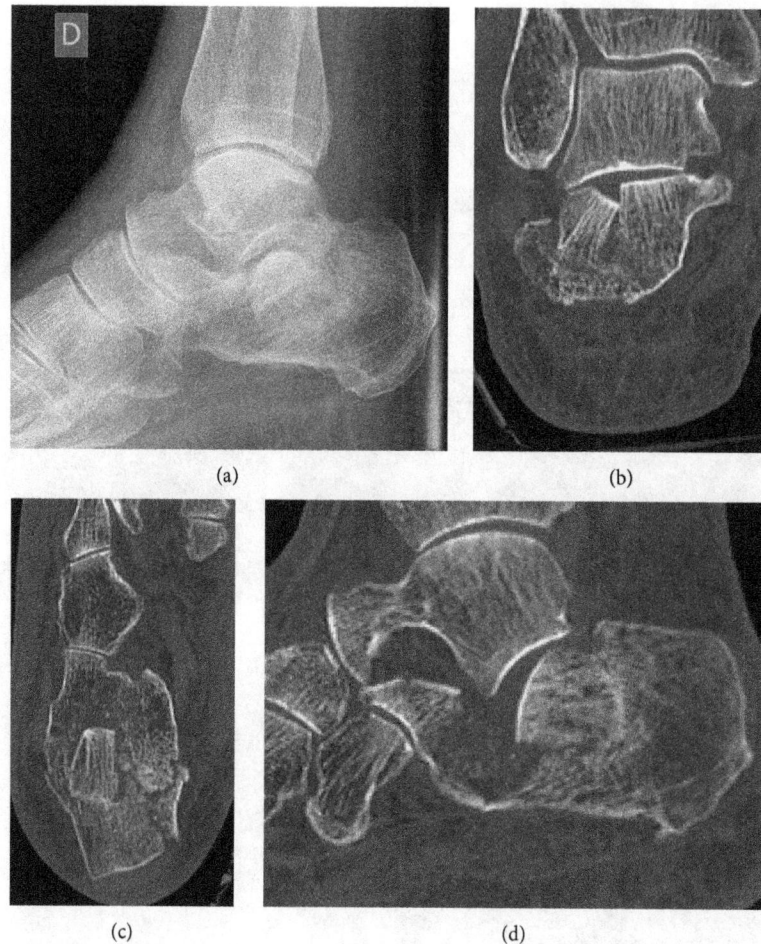

FIGURE 5: Preoperative radiographs and CT scan of the right foot, confirmed a bony destructive Sanders type IIIBC fracture with a Boehler's angle of less than 5 degrees.

3. Discussion

Nowadays, the still remaining challenges for the orthopaedic surgeon are the approach and reduction of the calcaneal fracture. Using our described technique, we performed a minimally invasive approach, to decrease soft-tissue damage. Postoperatively, the results were good about pain and motion in the two cases. Malawski and Pomianowski had the same results described in a case reported in 2013 [10]. They used a similar technique for the reduction, with a screw into the talus and calcaneus each, but inserted medially. However, they performed the reduction of the anterior facet by additional maneuvers. Clinically, at 6 months after surgery, normal hindfoot alignment was observed as well as normal range of motion of the ankle joint. The X-rays revealed a fracture union with good shape, but the Boehler's angle decreased to 19 degrees (versus 24 postoperative). According to the Creighton-Nebraska, AOFAS, and Maryland Foot Scores, very good results were observed.

The main argument in favour of our technique is the initial reduction. Thanks to the Schanz screws distraction and the balloon, the intra-articular part of the calcaneal fracture was well reduced, even for the bony destructive fracture.

Thanks to our spine surgery experience, we could similarly utilize an inflatable balloon in corporeal vertebral fracture reductions, according to the balloon kyphoplasty (BK) technique, which is a modified vertebroplasty technique. Vertebroplasty is the standard treatment employed for vertebral compression fractures (VCFs) due to osteoporosis. BK is a minimally invasive procedure that aims to relieve pain, restore vertebral height, and correct kyphosis of the spine. During this procedure, an inflatable bone tamp is inserted into the collapsed vertebral body so as to reduce the fracture. We made use of the procedure with the same objectives, adapted to the calcaneal fracture, to perform the surgery. The devices are well known, their advantages and their own issues. The outcomes described by the Ontario Health Technology [11] showed that BK to treat pain associated with VCFs due to osteoporosis was as effective as vertebroplasty at relieving pain, and it restores the height of the affected vertebra and results in lower fracture rates in other vertebrae compared with vertebroplasty and in fewer neurological complications due to cement leakage compared with vertebroplasty. These results were experienced by the retrospective study from Lee et al. [12], which reported a significantly better quality of life in the group treated by

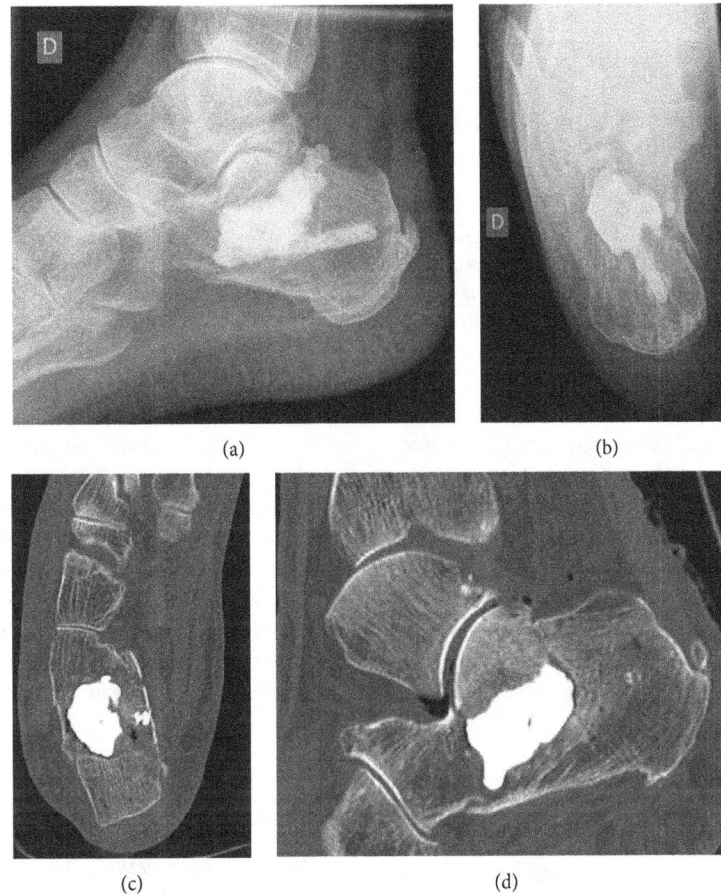

(a)　　　　　　　　　　　　　　(b)

(c)　　　　　　　　　　　　　　(d)

FIGURE 6: On the upper part, postoperative radiographs showed a Boehler''s angle from 33 degrees. On the lower part, postoperative CT scan showed satisfying alignment of the bone fragments, with presence of a discrete diastasis at the level of the posterior subtalar fracture, but without irregularity of the articular surface.

kyphoplasty than in the group treated by vertebroplasty, especially regarding mobility, pain, anxiety, and depression.

An in vitro cadaveric specimens' study from Broome and colleagues assessed the balloon-assisted technique in other indications than VCFs [13]. They assessed 6 proximal tibias and 6 distal radii with a fine-cut microcomputed tomography after creating intra-articular depression fractures and treated them by using a balloon-assisted technique, compared with conventional metal tamp. They showed that the inflatable bone tamp was successful in reducing all distal radius fractures without intra-articular complication, such as overreduction or penetration into the joint, and was even superior to the conventional technique when comminution was present at the articular surface, with minimal residual deformity.

The main limit of our technique was the difficulty to maintain the fracture reduction. The 2-month consultation revealed a partial leakage of postoperative Boehler's angle, despite the respect of no weight-bearing on the foot in case 1. This could be explained by the initial comminution of the fracture, which made the stabilization more difficult, and probably a continuous passive traction by the sural triceps. We supposed that the fracture needed a stronger way to stabilize it, compensating the potential lever arm created by the muscles of the calf, evaluated at 2535 N while walking [14].

But the comminution prevented from doing it with additional screws or K-wires. Probably, another choice would have been to put more cement inside the bone defect, until a partial overcorrection. However, this concept was not supported by the outcomes of Persson's study in 2014 which concluded to avoid surgical overcorrection of the Boehler's angle [15].

Balloon kyphoplasty to treat calcaneal fractures was one of the few described methods in the literature (Table 1). The first publishing was made by Bano et al. in 2009 through a single case [16]. They used a Medtronic inflatable balloon and manometer and made use of calcium phosphate cement. As a result, they showed no complication, full weight-bearing after 7 days, bone recovery after 12 months, and a good Maryland Foot Score with a CT scan revealing no loss of the fracture reduction at the 2-year follow-up.

Gupta et al. directed a study [17] which showed, through a 11 case series, that patients have demonstrated good outcomes in pain (Analogic Visual Scale ranging from 0 to 5, at 10 months) and motion without evidence of postoperative complications such as wound dehiscence, infection, or loss of reduction.

Two studies were conducted by Jacquot and colleagues and firstly published in 2011 [18] on 4 first cases. They showed a good clinical result on all patients and no need for

TABLE 1: Literature review of balloon calcaneoplasty procedures.

Author, year	Number of cases	Balloon technique	Relevant results
Bano et al., 2009 [16]	1 case	CaP cement	No loss of reduction after 2 years
Gupta et al., 2011 [17]	11 cases	$CaSO_4$ cement + graft	Good results on pain and cutaneous complications
Jacquot and Atchabahian, 2011 [18]	4 cases	PMMA cement	Good clinical results after 3 years, displacement < 1 mm
Jacquot et al., 2013 [19]	10 cases	PMMA cement	Mean Boehler angle 15°, 1 subtalar arthritis
Mauffrey et al., 2012 [20]	1 case	Cement + cannulated screw	No complication, good radiological consolidation
Biggi et al., 2013 [21]	11 cases	9 PMMA, 2 CaP cement	Mean Boehler angle 22.97°, 1 subtalar arthritis
Vittore et al., 2014 [22]	20 cases	Ca3P cement + KW 7 days	Mean Boehler angle 25°, 1 subtalar arthritis

CaP = calcium phosphate; CaSO4 = calcium sulfate; PMMA = polymethyl methacrylate; Ca3P = calcium triphosphate; KW = Kirschner wires.

further surgery. They had no pain at the 3-year follow-up for two of them and occasional weather-related pain for the two remaining. They all returned to work and life activities without any limitation. They used a minimally cutaneous approach and then reported no soft-tissue complication. They demonstrated that balloon kyphoplasty to treat calcaneal fractures on a limited series of patients without any risk factors of poor outcome is feasible and may be promising. Later, they published their five-year experience study on 10 patients, and among them one was a bilateral, thus totaling 11 calcaneal fractures [19]. They reported a mean AOFAS score of 84.5 (range from 27 to 100), with a mean Boehler's angle of 15.9 degrees, nearby our radiological results. Only one patient had a poor AOFAS score (27) because of subtalar osteoarthritis. Finally, all patients resumed their work activities at the same level than before the occurrence of the fracture.

Mauffrey and colleagues, in 2012, published their balloon reduction technique through one case of a calcaneal fracture classified Sanders type IV [20]. They described the procedure and pitfalls (top door effect, balloon burst, and cement extravasation) that the surgeon needs to consider.

Furthermore, Biggi et al. [21] published about 11 cases of percutaneous calcaneoplasty. They performed a balloon-assisted reduction and used PMMA cement on 9 cases and calcium phosphate cement on 2 cases. They obtained a postoperative mean Boehler angle of 22.97°, with a mean preoperative angle of 9.91°. Their AOFAS scores after an average of 24 months were excellent in six cases, good in four, and fair in one due to subtalar arthritis.

Finally, Vittore et al. published their results about 20 fractures of the os calcis, treated by a balloon-assisted reduction and a calcium phosphate cement fixation, helped by Kirschner wires [22]. The wires were removed at the seventh day after surgery, and then full weight-bearing was allowed. They showed a mean postoperative Boehler's angle of 25.05 degrees (range from 8 to 36). They reported that AOFAS scores ranged as follows: 4 excellent, 7 good, 6 fair and 3 poor. One patient had secondary subtalar arthritis. They concluded that their approach was associated with pain relief at the first postoperative day, early mobilization, and the tricalcium phosphate cement is a resorbable bone substitute that allows a fair bone stock for hindfoot fusion procedure.

More evidence is needed, despite the good clinical results of the technique described as promising by several authors on short series. A prospective trial with a large sample of patients would be required to assess these options. We advocate the use of the Schanz distractor and the balloon-assisted technique to reduce and treat intra-articular calcaneal fractures, because it provides a good reduction, especially of the intra-articular part which is the most important for the future mobility of the hindfoot and recovering of the gait, and it provides a minimally invasive approach, indicator of a low risk of soft-tissue complications. However, the stabilization of the fracture, on radiological results, remains a concern which should be addressed in further refinements of the technique.

Consent

The young patient gave his written and signed consent for publication. The old patient was already deceased, so her family gave her oral consent for publication.

Conflicts of Interest

The authors declare that they have no conflicts of interest.

References

[1] R. Sanders and M. Clare, *Calcaneus Fractures, Rockwood and Green's Fractures in Adults*, vol. 1, Lippincott Williams & Wilkins, Philadelphia, PA, USA, 7th edition, 2010.

[2] R. R. Ramos, C. D. C. de Castro Filho, R. R. Ramos et al., "Surgical treatment of intra-articular calcaneal fractures: description of a technique using an adjustable uniplanar external fixator," *Strategies in Trauma and Limb Reconstruction*, vol. 9, no. 3, pp. 163–166, 2014.

[3] D. Griffin, N. Parsons, E. Shaw et al., "Operative versus non-operative treatment for closed, displaced, intra-articular fractures of the calcaneus: randomised controlled trial," *BMJ*, vol. 349, p. g4483, 2014.

[4] R. Sanders, "Current concepts review-displaced intra-articular fractures of the calcaneus*," *Journal of Bone and Joint Surgery*, vol. 82, no. 2, pp. 225–250, 2000.

[5] *Pool SSAA, LAA 2005–2009, état +4 ans, auteur: szt/VTS*, https://www.unfallstatistik.ch/f/publik/publikationen_f.htm.

[6] Q. Wang, X. Li, Y. Sun, L. Yan, C. Xiong, and J. Wang, "Comparison of the outcomes of two operational methods

used for the fixation of calcaneal fracture," *Cell Biochemistry and Biophysics*, vol. 72, no. 1, pp. 191–196, 2015.

[7] A. Battaglia, P. Catania, S. Gumina, and S. Carbone, "Early minimally invasive percutaneous fixation of displaced intra-articular calcaneal fractures with a percutaneous angle stable device," *Journal of Foot and Ankle Surgery*, vol. 54, no. 1, pp. 51–56, 2015.

[8] C. X. Lin, Z. Y. Shi, Y. M. Xu et al., "Treatment of calcaneal fractures by fixation of Kirschner needle and thread cancellous bone screw through sinus tarsi interstice," *Zhongguo gu Shang = China Journal of Orthopaedics and Traumatology*, vol. 27, no. 7, pp. 551–554, 2014.

[9] K. J. Wallin, D. Cozzetto, L. Russell, D. A. Hallare, and D. K. Lee, "Evidence-based rationale for percutaneous fixation technique of displaced intra-articular calcaneal fractures: a systematic review of clinical outcomes," *Journal of Foot and Ankle Surgery*, vol. 53, no. 6, pp. 740–743, 2014.

[10] P. Malawski and S. Pomianowski, "Minimally invasive reposition of intraarticular calcaneal fractures: a case report," *Polish Orthopedics and Traumatology*, vol. 78, pp. 193–200, 2013.

[11] Medical Advisory Secretariat, "Balloon kyphoplasty: an evidence-based analysis," *Ontario Health Technology Assessment Series*, vol. 4, no. 12, pp. 1–45, 2004.

[12] S. K. Lee, S. H. Lee, S. P. Yoon, Y. T. Lee, G. Jang, S. Y. Lim et al., "Quality of life comparison between vertebroplasty and kyphoplasty in patients with osteoporotic vertebral fractures," *Asian Spine Journal*, vol. 8, no. 6, pp. 799–803, 2014.

[13] B. Broome, C. Mauffrey, J. Statton, M. Voor, and D. Seligson, "Inflation osteoplasty: in vitro evaluation of a new technique for reducing depressed intra-articular fractures of the tibial plateau and distal radius," *Journal of Orthopaedics and Traumatology*, vol. 13, no. 2, pp. 89–95, 2012.

[14] M. S. Orendurff, A. D. Segal, M. D. Aiona, and R. D. Dorociak, "Triceps surae force, length and velocity during walking," *Gait & Posture*, vol. 21, no. 2, pp. 157–163, 2005.

[15] J. Persson, S. Peters, S. Haddadin, P. F. O'Loughlin, C. Krettek, and R. Gaulke, "The prognostic value of radiologic parameters for long-term outcome assessment after an isolated unilateral calcaneus fracture," *Technology and Health Care*, vol. 23, no. 3, pp. 285–298, 2014.

[16] A. Bano, D. Pasku, A. Karantanas, K. Alpantaki, X. Souvatzis, and P. Katonis, "Intra-articular calcaneal fracture: closed reduction and balloon-assisted augmentation with calcium phosphate cement," *Cases Journal*, vol. 2, no. 1, p. 9290, 2009.

[17] A. K. Gupta, G. S. Gluck, and S. G. Parekh, "Balloon reduction of displaced calcaneus fractures: surgical technique and case series," *Foot and Ankle International*, vol. 32, no. 2, pp. 205–210, 2011.

[18] F. Jacquot and A. Atchabahian, "Balloon reduction and cement fixation in intra-articular calcaneal fractures: a percutaneous approach to intra-articular calcaneal fractures," *International Orthopaedics*, vol. 35, no. 7, pp. 1007–1014, 2011.

[19] F. Jacquot, T. Letellier, A. Atchabahian, L. Doursounian, and J. M. Feron, "Balloon reduction and cement fixation in calcaneal articular fractures: a five-year experience," *International Orthopaedics*, vol. 37, no. 5, pp. 905–910, 2013.

[20] C. Mauffrey, J. R. Bailey, D. J. Hak, and M. E. Hammerberg, "Percutaneous reduction and fixation of an intra-articular calcaneal fracture using an inflatable bone tamp: description of a novel and safe technique," *Patient Safety in Surgery*, vol. 6, no. 1, p. 6, 2012.

[21] F. Biggi, S. Di Fabio, C. D'Antimo, F. Isoni, C. Salfi, and S. Trevisani, "Percutaneous calcaneoplasty in displaced intraarticular calcaneal fractures," *Journal of Orthopaedics and Traumatology*, vol. 14, no. 4, pp. 307–310, 2013.

[22] D. Vittore, G. Vicenti, G. Caizzi, A. Abate, and B. Moretti, "Balloon-assisted reduction, pin fixation and tricalcium phosphate augmentation for calcanear fracture," *Injury*, vol. 45, pp. S72–S79, 2014.

29

Minimally Invasive Plate Osteosynthesis for a Distal Radius Fracture with Forearm Skin Problem

Kiyohito Naito [D],[1] Yoichi Sugiyama,[1] Mayuko Kinoshita,[1] Ahmed Zemirline,[2] Chihab Taleb,[3] Thitinut Dilokhuttakarn,[1,4] Philippe Liverneaux [D],[5] and Kazuo Kaneko[1]

[1]*Department of Orthopaedics, Juntendo University School of Medicine, Tokyo, Japan*
[2]*Centre de la Main de Bretagne, Centre Hospitalier de Saint Grégoire, Saint-Grégoire, France*
[3]*Unité de Chirurgie de la Main et du Poignet, Groupe Hospitalier de Mulhouse, Mulhouse, France*
[4]*Department of Orthopedics, Srinakharinwirot University, Nakhon Nayok, Thailand*
[5]*Department of Hand Surgery, SOS Main, CCOM, University Hospital of Strasbourg, FMTS, University of Strasbourg, Icube CNRS 7357, 10 Avenue Baumann, 67400 Illkirch, France*

Correspondence should be addressed to Kiyohito Naito; knaito@juntendo.ac.jp

Academic Editor: Werner Kolb

In this study, we performed osteosynthesis for a distal radius fracture using a minimally invasive approach for a patient with skin disorder of the forearm and obtained favorable results. This case report may provide new findings confirming the usefulness of this surgical approach for distal radius fractures. Blister formation on the right forearm was observed in a 53-year-old female who was diagnosed with a distal fracture of the right radius and underwent splinting in a local hospital, and she was referred to our hospital 2 days after the injury. Minimally invasive locking plate osteosynthesis was performed, and there was no skin lesion at this incision site. Postoperatively, there were no complications in soft tissues and the operative scar was almost unrecognizable. We reported volar locking plate osteosynthesis using the minimally invasive approach in a patient with skin disorder of the forearm. Such patients are rarely encountered. However, this minimally invasive approach is extremely useful for utilizing the advantages of volar locking plate fixation without being affected by the soft tissue environment.

1. Introduction

In recent years, there have been some studies on a minimally invasive approach in volar locking plate osteosynthesis for distal radius fractures [1, 2]. The feasibility of plate fixation using the Henry approach (10 mm) was already reported [3].

In this study, we performed osteosynthesis for a distal radius fracture using a minimally invasive approach for a patient with skin disorder of the forearm and obtained favorable results. This case report may provide new findings confirming the usefulness of this surgical approach for distal radius fractures.

2. Case Presentation

A 53-year-old female with no previous history visited a local hospital due to right wrist pain and swelling caused by falling. She was diagnosed with a distal fracture of the right radius, underwent splinting, and returned home. When she visited the local hospital again 2 days after the injury, blister formation on the right forearm was observed, and she was referred to our hospital. The blister was observed along the splint application area (Figure 1) and was considered to be due to the heat and stuffiness of the splint. Plain X-ray examination revealed a distal radius fracture accompanied by dorsal displacement of the distal bone fragment (AO classification:

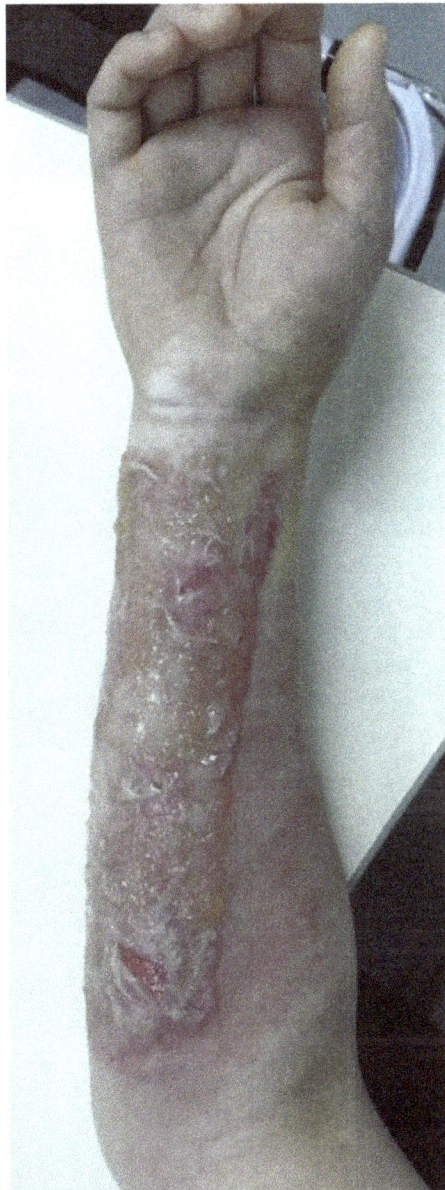

FIGURE 1: The forearm skin state on her visit to our hospital. Skin disorder accompanied by blister formation was observed on the right forearm. The blistering was present along the splint application area.

type A2) (Figures 2(a) and 2(b)). Based on the skin condition, we considered conservative treatment by external fixation using a splint or cast to be difficult, and surgery after improvement of the skin state would be more invasive due to bone union and, therefore, planned minimally invasive locking plate osteosynthesis.

As we previously reported, surgery was performed using the Henry approach through a 10 mm incision starting from 15 mm proximal to the radial styloid process at 9 days after injury [3]. In this patient, there was no skin lesion at this incision site, which allowed this surgical technique (Figure 3(a)). After reduction of the distal bone fragment using a Kirschner wire, osteosynthesis was performed using a volar locking plate (Acu-Loc 2 proximal plate standard, Nihon Medical Next, Osaka Japan) (Figures 3(b) and 3(c)). After the

operation, a favorable alignment was obtained (Figures 3(d) and 3(e)). The wrist was immobilized postoperatively in a bulky dressing without an arm splint until the tissue swelling had decreased.

All muscles, vessels, and nerves of the anterior compartment—except the radial artery—were retracted ulnarly. The pronator quadratus was incised transversely at its distal portion and dissected off the periosteum using a periosteal elevator preserving its ulnar and radial insertions. Therefore, active finger motion was encouraged immediately after the operation and wrist mobilization was started as soon, and as much, as pain allowed. Moreover, this approach can avoid the median nerve damages during the surgery.

Six months after the operation, favorable union of the radius was obtained. The wrist range of motion was as follows: flexion, 70°; extension, 65°; pronation, 85°; and supination, 85°. The visual analogue scale (VAS) was 1/10, and the quick disabilities of the arm, shoulder, and hand (Q-DASH) score was 20.45/100. The Mayo wrist score was 85/100 (excellent). The state of the forearm skin and surgical wound favorably improved (Figure 4), and she returned to her preinjury job.

3. Discussion

Previous studies on volar locking plate osteosynthesis using the minimally invasive approach for distal radius fractures have demonstrated some advantages (the patients' satisfaction level and aesthetically pleasing wound healing) of this technique, but clinical results were similar to those after conventional surgical methods [3, 4]. Authors have reported that there is a wide acceptable range of the reduced position, and anatomical reduction is not always required [5–7]. We have actively used the minimally invasive approach and believe that the advantages of this approach should be reevaluated.

In general, distal radius fractures are conservatively treated by manual reduction and casting [8]. However, this conservative treatment is not indicated for limbs with skin lesions. We previously treated distal radius fractures in limbs containing shunts in dialysis patients with skin fragility using volar locking plate as well as this case [9]. In patients with skin fragility, conservative treatment by splinting or casting is difficult [10, 11]. In addition, percutaneous pinning or external fixation may increase aggravation of skin lesions and infection [12]. Of course, it was also possible to place an external fixator. But, discharge from pin site may continue and this can lead to infection. When priority is given to the avoidance of soft tissue damage, volar locking plate fixation is the only method with fixation force allowing early joint motion at present. From our experience with distal radius fractures patients in limbs containing shunts, we learned that volar locking plate fixation for distal radius fractures is useful and possible by protective manipulation of soft tissue including the skin during operation [9]. This experience was applied to the present case. As shown in Figures 3(a) and 3(b), this surgical technique was possible because there was no skin lesion 15–25 mm proximal to the radial styloid process, which was the skin incision site for the insertion of a volar locking plate.

(a)   (b)

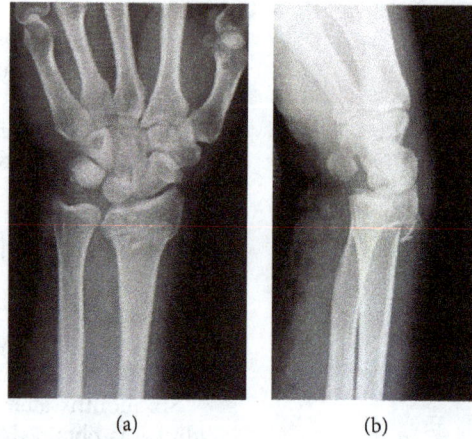

FIGURE 2: Plain X-ray films on her visit to our hospital. (a) Frontal plain X-ray image. (b) Lateral plain X-ray image. Plain X-ray images showed a distal radius fracture accompanied by dorsal displacement of the distal bone fragment. Due to the skin state, conservative treatment by external fixation, such as splinting and casting, was difficult. Surgery after improvement of the skin state was considered to be more invasive due to bone union. Therefore, osteosynthesis using a minimally invasive approach was planned.

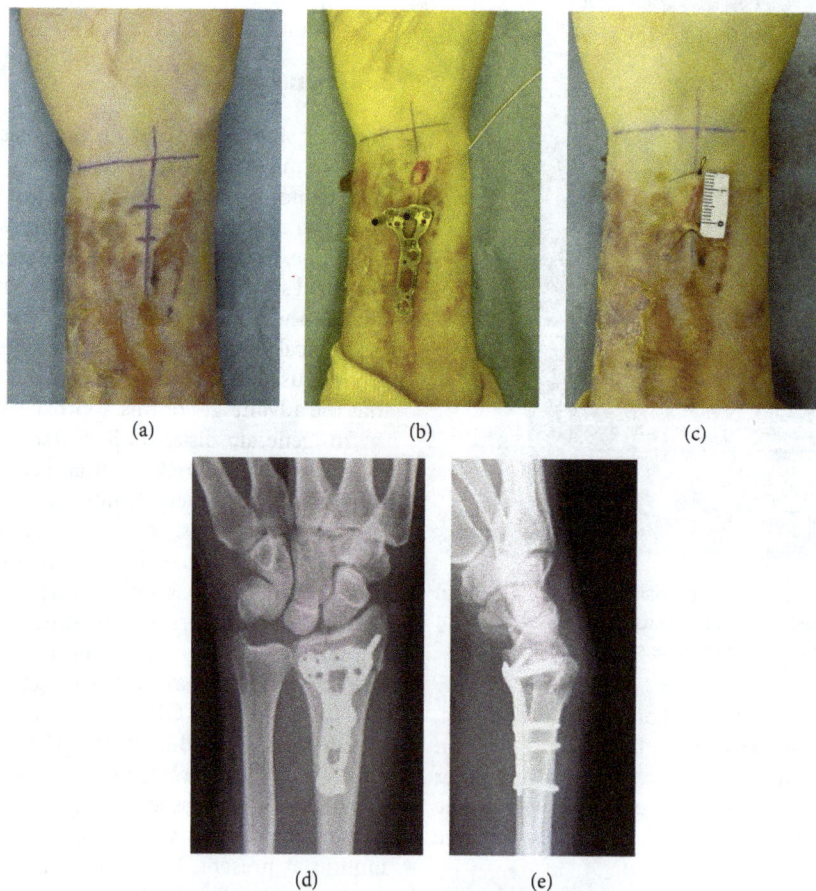

(a)   (b)   (c)

(d)   (e)

FIGURE 3: Findings during operation. (a) Skin incision design. This surgical technique could be performed because there was no skin lesion at the skin incision site. (b, c) Volar locking plate fixation. After reduction of the distal bone fragment using a Kirschner wire, osteosynthesis was performed using a volar locking plate (Acu-Loc 2 proximal plate standard, Nihon Medical Next, Osaka, Japan). (d, e) Plain X-ray images after volar locking plate fixation ((d): frontal image, (e): lateral image). Fixation in a favorably reduced position is observed.

We speculated about the development of the skin disorder in this patient. Some patients with skin disorders due to splinting and casting have been reported [10, 13]. Blister formation and burns at moderate temperatures are widely known and have recently been applied to the production of animal models of burn injury [14]. We speculate that the

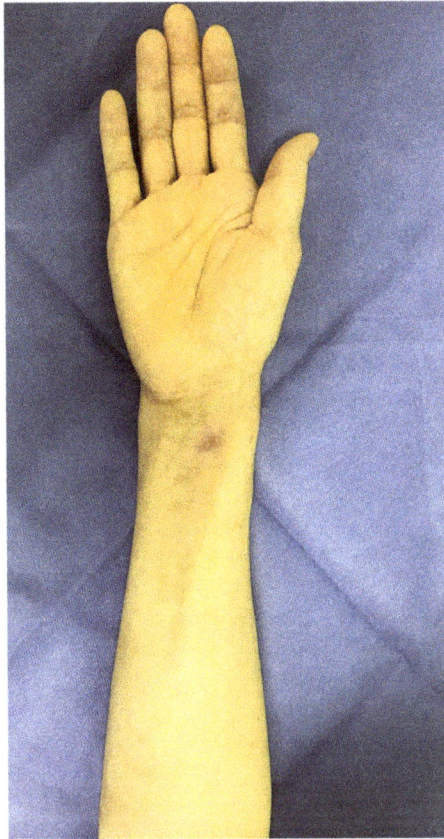

FIGURE 4: Forearm skin state 6 months after the operation. The forearm skin state and surgical wound favorably improved, and she returned to her preinjury job without any problems in daily life.

moisture from the used splint could not be adequately removed, and heat generated by the splint caused blister formation in this patient. Although close examination was performed for suspected contact dermatitis and allergic reactions, no abnormality was detected. Close examination for metal allergy was also performed before surgery to confirm that the implant used in this study could be safely used. During the clinical course of this patient, no aggravation of the skin disorder was observed, and the skin state steadily improved after removal of the physical stimulus.

We reported volar locking plate osteosynthesis using the minimally invasive approach in a patient with skin disorder of the forearm. Such patients are rarely encountered. However, this minimally invasive approach is extremely useful for utilizing the advantages of volar locking plate fixation without being affected by the soft tissue environment. This operative procedure is used in relatively stable fracture type. Fracture types which the authors believe this indication are A2 and A3 (extra-articular fractures) and C1 and C2 (complete articular fractures) according to AO classification. Even if type C1 or C2 fractures, the fractures that involve the depressed intra-articular fragment which is needed to the intramedullary reduction to perform osteosynthesis by this technique are not suitable. Moreover, type B fractures (partial articular fractures) are also unsuitable in our consideration [3].

Consent

Written informed consent was obtained from the patient for publication of this case report and any accompanying images.

Conflicts of Interest

Philippe Liverneaux has conflicts of interest with Newclip Technics and Argomedical. Chihab Taleb has conflicts of interest with Newclip Technics and Arthrex. The other authors declare that they have no conflict of interest.

References

[1] C. Taleb, A. Zemirline, F. Lebailly et al., "Minimally invasive osteotomy for distal radius malunion: a preliminary series of 9 cases," *Orthopaedics & Traumatology: Surgery & Research*, vol. 101, no. 7, pp. 861–865, 2015.

[2] A. Zemirline, K. Naito, F. Lebailly, S. Facca, and P. Liverneaux, "Distal radius fixation through a mini-invasive approach of 15 mm. Part 1: feasibility study," *European Journal of Orthopaedic Surgery & Traumatology*, vol. 24, no. 6, pp. 1031–1037, 2014.

[3] K. Naito, A. Zemirline, Y. Sugiyama, H. Obata, P. Liverneaux, and K. Kaneko, "Possibility of fixation of a distal radius fracture with a volar locking plate through a 10 mm approach," *Techniques in Hand & Upper Extremity Surgery*, vol. 20, no. 2, pp. 71–76, 2016.

[4] F. Lebailly, A. Zemirline, S. Facca, S. Gouzou, and P. Liverneaux, "Distal radius fixation through a mini-invasive approach of 15 mm. PART 1: a series of 144 cases," *European Journal of Orthopaedic Surgery & Traumatology*, vol. 24, no. 6, pp. 877–890, 2014.

[5] H. C. Chang, S. C. Tay, B. K. Chan, and C. O. Low, "Conservative treatment of redisplaced Colles' fractures in elderly patients older than 60 years old- anatomical and functional outcome," *Hand Surgery*, vol. 06, no. 02, pp. 137–144, 2001.

[6] N. D. Clement, A. D. Duckworth, C. M. Court-Brown, and M. M. McQueen, "Distal radial fractures in the superelderly: does malunion affect functional outcome?," *ISRN Orthopedics*, vol. 2014, Article ID 189803, 7 pages, 2014.

[7] A. J. Kelly, D. Warwick, T. P. K. Crichlow, and G. C. Bannister, "Is manipulation of moderately displaced Colles' fracture worthwhile? A prospective randomized trial," *Injury*, vol. 28, no. 4, pp. 283–287, 1997.

[8] N. Kodama, Y. Takemura, H. Ueba, S. Imai, and Y. Matsusue, "Acceptable parameters for alignment of distal radius fracture with conservative treatment in elderly patients," *Journal of Orthopaedic Science*, vol. 19, no. 2, pp. 292–297, 2014.

[9] Y. Sugiyama, K. Naito, Y. Igeta, H. Obata, K. Kaneko, and O. Obayashi, "Treatment strategy for distal radius fractures with ipsilateral arteriovenous shunts," *The Journal of Hand Surgery*, vol. 39, no. 11, pp. 2265–2268, 2014.

[10] M. Fujii, T. Shimizu, T. Nakamura, F. Endo, S. Kohno, and T. Nabe, "Inhibitory effect of chitosan-containing lotion on scratching response of hairless mice with atopic dermatitis-

like dry skin," *Biological and Pharmaceutical Bulletin*, vol. 34, no. 12, pp. 1890–1894, 2011.

[11] S. Ishiguro, Y. Oota, A. Sudo, and A. Uchida, "Calcium phosphate cement-assisted balloon osteoplasty for a Colles' fracture on arteriovenous fistula forearm of a maintenance hemodialysis patient," *The Journal of Hand Surgery*, vol. 32, no. 6, pp. 821–826, 2007.

[12] A. Kapandji, "Intra-focal pinning of fractures of the distal end of the radius 10 years later," *Annales de Chirurgie de la Main*, vol. 6, no. 1, pp. 57–63, 1987.

[13] A. S. Boyd, H. J. Benjamin, and C. Asplund, "Principles of casting and splinting," *American Family Physician Journal*, vol. 79, no. 1, pp. 16–22, 2009.

[14] S. Güzey, A. D. Dal, I. Sahin, M. Nisanci, and I. Yavan, "A new experimental burn model with an infrared heater," *Ulusal Travma ve Acil Cerrahi Dergisi*, vol. 22, no. 5, pp. 412–416, 2015.

30

Management of Patella Dislocation in Say-Barber-Biesecker-Young-Simpson's Syndrome: A Report of Two Cases

Meni Mundama ⓘ**, Serge Ayong, and Renaud Rossillon**

Department of Orthopaedic Surgery, Clinique Saint-Pierre Ottignies, Avenue Reine Fabiola 9, 1340 Ottignies, Belgium

Correspondence should be addressed to Meni Mundama; meni.mundama@gmail.com

Academic Editor: Athanassios Papanikolaou

Say-Barber-Biesecker-Young-Simpson's syndrome is one of the Ohdo-like syndromes. It is a very rare congenital condition that is commonly defined by its main clinical features that are blepharophimosis, ptosis, mental retardation, and delayed motor development. They are often associated with skeletal manifestations that are joint laxity, long thumbs and toes, and hypoplastic and/or dislocated patellae. To our knowledge, the available literature does not report any case where attention is drawn to management of skeletal aspect of this specific syndrome, especially surgically. We report 2 cases of SBBYS syndrome with patellar dislocation that we followed for 11 years. One case (with bilateral dislocation) was managed conservatively, and the other (with unilateral dislocation) underwent conservative and surgical treatment. Both had good functional outcome at follow-up. This experience shows that patellar abnormality in this condition can be efficiently addressed conservatively and/or surgically with satisfying results.

1. Introduction

Say-Barber-Biesecker-Young-Simpson (SBBYS) variant of Ohdo's syndrome is a very rare condition known to feature blepharophimosis, ptosis, mental retardation, delayed motor milestones, impaired speech, dental abnormalities, and hearing dysfunction. Cryptorchidism and scrotal hypoplasia are reported in male patients. Some skeletal characteristics are usually associated: joint laxity, abnormally long thumbs and great toes, and dislocated or hypoplastic patellae. At birth, early signs are hypotonia and feeding problems. Other features of variable frequency are described, such as cardiac defects and abnormal thyroid structure or function [1, 2].

This condition is related to KAT6B gene mutation (OMIM# 603736) [2].

To our knowledge, among SBBYS syndrome cases with patellar dislocation, no surgical case has been reported to date.

For more than 11 years, we followed two boys with SBBYS syndrome presenting patellar dislocation. Initially, both were managed conservatively. One patient finally underwent a surgical procedure aiming to optimise his walking and standing function. We have no records of earlier publication on any of the two cases.

2. Case Presentation

2.1. Case 1. Patient 1 is a boy born in 2002, followed by the senior author since age 3 (Table 1). He then featured bilateral blepharophimosis and ptosis, dental abnormalities, hypogonadism, and heart defects (pathologic valve and interatrial communication). He had psychomotor delay and presented skeletal anomalies: left side metatarsus adductus with reducible hindfoot valgus and bilateral reducible patellar dislocations. Joint hyperlaxity was also noticed, especially regarding both hips. The spine and pelvis were normal.

Genetical tests were performed when the patient was 11 and confirmed the KAT6B gene mutation which however was missing in both parents. The precision about the mutation was

TABLE 1: Patients' data.

Case	Birth	Age at 1st consultation (year)	Skeletal features	Management	Age at operation	Postop follow-up	Global follow-up (year)	Results
1	2002	3	Bilateral patella dislocation	Nonsurgical	—	—	11	Satisfactory walking function
2	2002	3	Unilateral patella dislocation	Nonsurgical and surgical	13	14 months	11	Satisfactory standing function; starting walking

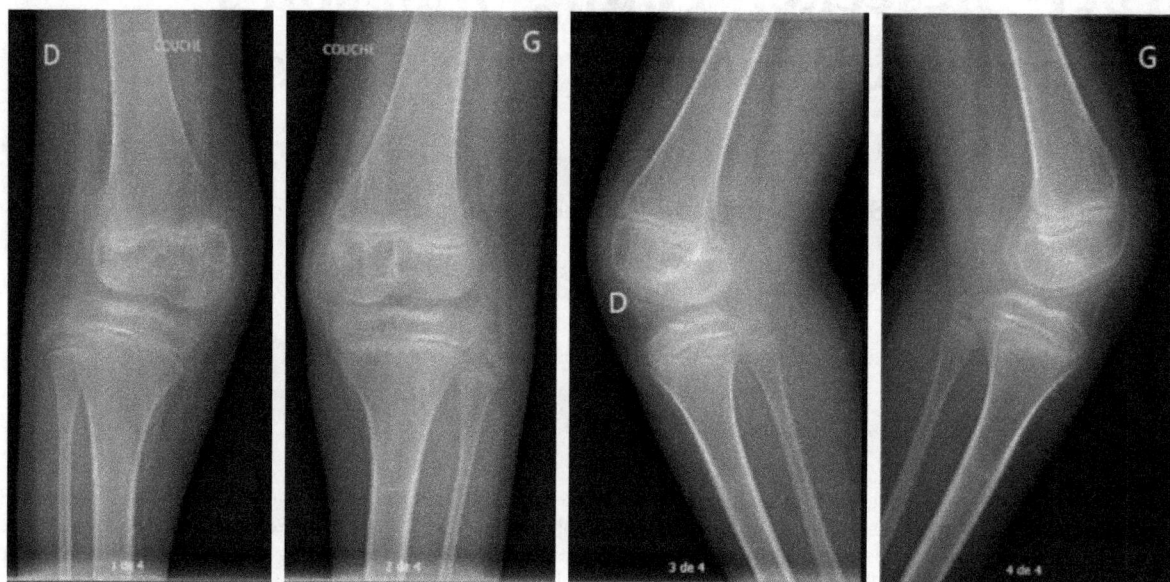

FIGURE 1: Patient 1: knee X-rays at follow-up (age 15).

NM_012330.3 (KAT6B): c.4205_4206delCT, classified as OMIM# 603736.

Although his knees were unstable, they allowed a functionally normal femorotibial axis in extension. Conservative management plan was implemented and consisted of physiotherapy, foot-ankle orthosis to correct foot deformity, especially on the left side, and knee orthosis to stabilise limbs axis during standing and walking. He used a K-walker up to age 8. The orthosis was withdrawn at age 12.

After 11 years of observation, the patellar dislocation had evolved from reducible to permanent, inducing a femorotibial subluxation with tibia external rotation in flexion (Figure 1). There was a discrete valgus in extension but enough stability for standing and walking. The left foot axis was normal.

2.2. Case 2. The second patient is the same age and was followed since age 3 as well (Table 1). He had a mask-like face with blepharophimosis and ptosis, dental anomalies, and psychomotor delay. His musculoskeletal anomalies were initially bilateral: crossed toes and valgus hindfoot, patellar hypoplasia, femorotibial subluxation, and excessive femoral anteversion. His spine and pelvis were normal.

A genetic workup confirmed the KAT6B gene mutation in the patient, but the parents were not tested. The mutation was classified as OMIM# 603736 with the description that

follows: NM_012330.3(KAT6B): c.4775_4794dupCCACGC TCGACGATTGCCA.

Initial management was conservative. It included physiotherapy, verticalization by NF-Walker and parapodium, KAFO-type leg brace, and seating shell.

At age 7, he could stand up with assistance and make few steps using a NF-walker. At age 11, patellae were palpated in a partially dislocated position on both sides. One year later, left patella remained unchanged but complete and permanent dislocation had occurred on the right side with pain, increased instability, and reluctance to stand on the right lower limb, hence losing the little walking progress he had obtained. Clinical and CT scan (Figure 2) workups of the right knee showed then an extension deficit of about 30°, patella luxation, and tibial external rotation of about 90°.

Surgery on the right knee was then proposed in order to regain walking function. It was conducted in two steps: first, an extensive lateral retinaculum release allowing patella reduction, then MPFL double-bundle reconstruction using tendon allograft, associated to Krogius tenoplasty (Figure 3). Peroperative assessment of the knee showed a correctly centered patella and a good range of motion (ROM: 0°–100°).

Postoperative plan was cast for 6 weeks followed by gradual mobilisation.

At cast withdrawal, the ROM quickly deteriorated, resulting in extension deficit of 30° at 8 weeks. Physiotherapy

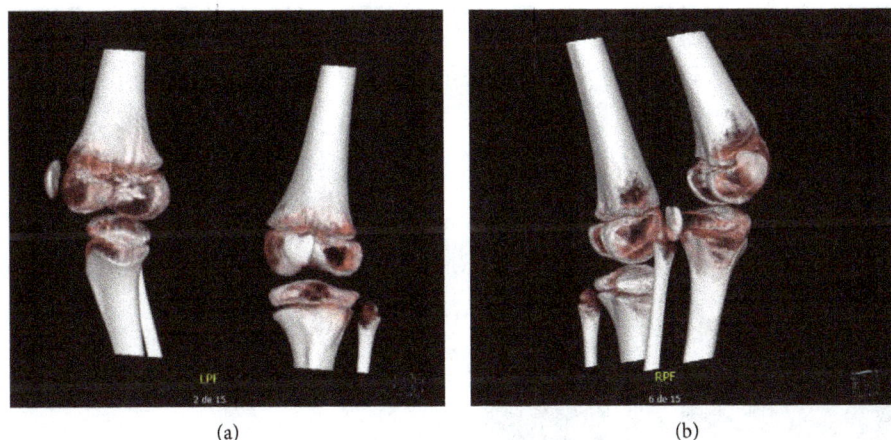

FIGURE 2: Patient 2: preoperative CT scan 3D reconstructions showing patella subluxation and femorotibial rotation (a) and normal state (b).

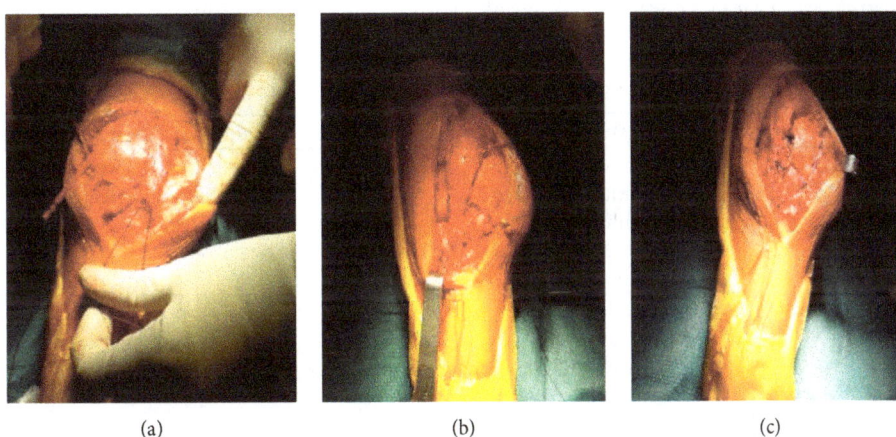

FIGURE 3: Peroperative pictures: after LLR and MPFL tenoplasty with allograft (a); a portion of vastus medialis was individualised and translocated to the lateral aspect of the patella (Krogius tenoplasty) (b); final sutures (c).

was attempted but remained inefficient at 12 months postoperative.

At this point, botulinum toxin injection was performed in a hamstring muscle group as follows: 450 Units (U) of Dysport® were divided into 3 injections of 100 U in the biceps femoralis and 3 injections of 50 U in semitendinous. We associated cast in maximal extension.

Checkups and cast changing were performed at week 1, week 2, week 4, and week 8 after injection. Extension limitation evolved respectively from −25°, −15°, −8°, to −4°. Standing and walking ability improved along with extension regain. He was able to perform a few steps at week 8. His patella kept a centered position on X-ray (Figure 4) and physical checks at last follow-up.

3. Discussion

SBBYS syndrome (OMIM# 603736) is a rare condition. According to Orphanet database's latest report, less than 20 cases have been described in the literature.

The diagnosis is based on clinical features and genetic testing. The clinical workup has been well summarised by Campeau and Lee considering major and minor criteria (Table 2)

[3]. Based on this reference, we observed in our both cases at least 2 major criteria and 3 minor criteria, which correlate to the diagnosis of SBBYS variant of Ohdo's syndrome.

Both patients were genetically tested and confirmed a KAT6b gene mutation classified OMIM# 603736, confirming the SBBYS/Ohdo. In one case, parents were also checked and were negative. This is in accordance with recent literature recognising the condition to be caused by de novo dominant mutation of KAT6b gene [4], although rare family recurrence cases exist and are explained by possible gonadal mosaicism [2, 5].

Hypoplastic dislocated patellae were featured in both cases. The management was guided by functional state. The first patient was affected on both sides but with good axial alignment and walking function, which advocated non-surgical option. The results were good at follow-up.

Conservative treatment with brace and physiotherapy was unsuccessful on the right side in Patient 2 resulting in loss of walking and standing function, which indicated surgical treatment. It was a combined procedure including lateral retinacular release (LRR), double-bundle medial patellofemoral ligament (MPFL) reconstruction, and a vastus medialis tenoplasty according to the Krogius technique.

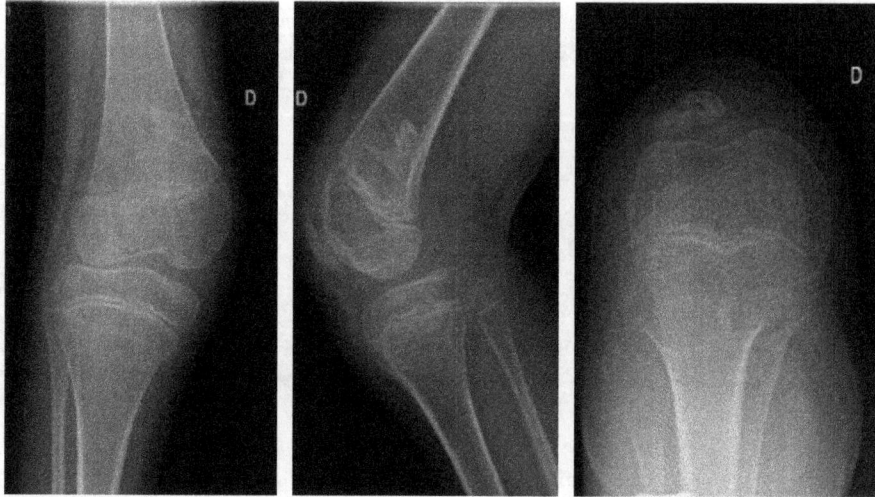

FIGURE 4: Patient 2: X-ray at follow-up. The patella is centered.

TABLE 2: Clinical diagnosis guide by Campeau et al. [3].

Category	Features	Likelihood to have the syndrome
Major features	Long thumbs/great toes Immobile mask-like face Blepharophimosis/ptosis Lacrimal duct anomalies Patellar hypoplasia/agenesis	(i) Two major features, or (ii) One major feature and two minor features
Minor features	Congenital heart defect Dental anomalies Hearing loss Thyroid anomalies Cleft palate Genital anomalies Hypotonia Global developmental delay/intellectual disability	(i) Two major features, or (ii) One major feature and two minor features

Trochleoplasty and tibial tubercle transposition were not considered because physis was still open.

Isolated LRR has failed to show long-term benefit in case of patellar instability. It has then been suggested as an adjunct to patellar realignment procedures [6].

MPFL is the most important medial structure to control patellar stability throughout flexion as it has been shown to contribute more than 50% of forces that prevent lateral displacement of the knee extensor mechanism. Medial soft structure reconstruction is then crucial in patellar realignment surgery [6].

In our case, MPFL reconstruction was impossible without LRR. Despite the possibility of the single-bundle technique to minimize the number of tunnels in the hypoplastic patella, we decided to use the double-bundle MPFL technique because it has proven better efficiency [7].

Krogius tenoplasty as sole procedure has been reported to be ineffective in cases with joint laxity [8]. In our case, it was useful in filling the lateral defect created by LRR.

The combination of serial casting and toxinum botulinum injection has shown good results in children with cerebral palsy [9]. We referred to this principle to manage the extension deficit of our Patient 2, and it resulted in good improvement after 8 weeks.

4. Conclusion

We have observed that in a case of SBBYS variant of Ohdo's syndrome, patella dislocation can be treated either conservatively or surgically with satisfying results. Considering functional preservation, bilateral dislocation can keep good function with conservative treatment, but unilateral dislocation can necessitate surgical correction to maintain or acquire walking and standing abilities.

Conflicts of Interest

The authors declare that there are no conflicts of interest regarding the reported cases.

References

[1] J. Clayton-Smith, M. Krajewska-Walasek, A. Fryer, and D. Donnai, "Ohdo-like blepharophimosis syndrome with distinctive facies, neonatal hypotonia, mental retardation and

hypoplastic teeth," *Clinical Dysmorphology*, vol. 3, no. 2, pp. 115–120, 1994.

[2] J. Clayton-Smith, J. O'Sullivan, S. Daly et al., "Whole-exome-sequencing identifies mutations in histone acetyltransferase gene KAT6B in individuals with the Say-Barber-Biesecker variant of Ohdo syndrome," *American Journal of Human Genetics*, vol. 89, no. 5, pp. 675–681, 2011.

[3] P. M. Campeau and B. H. Lee, "KAT6B-related disorders," in *Gene Reviews (R)*, R. A. Pagon, Ed., University of Washington, Seattle, WA, USA, 1993.

[4] P. M. Campeau, J. T. Lu, B. C. Dawson et al., "The KAT6B-related disorders genitopatellar syndrome and Ohdo/SBBYS syndrome have distinct clinical features reflecting distinct molecular mechanisms," *Human Mutation*, vol. 33, no. 11, pp. 1520–1525, 2012.

[5] T. Gannon, R. Perveen, H. Schlecht et al., "Further delineation of the KAT6B molecular and phenotypic spectrum," *European Journal of Human Genetics*, vol. 23, no. 9, pp. 1165–1170, 2015.

[6] A. D. Iliadis, "The operative management of patella malalignment," *Open Orthopaedics Journal*, vol. 6, no. 1, pp. 327–339, 2012.

[7] C. H. Wang, L.-F. Ma, J.-W. Zhou et al., "Double-bundle anatomical versus single-bundle isometric medial patellofemoral ligament reconstruction for patellar dislocation," *International Orthopaedics*, vol. 37, no. 4, pp. 617–624, 2013.

[8] F. C. Bauer, T. Wredmark, and B. Isberg, "Krogius tenoplasty for recurrent dislocation of the patella: failure associated with joint laxity," *Acta Orthopaedica Scandinavica*, vol. 55, no. 3, pp. 267–269, 1984.

[9] A. I. Dai and A. T. Demiryurek, "Serial casting as an adjunct to botulinum toxin type a treatment in children with cerebral palsy and spastic paraparesis with scissoring of the lower extremities," *Journal of Child Neurology*, vol. 32, no. 7, pp. 671–675, 2017.

31

Extensor Tendons Rupture after Volar Plating of Distal Radius Fracture Related to a Dorsal Radial Metaphyseal Bone Spur

M. O. Abrego ⓘ, F. L. De Cicco, J. G. Boretto, G. L. Gallucci, and P. De Carli

Trauma and Orthopedics Institute "Carlos E. Ottolenghi", Italian Hospital of Buenos Aires, Buenos Aires, Argentina

Correspondence should be addressed to M. O. Abrego; mariano.abrego@hospitalitaliano.org.ar

Academic Editor: Andreas Panagopoulos

Extensor tendon ruptures due to volar plating in distal radius fractures have mostly been described in relation with technique failures such as screw prominence and drill penetration. We report the case of a 71-year-old female with a C2 distal radius fracture with severe dorsal metaphyseal comminution. The patient underwent surgical treatment with reduction of the large fragments and fixation with a volar locking plate; the small dorsal metaphyseal nonarticular fragments were not reduced. Six months later, the patient developed extensor digitorum communis (EDC) rupture and extensor indicis proprius (EIP) laceration in coincidence with the dorsal comminution turned into a bony spur. The possible association between the extensor tendon injury and the dorsal residual metaphyseal bony spur in the distal radius fractures is unusual but should be taken into account in fracture patterns presenting dorsal comminution.

1. Introduction

Volar plating is established as the gold standard treatment for distal radius fractures [1]. Even fractures involving dorsally displaced fragments can be treated with volar plates, decreasing the high rates of extensor tendons injuries due to dorsal plating [2]. Nevertheless, extensor tendinous complications following volar plating have been reported. Reported complications are irritation, adhesion, tenosynovitis, laceration, and even tendon rupture [3]. They are mostly associated with screw prominence and drill penetration of the dorsal cortex during screw fixation [4]. Extensor tendons rupture due to dorsal metaphyseal bony spur as a consequence of dorsal comminution is unlikely to happen. We present a case of rupture and laceration of extensor digitorum communis and extensor indicis proprius, respectively, as a complication of a distal radius fracture treated with a volar locking plate and in coincidence with dorsal metaphyseal exostoses secondary to dorsal metaphyseal comminution.

2. Case Report

A 71-year-old right hand dominant female patient with no comorbidities was admitted in our institution after suffering a fall from her own height. Plain radiographs and CT scan were performed. The patient had a C2 fracture according to AO/ASIF classification with dorsal metaphyseal comminution (Figure 1). Seven days later, the patient underwent surgical treatment: using a volar approach, open reduction and internal fixation with volar locking plate was performed. Drilling was performed only through the volar cortex without violating dorsal cortex as we usually do when performing this technique, in order to avoid extensor tendon erosion. Attention was specially paid to restoration of the articular surface and radial bone angles. Dorsal fragments from metaphyseal comminution were left in site, maintained by the dorsal periosteum. Postoperative X-rays showed adequate fracture reduction. However, dorsal metaphyseal fragments were larger than usual and displaced in a perpendicular plane in relation with the dorsal radial cortex (Figure 2). The patient was splinted for 15 days and then moved onto a removable wristband, starting rehabilitation protocol. Three-month follow-up showed that the patient's wrist had full-range motion, no pain, and the Disabilities of the Arm, Shoulder and Hand (DASH) score of 37.

Six months after surgery, the patient's DASH score improved to 9, maintaining a full range of motion, but she addressed dorsal wrist tenderness, with incomplete extension

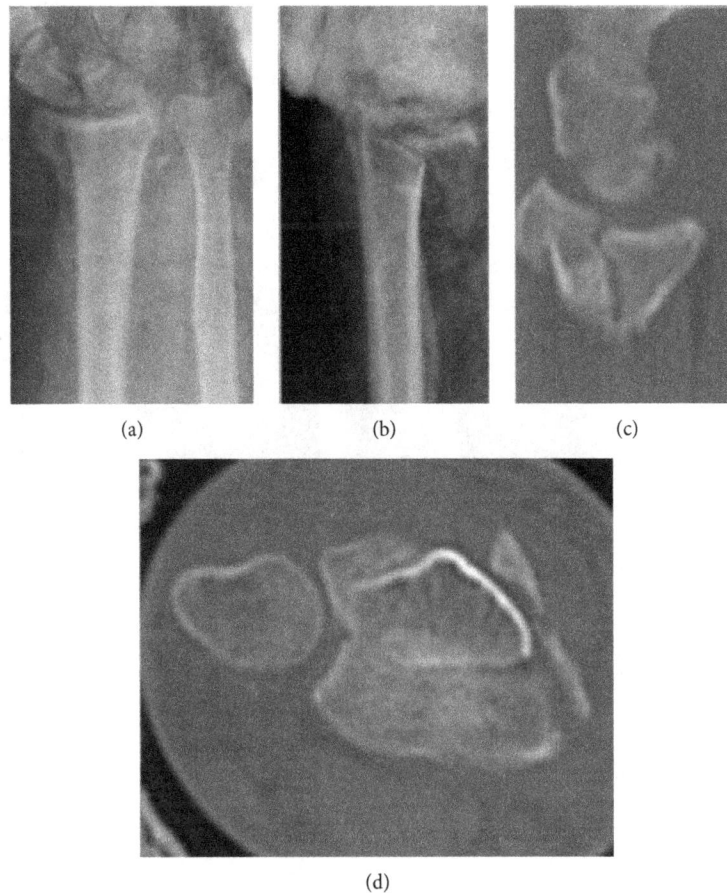

FIGURE 1: Preoperative X-rays, anteroposterior and lateral view of the 23C2 fracture (a, b). CT scan showing articular damage (c, d).

of the index finger. Her Visual Analogue Scale (VAS) for pain at rest was 1 but increased to 4 with activity. Normal "tenodesis effect" was reported, but the patient could not further extend her index finger with the hand on top of a table, as she could do with the other three ulnar fingers.

Musculoskeletal ultrasound showed the presence of tenosynovitis of the fourth compartment and thinning of the index extensors at the radioulnar space, compatible with tendon rupture. New X-rays and CT scan showed sequel bone spicules at the dorsal epiphysis of the radius (Figure 3). Fracture was already consolidated, and there was no screw protrusion through the dorsal radial cortex. Surgical exploration was performed. A dorsal longitudinal approach through Lister's tubercle and third compartment with extensor retinaculum exposure was done. Extensor pollicis longus was unscathed. The fourth compartment was explored, with evidence of EDC rupture and EIP laceration (Figure 4). Large bone spurs from the dorsal radius were observed below the tendon plane in relation to Lister's tubercle, generating friction with the extensor apparatus. We confirmed no screws were prominent through the dorsal cortex. Dorsal bone spurs were resected, and tenodesis of EDC to the middle finger tendon was performed. A retinacular flap was designed to protect the tendons from the underlying bone. Volar plate was removed using the previous volar approach, and fracture consolidation was evidenced.

The patient underwent physiotherapy rehabilitation, wearing a dynamic elastic band splint. At three-month follow-up, the patient had complete flexion and extension of the fingers, with some slight extensor plus noted as she fully flexed her wrist while her fingers were passively flexed.

3. Discussion

Reported volar plating complications reach up to 36% [5, 6]. Tendinous injury secondary to distal radius plating has been strongly related with implant failure (plate positioning, screw length and orientation, and drill violation of dorsal cortex). During a previous study in our institution [7], among 992 consecutive patients treated with volar locking plate, 1.3% developed extensor tendonitis, with no extensor ruptures. Four patients had dorsal tendon irritation related to screw protrusion and 4 patients without dorsal screw protrusion.

According to reports, extensor pollicis longus (EPL) remains the most frequently injured extensor tendon involving distal radius volar plating. Furthermore, EPL rupture without evidence of trauma or pathologic condition has been reported to be caused by a prominent and sharp Lister's tubercle [8]. On the other hand, EDC and EIP injury is much less common [9–11].

According to Wei et al. [12] metaanalysis, the volar approach is more related to neuropathy and carpal tunnel

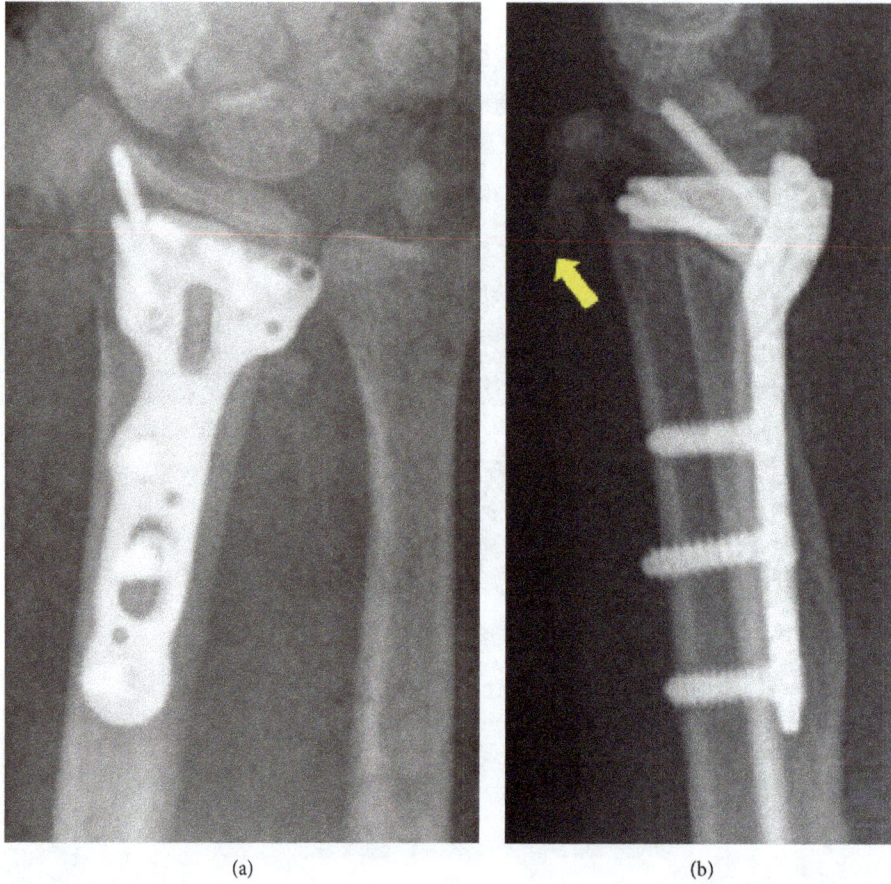

(a)   (b)

FIGURE 2: Immediate postoperative X-rays showing internal fixation (a). Lateral view showing dorsal metaphyseal comminution (arrow) (b).

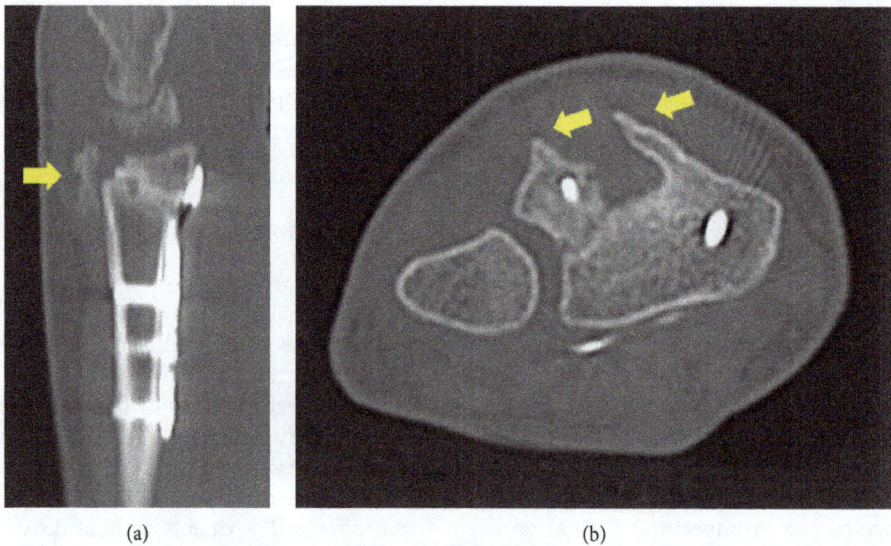

(a)   (b)

FIGURE 3: CT scan performed at 6-month follow-up. The arrows show dorsal bone spur.

syndrome, while tendon injuries appear to have a stronger relation with the dorsal approach. Azzi et al. [13] showed in their systematic review that tendon rupture involving volar approaches was 1.5%, without differentiating between flexors or extensors. They also report that 0.8% were EPL injuries, while EDC injuries represented only 0.02%. When intra-surgical fluoroscopy or immediate postoperative X-rays reveal some sort of risk factors (screw prominences or misplaced implant) for tendinous injury, early hardware removal is recommended [6].

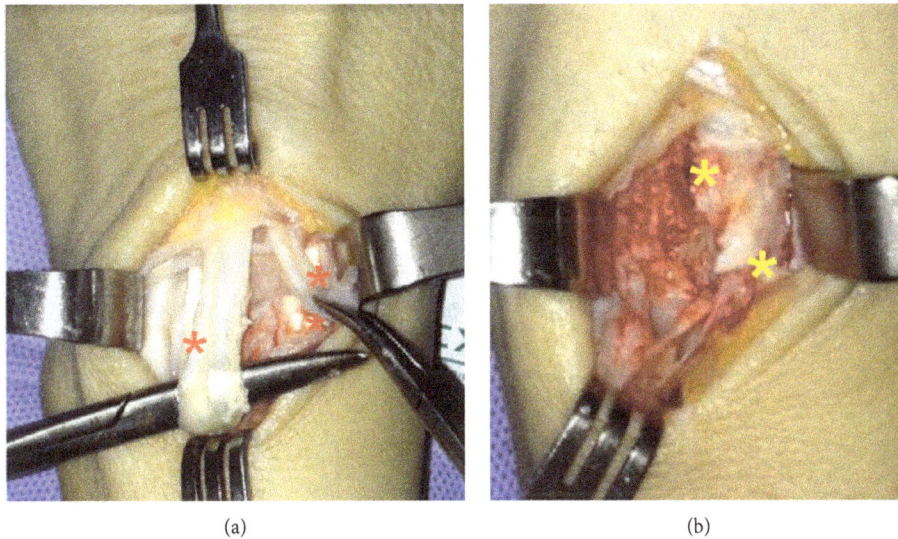

(a)   (b)

FIGURE 4: EDC laceration and EIP rupture (a). Dorsal exostoses (b).

Surgical techniques for treatment of distal radius fractures dismiss the importance of reduction of metaphyseal dorsal fragments. This condition is indeed a cause of fracture instability when present, but they are usually left in place and have no clinical or imaging implications. We found no reports in medical literature addressing extensor tendon injuries (especially EDC and EIP) as a complication of volar plating for distal radius fracture due to dorsal exostoses. Though we cannot affirm that the cause of tendon rupture in the index case is attrition by dorsal bone spurs, the described complication suggests that hand surgeons should be aware in distal radius fracture with dorsal metaphyseal comminution. Small dorsal fragments maintained by the dorsal periosteum usually have no further sequel if left in place and need no reduction maneuvers. If these fragments protrude dorsally or seem to be rotated perpendicular to the dorsal cortex, the extensor tendons could be in danger and at least attempts for percutaneous reduction could be indicated to avoid future bone spurs formation.

Disclosure

All authors certify that their institution has approved the reporting of this case.

Conflicts of Interest

All authors declare that there are no conflicts of interest regarding the publication of this paper.

Acknowledgments

The study was performed at the Italian Hospital of Buenos Aires, Argentina.

References

[1] K. C. Chung, M. J. Shauver, and J. D. Birkmeyer, "Trends in the United States in the treatment of distal radial fractures in the elderly," *Journal of Bone and Joint Surgery*, vol. 91, pp. 1868–1873, 2009.

[2] D. H. Wei, N. M. Raizman, C. J. Bottino, C. M. Jobin, R. J. Strauch, and M. P. Rosenwasser, "Unstable distal radial fractures treated with external fixation, a radial column plate, or a volar plate. A prospective randomized trial," *Journal of Bone and Joint Surgery*, vol. 91, pp. 1568–1577, 2009.

[3] S. D. McKay, J. C. MacDermid, J. H. Roth, and R. S. Richards, "Assessment of complications of distal radius fractures and development of a complication checklist," *Journal of Hand Surgery*, vol. 26, no. 5, pp. 916–922, 2001.

[4] L. M. Berglund and T. M. Messer, "Complications of volar plate fixation for managing distal radius fractures," *Journal of the American Academy of Orthopaedic Surgeons*, vol. 17, no. 6, pp. 369–377, 2009.

[5] R. Thorninger, M. L. Madsen, D. Wæver, L. C. Borris, and J. H. D. Rölfing, "Complications of volar locking plating of distal radius fractures in 576 patients with 3.2 years follow-up," *Injury*, vol. 48, no. 6, pp. 1104–1109, 2017.

[6] M. Rampoldi and S. Marsico, "Complications of volar plating of distal radius fractures," *Acta Orthopaedica Belgica*, vol. 73, no. 6, pp. 714–719, 2007.

[7] I. Rellán, G. L. Gallucci, J. G. Boretto, A. Donndorff, and P. De Carli, "Secondary tendinopathy after distal radius volar plate fixation: results of 8 years' experience," *Hand*, vol. 11, no. 1, p. 38S, 2016.

[8] G. L. Gallucci, N. Pacher, J. G. Boretto, and P. De Carli, "Bilateral rupture of the extensor pollicis longus tendon. a case report," *Chirurgie de la Main*, vol. 32, no. 3, pp. 186–188, 2013.

[9] P. C. Rhee, D. G. Dennison, and S. Kakar, "Avoiding and treating perioperative complications of distal radius fractures," *Hand Clinics*, vol. 28, no. 2, pp. 185–198, 2012.

[10] Y. Hirasawa, Y. Katsumi, T. Akiyoshi, K. Tamai, and T. Tokioka, "Clinical and microangiographic studies on rupture of the EPL tendon after distal radial fractures," *Journal of Hand Surgery*, vol. 15, pp. 51–57, 1990.

[11] B. Helal, S. C. Chen, and G. Iwegbu, "Rupture of the extensor pollicis longus tendon in undisplaced Colles' type of fracture," *Hand*, vol. 14, no. 1, pp. 41–47, 1982.

[12] J. Wei, T. B. Yang, W. Luo, J. B. Qin, and F. J. Kong, "Complications following dorsal versus volar plate fixation of distal radius fracture: a meta-analysis," *Journal of International Medical Research*, vol. 41, no. 2, pp. 265–275, 2013.

[13] A. J. Azzi, S. Aldekhayel, K. S. Boehm, and T. Zadeh, "Tendon rupture and tenosynovitis following internal fixation of distal radius fractures: a systematic review," *Plastic and Reconstructive Surgery*, vol. 139, no. 3, pp. 717e–724e, 2017.

32

Case Report of an Acute Complex Perilunate Fracture Dislocation Treated with a Three-Corner Fusion

Graeme Matthewson ⓘ,[1] **Samuel Larrivee,**[1] **and Tod Clark**[2]

[1]*University of Manitoba, S013-750 Bannatyne Avenue, Winnipeg, MB, Canada R3E 0W2*
[2]*Pan Am Clinic Foundation, 75 Poseidon Bay, Winnipeg, MB, Canada R3M 3E4*

Correspondence should be addressed to Graeme Matthewson; graememmatthewson@icloud.com

Academic Editor: Athanassios Papanikolaou

Perilunate fracture dislocations are a rare but devastating injury, which is often missed on initial presentation leading to significant delays in treatment. With the delay in treatment and a high energy mechanism of injury, patients are at increased risk of developing complex regional pain syndrome following trauma. In this report, we review the case of a 57-year-old left-hand dominant female who presented to a clinic with a five-and-a-half-week-old transtriquetral, perilunate fracture dislocation with comminution of the scaphoid facet. Due to the increased likelihood of a secondary procedure and low probability of a satisfactory outcome with open reduction internal fixation secondary to the loss of the scaphoid articulation, a salvage procedure was deemed her best option. To our knowledge, this is the first case reported in the literature in which a scaphoidectomy, triquetromy, and midcarpal fusion (three-corner fusion) was performed in the acute setting for a perilunate fracture dislocation.

1. Introduction

Perilunate injuries are relatively rare, accounting for only 7% of pathologies to the carpus. However, a staggering number of these injuries are not diagnosed, with up to 25% of perilunate dislocations being missed on initial presentation [1–3]. The importance of identifying these injuries is highlighted by the significant complications produced by missed or improperly treated injuries including median nerve injury, chronic carpal instability, avascular necrosis of the malreduced lunate, complex regional pain syndrome, unreliable return of function, and posttraumatic arthrosis requiring a secondary procedure [2–5]. In addition to patient factors, surgical complications are increased due to extensive fibrosis and scarring and the inability to achieve an anatomic reduction of the carpal bone complex [4]. Here, we present a case of a 57-year-old female who suffered a complex perilunate fracture dislocation treated by scaphoidectomy, triquetromy, and midcarpal fusion (three-corner fusion). To our knowledge, this is the first reported case in the literature for the treatment of an acute perilunate dislocation with this procedure.

2. Case Report

A 57-year-old left-hand dominant woman presented to the arthroplasty clinic for a consultation regarding her right knee osteoarthritis. On her visit, the consulting surgeon noticed an improperly placed below elbow cast which was well past her metacarpal phalangeal joints, greatly restricting movement of her left fingers. She was previously seen at a peripheral hospital approximately five weeks prior, after sustaining a fall on an outstretched hand (FOOSH) from standing height. Noting this, the consulting surgeon ordered an X-ray which revealed that the patient had a missed perilunate dislocation with a fracture of the triquetrum and a comminuted impaction fracture of the scaphoid facet (Figure 1). This prompted the surgeon to put in an immediate call to the senior author for an immediate consult.

In the clinic, the patient complained of considerable volar wrist pain with occasional numbness and tingling to the hand. Examination of the hand revealed significant swelling and hyperalgesia of the skin of the wrist and hand. She was otherwise neurovascularly intact to all nerve distributions. X-ray examination included an anteroposterior (AP) and

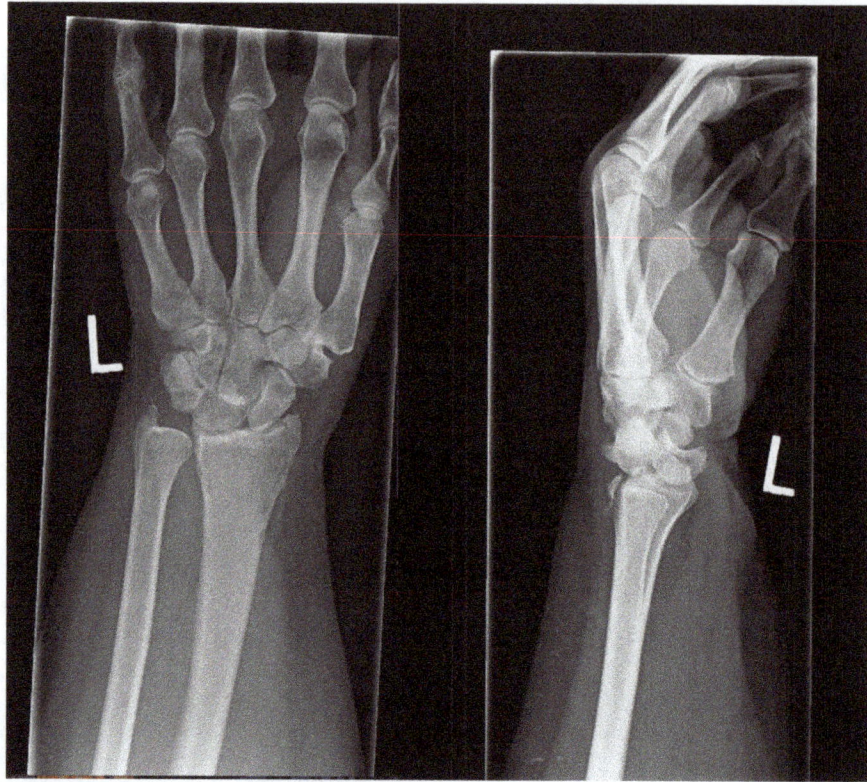

FIGURE 1: AP and lateral images of the initial radiographs taken in the peripheral hospital. Note the comminuted scaphoid facet, subtle triquetral fracture (AP) as well as the obvious perilunate dislocation (lateral).

lateral imaging of the left hand and wrist. On the anterior radiograph, there was an obvious disruption of Gilula's lines (see Figure 2 for comparison), as well as an impaction injury to the scaphoid facet (Figure 3), and fracture of the triquetrum. On the lateral X-ray, there was an obvious dorsal dislocation of the lunocapitate joint consistent with a perilunate fracture dislocation. Treatment options were discussed with the patient regarding open reduction internal fixation (ORIF) compared with a salvage procedure. Since the scaphoid facet was badly injured, the decision to perform an ORIF versus a salvage procedure was left until the status of the cartilage could be determined. A proximal row carpectomy and a three-corner fusion were discussed as salvage procedures in the acute setting. The patient agreed with the treatment plan, was placed into a well-fitting cast, and was booked for surgery for the following week.

The patient was brought to the operating room and was placed supine with the use of an arm board. The patient was prepped and draped in usual fashion, and an operative time out was performed. A dorsal approach to the wrist was used, utilizing a Berger ligamentous sparing capsulotomy (Figures 4 and 5). Once the carpus was exposed, it was evident that the second carpal row was dislocated dorsal to the lunate. Examination of the articular surfaces of the carpus revealed a healthy appearing lunate and lunate fossa with a significantly comminuted and impacted scaphoid facet. In addition, there was significant damage to the proximal capitate chondral surface. As the proximal capitate articulation is

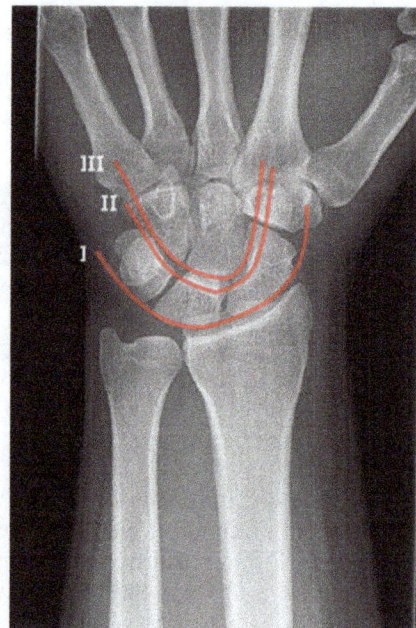

FIGURE 2: Radiograph demonstrating Gilula's lines. Line I represents the proximal articular surfaces of the proximal carpal row. Line II represents the distal articular surfaces of the first carpal row. Line III represents the proximal articular surfaces of the distal carpal row. Disruption of these lines is indicative of a boney (greater arc) or ligamentous (lesser arc) injury.

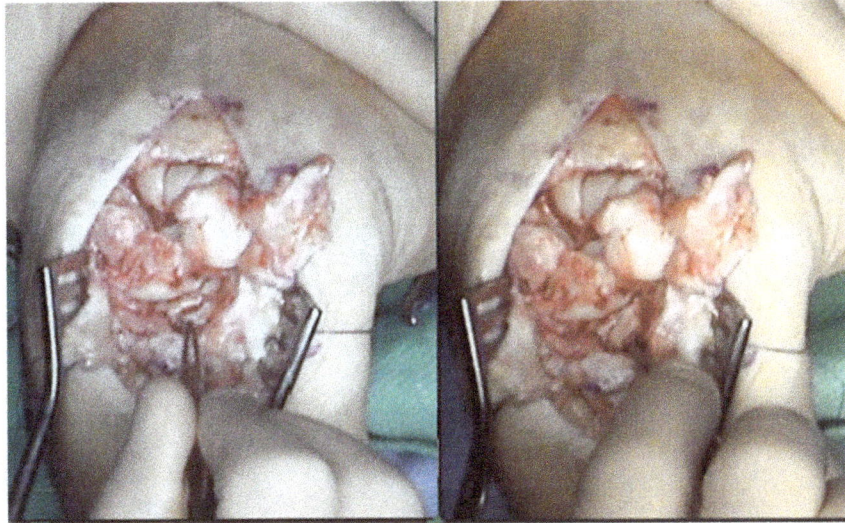

FIGURE 3: Examination of the comminuted scaphoid facet. (a) Obvious impaction injury. (b) Impaction fragment loose and nonadherent has a high likelihood of secondary arthrosis.

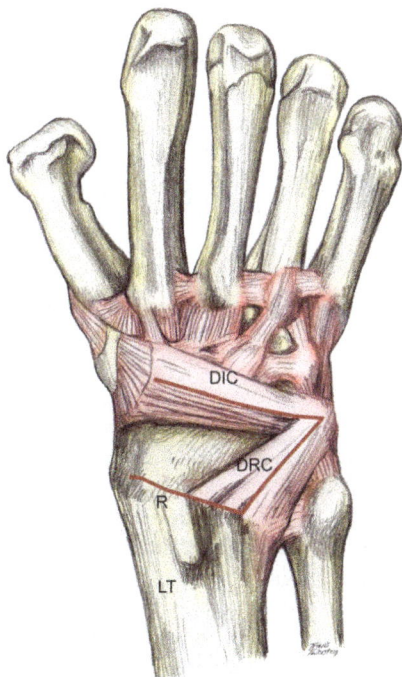

FIGURE 4: Illustration of the capsular incision used in the ligamentous sparing Berger capsulotomy. Note the radially based flap created. DRC: dorsal radiocarpal ligament. DIC: dorsal intercarpal ligament. The image was reprinted with a permission from Medscape Drugs & Diseases (https://emedicine.medscape.com/) and Perilunate Fracture Dislocations, 2017, available at https://emedicine.medscape.com/article/1240108-overview.

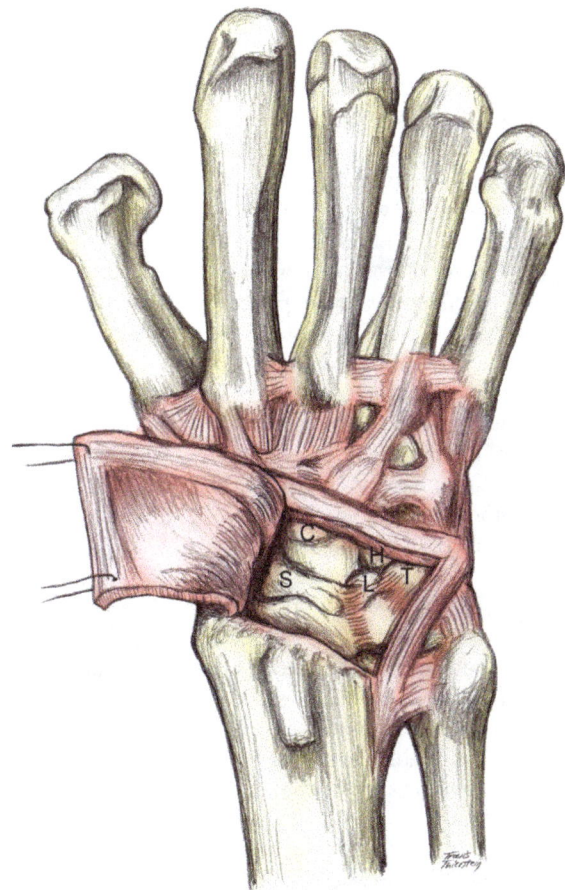

FIGURE 5: Visualization of the carpal bones once the radially based flap is lifted. S: scaphoid; C: capitate; L: lunate; T: triquetrum; H: hamate. The image was reprinted with permission from Medscape Drugs & Diseases (https://emedicine.medscape.com/) and Perilunate Fracture Dislocations, 2017, available at https://emedicine.medscape.com/article/1240108-overview.

key for optimal results in a proximal row carpectomy and with the significant chondral damage and comminution of the scaphoid facet, the decision was made to perform a three-corner fusion. The cartilage was removed from the distal aspect of the lunate and proximal aspects of the capitate

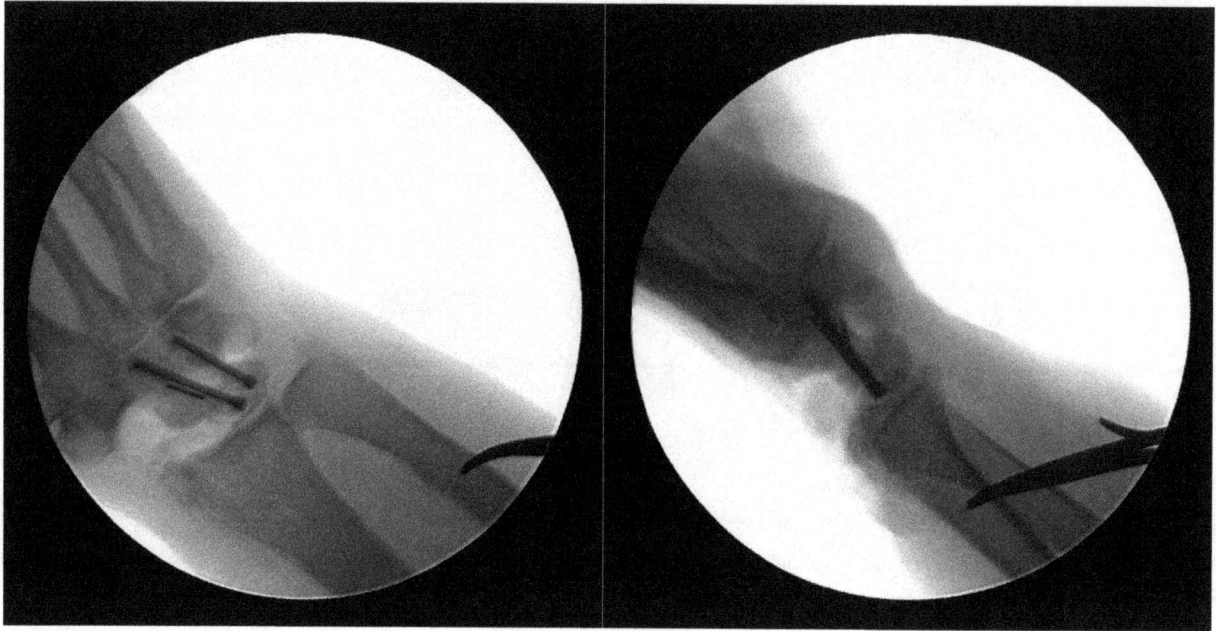

FIGURE 6: Intraoperative fluoroscopic images confirming screw position and proper alignment of the midcarpal fusion.

and hamate with a scalpel, and the articular surfaces were contoured using a 3 mm burr with copious irrigation to prevent thermal necrosis. K-wires were placed across the lunocapitate joint, with the position confirmed on fluoroscopy, and a 3 mm headless compression screw was used to affix the joint. This was followed by a lunohamate screw placed in a similar fashion. The final screw position was confirmed on imaging (Figure 6), followed by irrigation and closure of the wound. The patient was then placed in a volar slab and sent to recovery in a stable condition. Immobilization was maintained for a total of 6 weeks. Upon follow up, the patient's clinical course deteriorated with the development of postoperative complex regional pain syndrome. On the most recent follow up appointment at 12 weeks postoperatively, the patient began to have some relief of her symptoms following the implementation of an extensive physiotherapy and pain control protocol.

3. Discussion

The treatments of acute (defined as <6 weeks) [6] and chronic perilunate dislocations are considerably varied. Currently, most clinicians would opt to perform an ORIF in the acute and many times chronic setting. This would involve either the reconstruction of the scapholunate ligament or, if possible, primary repair, in addition to the pinning of the lunotriquetral joint and fixation of any fractures that occurred. However, particularly in the chronic setting, ORIF has had unreliable outcomes and high rates of secondary arthrosis with some authors reporting rates as high as 50–100% [3, 7]. With a mean incidence of 38%, a staggering number of perilunate injuries go on to develop posttraumatic arthrosis. In a retrospective review, Forli et al. [8] found in patients who suffered a perilunate injury that 11/18 cases had progressed to develop signs of posttraumatic degenerative changes with a minimum

of 10 years postsurgery, and some authors have reported the appearance of degenerative changes as early as few years from injury [9]. Of the patients showing radiographic change, 2 had excellent results, 2 had good results, 5 had fair results, and 2 had poor results according to the Mayo Wrist Score (MWS). Following this, Breyer et al. [10] retrospectively reviewed 37 patients who sustained either perilunate dislocation or perilunate fracture dislocation treated with ORIF at an average of 4 years. They found similar results with an excellent result in one patient, good results in 7 patients, fair results in 18 patients, and poor results in 11 according to the MWS. As referenced by Forli et al. [8], at this point, the literature fails to show a clear correlation between posttraumatic arthrosis and functional outcomes. This was corroborated by Kailu et al. [11], where they found that satisfactory results could be obtained up to 25 weeks from the time of injury. However, they also noted that the patients with substantial chondral damage had poor results, regardless of the timing of surgery. This led the authors to recommend a salvage procedure in the setting of significant cartilage damage. Due to the number of less than optimal results with ORIF, many authors have opted for salvage procedures as the primary operation, particularly in the setting of severe carpal trauma [12]. In a retrospective cohort analysis, Muller et al. [1] compared ORIF against proximal row carpectomy (PRC) for the treatment of acute perilunate dislocations. In their study, 13 patients were treated by ORIF while 8 patients were treated by PRC with an average follow up of 35 months. The results of this study showed that ORIF and PRC were quite comparable in the acute setting, with shorter surgical time and postoperative immobilization. With significant cartilage damage and comminution of the scaphoid facet, it was felt that the maintenance of the radioscaphoid joint would result in significant morbidity leading the surgeon to opt for a salvage procedure. Due to the damage to the capitate articular cartilage, the results from a PRC would have been considerably compromised in our patient. With the additional fracture to the triquetrum, the senior author decided to perform a three-corner fusion as an alternative to four-corner fusion, which has shown equivalent results, only with additional ROM in ulnar deviation [13]. Unfortunately, the patient went on to develop complex regional pain syndrome (CRPS). CRPS is a devastating and relatively uncommon condition with a predilection towards patients with injuries to the hand or wrist. While researchers have not clearly defined the precise cause of CRPS, they have been able to identify many of the contributing factors, including inflammation, central sensitization, sympathetic mediation, cortical reorganization, and neurogenic inflammation [5]. As all of these states are triggered and exacerbated by an untreated injury, delay in diagnosis for hand and wrist injuries inevitably increases the chances of developing this condition. Unfortunately, due to the significant ligamentous injury and fractures of the distal radius and triquetrum, in combination with the delay in diagnosis, our patient was at a significant risk of developing CRPS. This made performing only one procedure even more important with regard to long-term outcomes as to not expose the patient to a secondary procedure, risking a second insult, and subsequent episode of CRPS.

4. Conclusion

In summary, with the high rate of secondary pathology and an increased risk of complications with multiple procedures, performing a salvage surgery in the acute setting for severe perilunate fracture dislocations could prevent a patient from undergoing a secondary surgery. This case highlights the importance of prompt diagnosis of perilunate injuries, the negative consequences associated with missed injuries, and an alternative primary procedure to the traditional ORIF of perilunate fracture dislocations.

Conflicts of Interest

The authors declare that they have no conflicts of interest.

References

[1] T. Muller, J. J. Hidalgo Diaz, E. Pire, G. Prunières, S. Facca, and P. Liverneaux, "Treatment of acute perilunate dislocations: ORIF versus proximal row carpectomy," *Orthopaedics & Traumatology: Surgery & Research*, vol. 103, no. 1, pp. 95–99, 2017.

[2] R. C. Muppavarapu and J. T. Capo, "Perilunate dislocations and fracture dislocations," *Hand Clinics*, vol. 31, no. 3, pp. 399–408, 2015.

[3] G. Herzberg, J. J. Comtet, R. L. Linscheid, P. C. Amadio, W. P. Cooney, and J. Stalder, "Perilunate dislocations and fracture-dislocations: a multicenter study," *The Journal of Hand Surgery*, vol. 18, no. 5, pp. 768–779, 1993.

[4] M. S. Dhillon, S. Prabhakar, K. Bali, D. Chouhan, and V. Kumar, "Functional outcome of neglected perilunate dislocations treated with open reduction and internal fixation," *Indian Journal of Orthopaedics*, vol. 45, no. 5, pp. 427–431, 2011.

[5] A. Goebel, "Complex regional pain syndrome in adults," *Rheumatology*, vol. 50, no. 10, pp. 1739–1750, 2011.

[6] E. G. Huish Jr., M. A. Vitale, and A. Y. Shin, "Acute proximal row carpectomy to treat a transscaphoid, transtriquetral perilunate fracture dislocation: case report and review of the literature," *Hand*, vol. 8, no. 1, pp. 105–109, 2013.

[7] K. A. Hildebrand, D. C. Ross, S. D. Patterson, J. H. Roth, J. C. MacDermid, and G. J. W. King, "Dorsal perilunate dislocations and fracture-dislocations: questionnaire, clinical, and radiographic evaluation," *The Journal of Hand Surgery*, vol. 25, no. 6, pp. 1069–1079, 2000.

[8] A. Forli, A. Courvoisier, S. Wimsey, D. Corcella, and F. Moutet, "Perilunate dislocations and transscaphoid perilunate fracture-dislocations: a retrospective study with minimum ten-year follow-up," *The Journal of Hand Surgery*, vol. 35, no. 1, pp. 62–68, 2010.

[9] G. Herzberg and D. Forissier, "Acute dorsal trans-scaphoid perilunate fracture-dislocations: medium-term results," *Journal of Hand Surgery*, vol. 27, no. 6, pp. 498–502, 2002.

[10] J. M. Breyer, P. Vergara, A. Perez, P. Sotelo, and N. Prado, "Mid-term outcomes in perilunate dislocations: how often are poor results?," *The Hand*, vol. 11, Supplement 1, pp. 127S–128S, 2016.

[11] L. Kailu, X. Zhou, and H. Fuguo, "Chronic perilunate dislocations treated with open reduction and internal fixation: results of medium-term follow-up," *International Orthopaedics*, vol. 34, no. 8, pp. 1315–1320, 2010.

[12] E. O. van Kooten, E. Coster, M. J. M. Segers, and M. J. P. F. Ritt, "Early proximal row carpectomy after severe carpal trauma," *Injury*, vol. 36, no. 10, pp. 1226–1232, 2005.

[13] G. I. Bain, A. Sood, N. Ashwood, P. C. Turner, and Q. A. Fogg, "Effect of scaphoid and triquetrum excision after limited stabilisation on cadaver wrist movement," *Journal of Hand Surgery*, vol. 34, no. 5, pp. 614–617, 2009.

33

The Waterfall Fascia Lata Interposition Arthroplasty "Grika Technique" as Treatment of Posttraumatic Osteoarthritis of the Elbow in a High-Demand Adult Patient: Validity and Reliability

Giuseppe Rollo,[1] Roberto Rotini,[2] Denise Eygendaal,[3,4] Paolo Pichierri,[1] Ante Prkic,[3] Michele Bisaccia ⓘ,[5] Riccardo Maria Lanzetti ⓘ,[5] Domenico Lupariello,[6] and Luigi Meccariello ⓘ[1]

[1]Department of Orthopedics and Traumatology, Vito Fazzi Hospital, Lecce, Italy
[2]Shoulder and Elbow Unit, Rizzoli Orthopedic Institute, Bologna, Italy
[3]Upper Limb Unit, Department of Orthopedic Surgery, Amphia Hospital, Breda, Netherlands
[4]Department of Orthopedic Surgery, AMC, Amsterdam, Netherlands
[5]Orthopedics and Traumatology Unit, SM Misericordia Hospital, University of Perugia, Perugia, Italy
[6]Orthopedics and Traumatology Unit, Univerisity of Rome La Sapienza, Rome, Italy

Correspondence should be addressed to Riccardo Maria Lanzetti; riccardolanzetti@gmail.com

Academic Editor: Werner Kolb

Introduction. The elbow interposition arthroplasty is a very common procedure performed mainly on active young patients who need great functionality and for whom total joint replacement is contraindicated and arthrodesis is noncompliant. We are going to demonstrate a case of a 34-year-old male suffering from malunion of the distal humerus, elbow stiffness, and manifest signs of arthrosis of the dominant limb, treated with the IA Grika technique at a 5-year follow-up. *Patients and Methods*. The chosen criteria to evaluate the injured side and the uninjured side during the clinical and radiological follow-up were the objective function and related quality of life, measured by the Mayo Elbow Performance Score (MEPS), and postoperative complications. To assess flexion and supination forces and elbow muscular strength, a hydraulic dynamometer was used. *Results*. At a 5-year follow-up, the results were excellent as during the first year. *Conclusions*. The Grika technique is a valid and feasible option in the treatment of elbow injuries.

1. Introduction

Management of elbow arthritis in young patients poses a dilemma in treatment options. Elbow arthritis is a debilitating condition producing pain, stiffness, and functional loss [1]. Etiology varies from the rare primary elbow osteoarthrosis, to more common rheumatoid arthritis and posttraumatic osteoarthritis [1]. Surgery for osteoarthritis includes arthroscopic debridement, resection arthroplasty, interposition arthroplasty, ulnohumeral prosthesis, total elbow prosthesis, and arthrodesis [2]. The purpose of this case report is to describe and demonstrate how the Grika technique proved an excellent salvage option in the posttraumatic elbow osteoarthrosis in a young adult at a 5-year follow-up.

2. The Grika Surgical Technique

The surgical technique is based on our previous elbow trauma surgery experiences. We used a longitudinal posterior incision over the old scar and blunt dissection with careful hemostasis to approach the elbow joint (Figures 1(a) and 1(b)). First of all, the ulnar nerve was identified and left in situ without transposition (Figures 1(b) and 1(c)). Then we identified and opened the Kocher interval between the anconeus and the

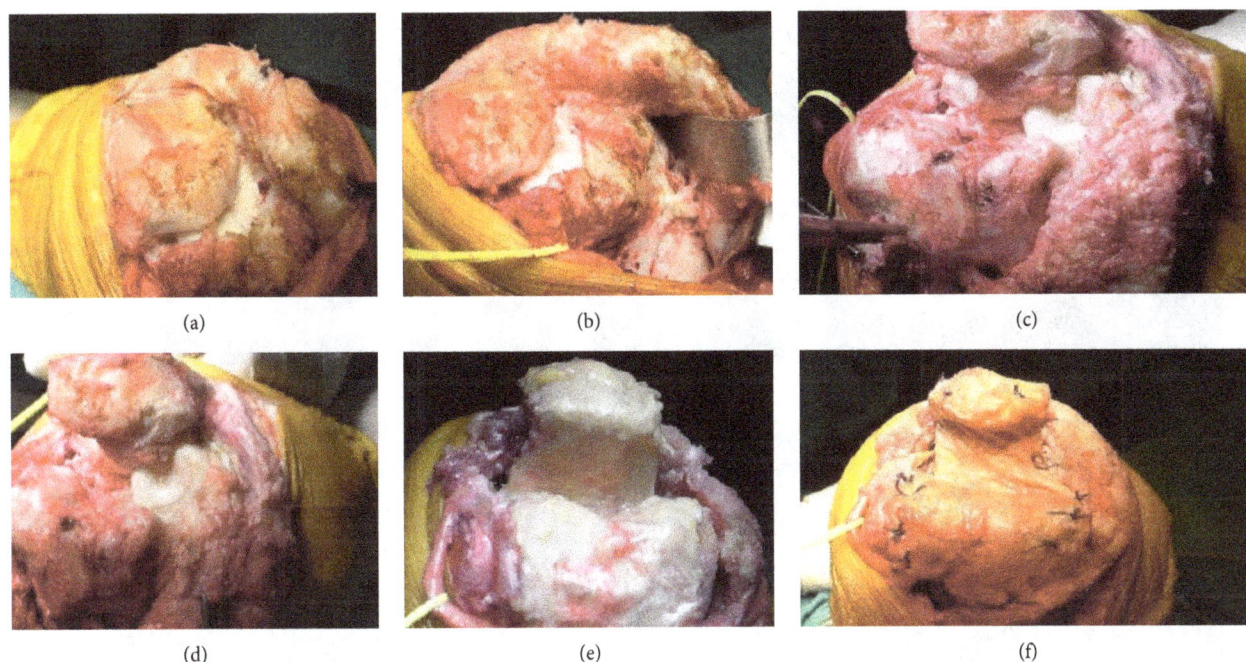

FIGURE 1: Peroperative situation. Posterior arthrotomy (a); marking and preservation of the ulnar nerve (yellow loop) (b); debridement of the ulnohumeral joint (c, d); good cartilage quality on the radial head (d); debrided ulnohumeral joint (e); interposition arthroplasty with sutured fascia lata graft, like a waterfall (f).

carpi ulnaris muscles. Both the lateral and medial collateral ligaments were released from the humerus. A release of the distal tendon of the brachial triceps was performed for complete overview of the elbow joint (Figures 1(c)–1(e)).

Arthrolysis and total synovectomy were performed to maximize range of motion (Figures 1(c)–1(e)) the head of the radius was assessed to have sufficient cartilage quality (Figure 1(d)). The allogeneic fascia lata was interposed like a waterfall from the olecranon over the coronoid process up to the posterior side of the humeral articular surface. Using no. 2 Vicryl (Johnson & Johnson, New Brunswick, NJ, USA), two transosseous Krackow locking stitches at the olecranon and humerus were placed along cascade sutures on all edges of the graft (Figure 1(f)).

After suturing the graft, we reduced the elbow and reinserted the medial and lateral collateral ligaments, strengthened with allograft iliotibial band, were sutured with two Krackow locking stitches using no. 2 Ethibond (Johnson & Johnson, New Brunswick, NJ, USA) into their physiological position. The tendon of the brachial triceps was reanchored with four Krackow locking stitches using no. 2 Ethibond (Johnson & Johnson, New Brunswick, NJ, USA).

After performing stability tests of the elbow and assessing the range of motion, we applied a hinged external elbow fixator (Orthofix, Verona, Italy), with 4 mm of extra distraction (Figure 2).

3. Case Presentation

A 34-year-old male patient was admitted to our center. He had malunion of the distal humerus of his dominant arm (Figure 3), accompanied with elbow stiffness (Figure 4), and evident signs of osteoarthritis were seen on radiographs (Figures 3(c) and 3(d)).

The study was approved by the hospital's Ethical Review Board, and it was conducted in accordance with the principles of the Declaration of Helsinki and its amendments. We fully informed the subject, and he gave his consent.

The patient underwent Grika interposition arthroplasty (see surgical technique paragraph and Figure 1) followed by a suitable rehabilitation protocol (see Rehabilitation Protocol and Figure 2). The external fixator which was used for initial support was removed 14 weeks after surgery.

The injured side (IS) and the noninjured side (NIS) were compared during the clinical follow-up. Function was evaluated with subjective quality of life measured by the Mayo Elbow Performance Score (MEPS) [3].

Objective function was evaluated by range of motion, flexion strength, and supination strength. A calibrated hydraulic dynamometer was used for the strength measurements. During these strength measurements, five measurements were taken by the same evaluator. The mean score of the last four was calculated as the first measurement was disregarded to avoid bias because of a learning curve caused by the patient's awareness.

At 1 year after surgery, both the MEPS and muscle strengths showed a difference in favor of the NIS. At 5 years of follow-up, the IS had a flexion strength of 98% of the NIS (28.9 N versus 29.5 N) and supination strength of 98% of that in the NIS (4.6 versus 4.7) and a MEPS of 100. Functional outcomes are shown in Figure 5.

The patient was monitored for any postoperative complications.

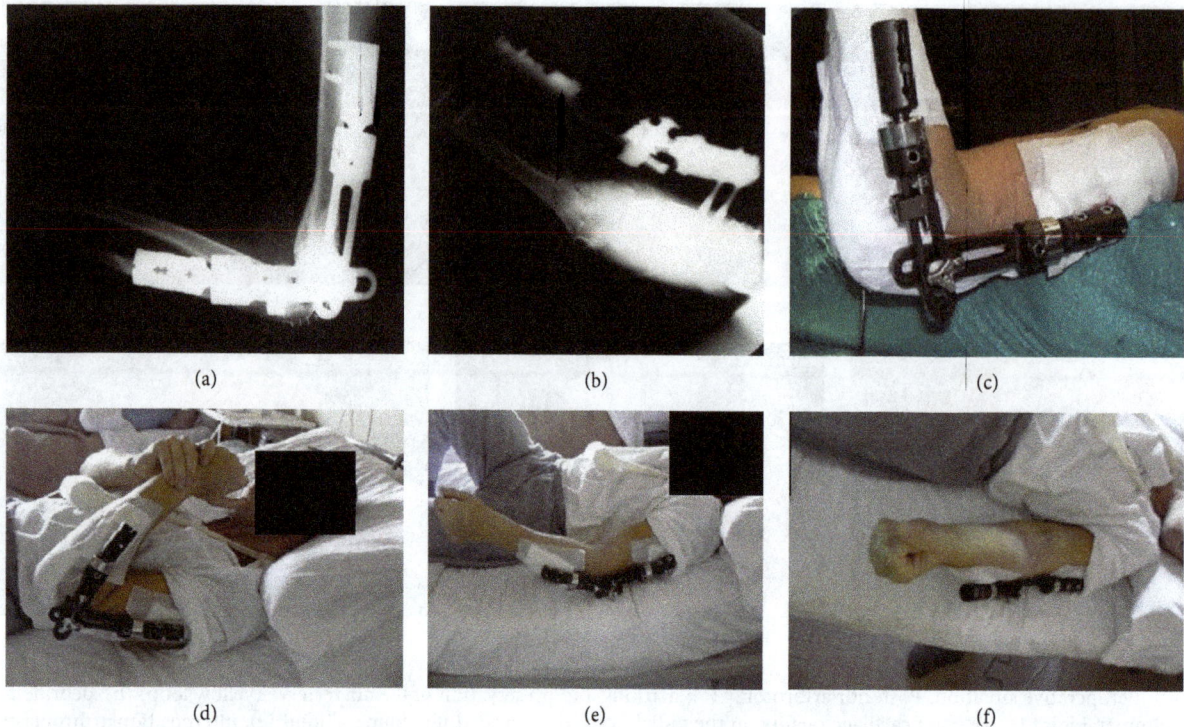

FIGURE 2: Postoperative situation. Postoperative radiographs after Grika interposition arthroplasty with hinged external fixator (a, b); active and passive motion during hospitalization (c–f).

4. Rehabilitation Protocol

4.1. Postoperative Recovery. *Assisted supination and pronation with elbow in 90 degrees of flexion with the arm horizontally. Shoulder range of motion as needed based on evaluation of the physiotherapist, avoiding excessive anteflexion.*

Week 1: active, pain-free flexion and extension combined with assisted passive motions.

> *Range of motion exercises*: Active and assisted passive elbow flexion from 45 degrees of flexion to full flexion and supination with the arm horizontally.

4.2. Strengthening Programme: Part 1. The patient wears a protective brace, except during rehabilitation. Single-plane flexion-extension is trained.

Week 2: submaximal pain-free biceps isometric contractions with elbow in 90 degrees of flexion.

Week 3: single-plane active pain-free elbow flexion, extension, supination, and pronation.

Week 4: pain-free active flexion; 30 degrees of flexion to full elbow flexion with HEEF.

Week 5: pain-free active flexion; 20 degrees of flexion to full elbow flexion with HEEF.

Week 6: pain-free active flexion; 10 degrees of flexion to full elbow flexion with HEEF.

> *Range of motion exercises*: active ROM elbow flexion and extension, pain-free.

4.3. Strengthening Programme: Part 2. Continuing pain-free single plane active elbow flexion, extension, supination, and pronation.

Week 7–11: full range of motion of HEEF and elbow; discontinue brace if adequate motor control without brace.

> *Range of motion exercises*: continue active ROM elbow flexion and extension, pain-free. May begin composite motions, that is, extension with pronation.

If at 8 weeks postoperatively the patient has significant range of motion deficits, physiotherapist may consider more aggressive management, after consultation with referring surgeon, to regain range of motion.

4.4. Strengthening Programme: Part 3. Elbow flexion, extension, supination, and pronation against resistance are progressively allowed.

Week 12: removal of HEEF.

After week 12: may start light upper extremity weight training. Initiate endurance program that simulates desired work activities and requirements.

5. Discussion

The purpose of interposition arthroplasty is to effectively reduce pain and improve functionality in young patients with elbow osteoarthritis without compromising future surgical options. Sears et al. suggested this requires an accurate evaluation of the compliance and the functional demands of the patients [2].

Ulnohumeral arthroplasty is performed for mild and moderate degeneration and may be carried out arthroscopically or open with good functional outcomes. However, the elbow may be at risk of intra-articular fractures

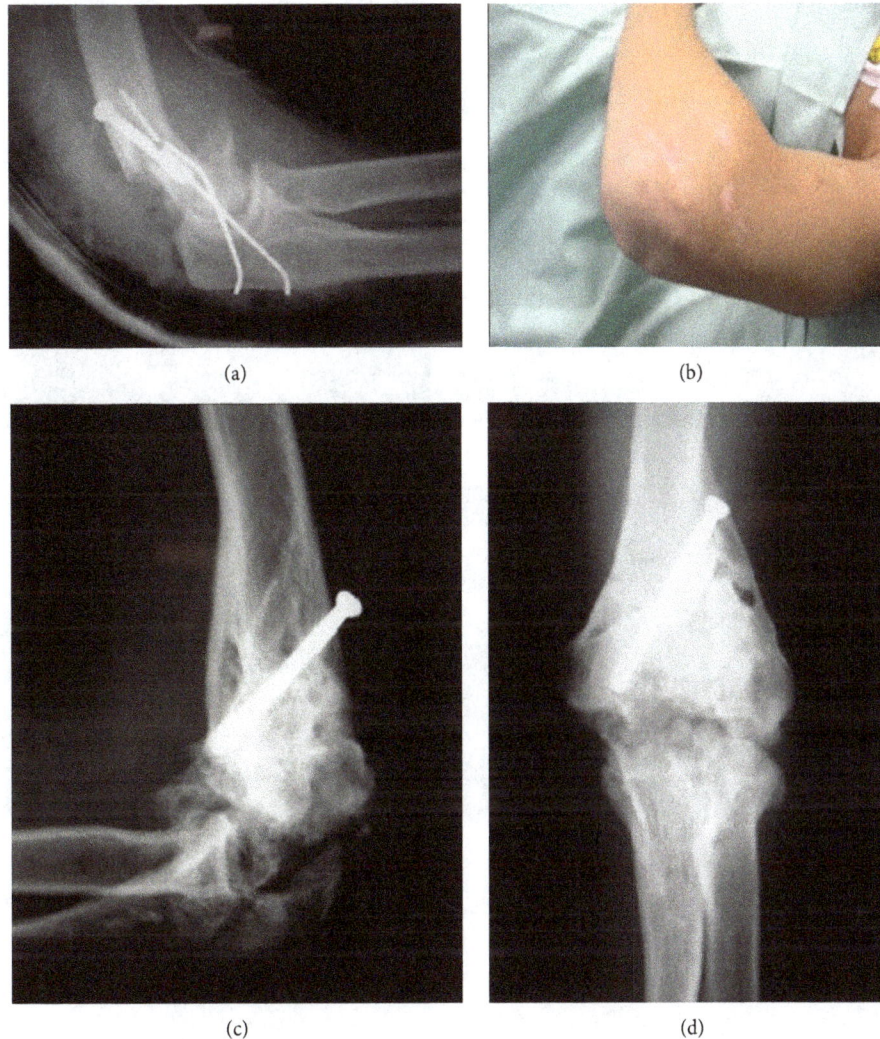

FIGURE 3: Direct postoperative radiograph showing the insufficient fracture fixation after previous surgery (a); the skin showing the scar following previous surgery (b); radiographs showing distal humeral malunion and generalized elbow joint osteoarthritis (c, d).

immediately after surgery, and a certain caution is required before resuming sports activities [4]. Total elbow arthroplasty is performed in patients with osteoarthritis, yet according to literature, it seems to be less favorable and with a greater risk of complications in younger and more demanding patients [5]. Resection arthroplasty and arthrodesis are not feasible for the young and demanding patient, as the consequent loss of function is highly disabling and therefore should be performed only as a last resort [1].

The interposition arthroplasty is one of the oldest reconstructive options for elbow arthritis and other joints, described for a variety of disorders [6]. For years, different elbow interposition tissues have been utilized, varying from synthetic grafts to Achilles tendon allografts [2], free rectus abdominis muscle flaps [7], scapular flaps [2, 6], and the anconeus muscle [6, 8, 9], with or without the addition of a hinged external fixator [1, 10, 11]. This procedure is considered as a salvage option in patients for whom conservative treatment failed, and total elbow arthroplasty is contraindicated [12].

In this specific case, our decision to return to the past, to the Vittorio Putti technique, is based on discoveries that interposition grafts microscopically form a zone with endothelial lined sacs [6, 13]. Melvin Henderson already in 1918 reported that the outcomes of interposition arthroplasty were better in the temporomandibular joint (93% of good outcomes), compared to the elbow (78%), the hip (57%), and the knee (15%) [6]. The high rate of failures in the lower limbs was probably caused by weight bearing [13]. In reexamining the scientific articles published by Vittorio Putti, it is interesting to notice his emphasis placed on the use of the fascia lata [6]. The preference of fascia lata originates from the composition of the fascia lata, as it is rich in collagen. The high collagen content seems to be a rational choice for grafting into osteoarthritic joints. The flap of the fascia lata, used by Putti and in our technique, has a considerable similarity with the small intestinal submucosa and decellularized dermis [1, 14, 15].

In contrast to the original Putti technique, we have used a cadaveric fascia lata allograft instead of an autologous

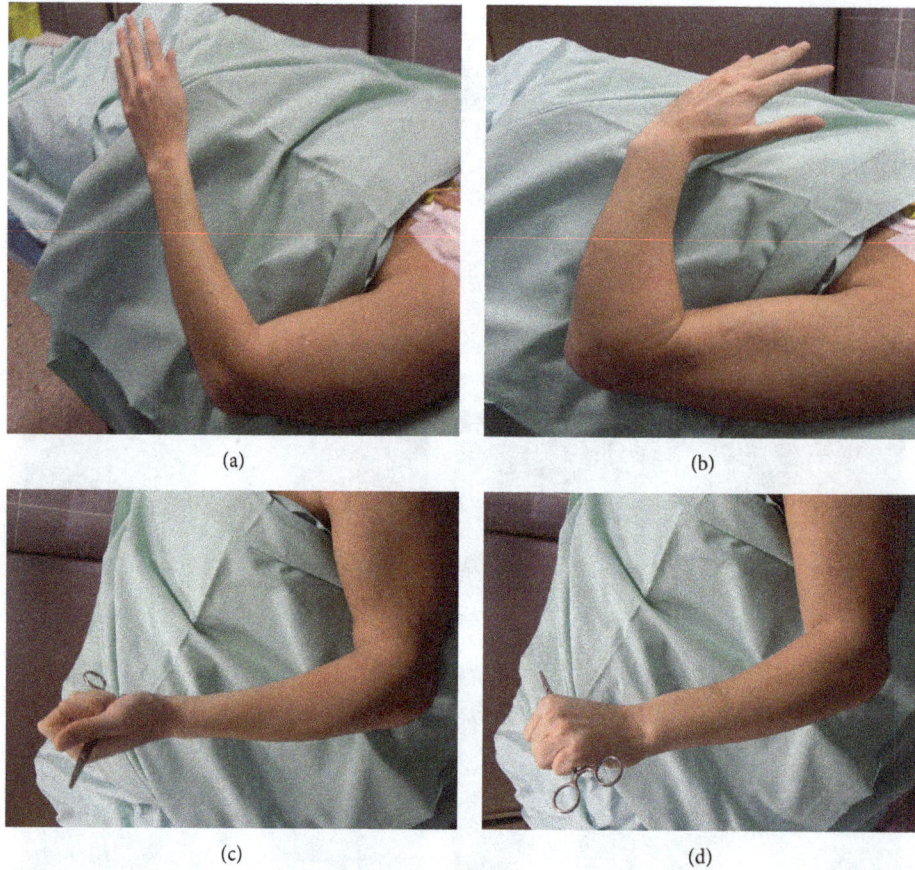

FIGURE 4: Preoperative situation and active elbow range of motion. Maximum of 80 degrees of flexion (a); no possibility of extension (b); sufficient pronation and supination (c, d).

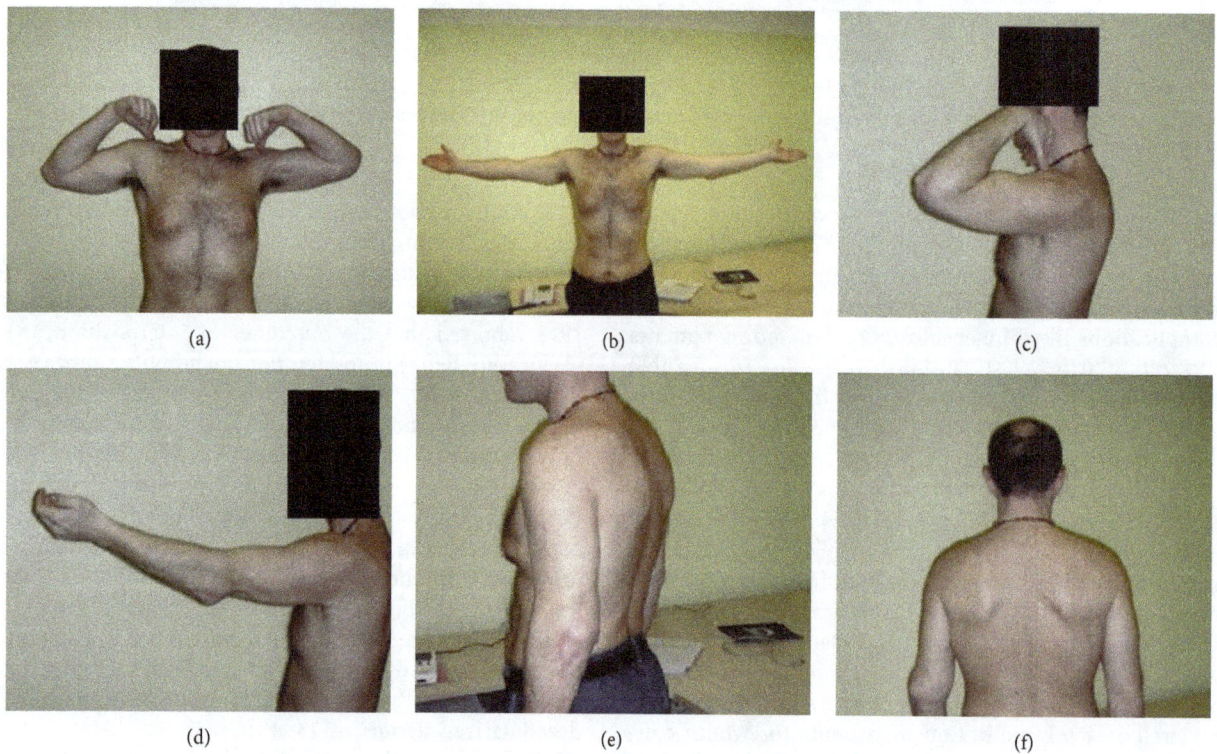

FIGURE 5: Final postoperateive situation at 5 years of follow-up (a–d). Valgus axial deviation (e, f).

graft. Using an autologous graft would result in donor site morbidity and allografts were not available in his time [16]. Another difference between our technique and that of Putti is that our cascade suturing not only fixates the interposition but also ensures covering of the entire joint. Besides, the cascade effect allows neovascularization of the fascia lata through the arterial vessels from the anterior capsule, which are the main protagonists of blood supply to this articular zone [17].

Furthermore, we have used iliotibial allografts to reconstruct the medial and lateral collateral ligaments. Trauma-surgical experience on the ankle and foot demonstrates that iliotibial band allografts showed excellent outcomes in 92% of the cases [18]. Additionally, Lindenhovius and Jupiter [19] describes surgically unblocking the rigid elbow usually necessitates the release of the posterior fascia of the medial collateral ligament, debridement of all calcifications and anterioposterior capsulotomy.

We have used a hinged elbow external fixation to protect the grafts from high-impact loads, as the use of the hinged elbow external fixator had good functional outcomes and good subjective results after extensive releases of the stiff elbow [11, 20]. Besides, distraction itself might have a positive influence on regeneration of the affected tissues [21–23].

6. Conclusion

This case report is to show the first 5-year result of our interposition arthroplasty technique. It also emphasizes that an old surgical technique can be a good solution when a surgical problem is presented which does not fit into standard care programs. This is comparable to the Grika language dialect of the senior author, which is a dialect in the south of Italy dating back to the ancient Greeks but still in use and actual.

Conflicts of Interest

The authors declare that there are no conflicts of interest regarding the publication of this paper.

References

[1] M. Laubscher, A. J. Vochteloo, A. A. Smit, B. C. Vrettos, and S. J. L. Roche, "A retrospective review of a series of interposition arthroplasties of the elbow," *Shoulder & Elbow*, vol. 6, no. 2, pp. 129–133, 2014.

[2] B. W. Sears, G. J. Puskas, M. E. Morrey, J. Sanchez-Sotelo, and B. F. Morrey, "Posttraumatic elbow arthritis in the young adult: evaluation and management," *Journal of the American Academy of Orthopaedic Surgeons*, vol. 20, no. 11, pp. 704–714, 2012.

[3] M. C. Cusick, N. S. Bonnaig, F. M. Azar, B. M. Mauck, R. A. Smith, and T. W. Throckmorton, "Accuracy and reliability of the mayo elbow performance score," *Journal of Hand Surgery*, vol. 39, no. 6, pp. 1146–1150, 2014.

[4] I. Degreef and L. De Smet, "The arthroscopic ulnohumeral arthroplasty: from mini-open to arthroscopic surgery," *Minimally Invasive Surgery*, vol. 2011, Article ID 798084, 5 pages, 2011.

[5] A. Prkic, C. Welsink, B. The, M. P. J. van den Bekerom, and D. Eygendaal, "Why does total elbow arthroplasty fail today? A systematic review of recent literature," *Archives of Orthopaedic and Trauma Surgery*, vol. 137, no. 6, pp. 761–769, 2017.

[6] N. Nicoli Aldini, A. Angelini, S. Pagani, R. Bevoni, M. Girolami, and M. Fini, "Past and present of interposition arthroplasties for joint repair with special tribute to the contribution by Vittorio Putti," *Knee Surgery, Sports Traumatology, Arthroscopy*, vol. 24, no. 12, pp. 4005–4011, 2014.

[7] R. Jaiswal, B. Busse, R. Allen, and D. Sahar, "Treatment of elbow osteomyelitis with an interposition arthroplasty using a rectus abdominis free flap," *Annals of Plastic Surgery*, vol. 74, no. 1, pp. S19–S21, 2015.

[8] B. F. Morrey and A. G. Schneeberger, "Anconeus arthroplasty: a new technique for reconstruction of the radiocapitellar and/or proximal radioulnar joint," *Journal of Bone and Joint Surgery-American Volume*, vol. 84, no. 11, pp. 1960–1969, 2002.

[9] Y. M. K. Baghdadi, B. F. Morrey, and J. Sanchez-Sotelo, "Anconeus interposition arthroplasty: mid- to long-term results," *Clinical Orthopaedics and Related Research*®, vol. 472, no. 7, pp. 2151–2161, 2014.

[10] V. Tan, A. Daluiski, and J. Capo, "Hinged elbow external fixators: indications and uses," *Journal of the American Academy of Orthopaedic Surgeons*, vol. 13, no. 8, pp. 503–514, 2005.

[11] N. C. Chen and A. Julka, "Hinged external fixation of the elbow," *Hand Clinics*, vol. 26, no. 3, pp. 423–433, 2010.

[12] A. Chauhan, B. A. Palmer, and M. E. Baratz, "Arthroscopically assisted elbow interposition arthroplasty without hinged external fixation: surgical technique and patient outcomes," *Journal of Shoulder and Elbow Surgery*, vol. 24, no. 6, pp. 947–954, 2015.

[13] J. Murphy, "The classic: ankylosis: arthroplasty–clinical and experimental. 1905," *Clinical Orthopaedics and Related Research*, vol. 466, no. 11, pp. 2573–2578, 2008.

[14] S. Szotek, J. Dawidowicz, B. Eyden et al., "Morphological features of fascia lata in relation to fascia diseases," *Ultrastructural Pathology*, vol. 40, no. 6, pp. 297–310, 2016.

[15] T. Mihata, M. H. McGarry, T. Kahn, I. Goldberg, M. Neo, and T. Q. Lee, "Biomechanical effect of thickness and tension of fascia lata graft on glenohumeral stability for superior capsule reconstruction in irreparable supraspinatus tears," *Arthroscopy: The Journal of Arthroscopic & Related Surgery*, vol. 32, no. 3, pp. 418–426, 2016.

[16] F. C. Akpuaka, C. B. Eze, and U. E. Anyaehie, "The use of the radial recurrent fasciocutaneous flap in interposition arthroplasty of elbow ankylosis case report and review of literature," *International Journal of Surgery*, vol. 95, pp. 315–318, 2010.

[17] G. Wavreille, C Dos Remedios, C. Chantelot, M. Limousin, and C. Fontaine, "Anatomic bases of vascularized elbow joint harvesting to achieve vascularized allograft," *Surgical and Radiologic Anatomy*, vol. 28, no. 5, pp. 498–510, 2006.

[18] Y. Zhang, "Discussion: Use of the fix and flap approach to complex open elbow injury: The role of the free anterolateral thigh flap," *Archives of Plastic Surgery*, vol. 39, no. 2, p. 137, 2012.

[19] A. L. C. Lindenhovius and J. B. Jupiter, "The Posttraumatic Stiff Elbow: A Review of the Literature," *Journal of Hand Surgery*, vol. 32, no. 10, pp. 1605–1623, 2007.

[20] Y. Zhou, C. J. yu, S. Chen et al., "Application of distal radius–positioned hinged external fixator in complete open release for severe elbow stiffness," *Journal of Shoulder and Elbow Surgery*, vol. 26, no. 2, pp. e44–e51, 2017.

[21] S. L. Cheng and B. F. Morrey, "Treatment of the mobile, painful arthritic elbow by distraction interposition arthroplasty," *Journal of Bone and Joint Surgery. British Volume*, vol. 82, no. 2, pp. 233–238, 2000.

[22] A. De Carli, R. M. Lanzetti, A. Ciompi et al., "Can platelet-rich plasma have a role in Achilles tendon surgical repair?," *Knee Surgery, Sports Traumatology, Arthroscopy*, vol. 24, no. 7, pp. 2231–2237, 2016.

[23] R. M. Lanzetti, A. Vadalà, F. Morelli et al., "Bilateral quadriceps rupture: results with and without platelet-rich plasma," *Orthopedics*, vol. 36, no. 11, pp. e1474–e1478, 2013.

34

Malposition of Cage in Minimally Invasive Oblique Lumbar Interbody Fusion

Chaiwat Kraiwattanapong ⓘ,[1] Vanlapa Arnuntasupakul,[2] Rungthiwa Kantawan,[3] Gun Keorochana,[1] Thamrong Lertudomphonwanit,[1] Pakkanut Sirijaturaporn,[1] and Methawut Thonginta[1]

[1]*Department of Orthopaedics, Ramathibodi Hospital, Mahidol University, Bangkok, Thailand*
[2]*Department of Anesthesiology, Ramathibodi Hospital, Mahidol University, Bangkok, Thailand*
[3]*Department of Nursing, Ramathibodi Hospital, Mahidol University, Bangkok, Thailand*

Correspondence should be addressed to Chaiwat Kraiwattanapong; chaiwatkrai@gmail.com

Academic Editor: Steven Vanni

Introduction. Minimally invasive oblique lumbar interbody fusion is one of the novel lateral lumbar interbody fusion techniques for which the successful early results have been reported. However, new complications were increasingly reported from ongoing studies. *Case Presentation.* We report a case of an unusual complication of minimally invasive oblique lumbar interbody fusion associated with contralateral nerve root compression due to deep and posterior position of polyetheretherketone cage and discussion of the operating technique for repositioning polyetheretherketone cage. *Conclusion.* Malposition of polyetheretherketone cage can cause contralateral nerve root compression and neurological complication. The surgical technique to proper pull the polyetheretherketone cage back into the acceptable position should be considered and well prepared.

1. Background

Minimally invasive lateral lumbar interbody fusion has gained popularity because of several advantages such as less blood loss, less tissue dissection, larger footprint of implant, maximizing load bearing on the cortical bone, and increasing more lordosis of the lumbar spine [1–4].

Minimally invasive oblique lumbar interbody fusion (MIS-OLIF) is one of the novel lateral lumbar interbody fusion techniques. This technique allows access to the intervertebral disc of lumbar spine via retroperitoneal space, between great vessels and psoas muscle. Mayer first described this minimally invasive anterior to psoas muscle technique for lumbar interbody fusion in 1977 [5]. Davis et al. reported an anatomical study of the oblique corridor at each lumbar disc level between the psoas muscle and great vessels and found the potential of the MIS oblique retroperitoneal approach to the L2–S1 discs [6]. Molinares et al. studied 133 MR images of the lumbar spine and reported the oblique corridors of L2–S1 discs between the psoas and the aorta or the left common iliac artery in 90% of the studied samples [7]. With the similar approach, but different instruments and implants, several studies of the MIS-OLIF in term of outcomes and complications have been reported. From the previous studies, complication of mini-open and MIS-OLIF range from 3.9%–48.3% [8–16]. Most of them are transient and completely recover by time. Few case reports published the special complications of MIS-OLIF such as ureteral injury, ventral dural injury [17–19]. This article presents an unusual complication of MIS-OLIF associated with contralateral nerve root compression due to deep and posterior position of MIS-OLIF polyetheretherketone (PEEK) cage and discusses the operating technique for removing MIS-OLIF PEEK cage.

2. Case Presentation

A 60-year-old woman presented with 1-year history of low back pain with lateral aspect of left leg pain and severe neurogenic claudication. There was no neurological deficit. Plain films showed narrowing of L4-L5 disc space and degenerative spondylolisthesis of L4-L5. MRI of L4-L5 showed a degenerative change of intervertebral disc, severe bilateral foraminal stenosis, and moderate central stenosis.

On the axial T1W image, the space between the left common iliac artery and the left psoas muscle was 18.98 mm at level of intervertebral disc space L4-L5 which almost obliterated prepsoas space at level of upper vertebral body of L5 (Figure 1). Her symptoms did not improve after conservative treatments. She was scheduled to perform MIS-OLIF with decompressive laminectomy and fixation with cortical bone trajectory screws at L4-L5.

Intraoperatively, after general anesthesia, the patient was put in right lateral decubitus position. Fluoroscopy was used to confirm true AP and true lateral of L4-L5 intervertebral disc space. Lateral retroperitoneal approach to lumbar spine was performed. Guide wire and sequential dilator were placed and then retractor blades and L4 stability pin were placed as usual. Unfortunately, when the retractor blades were distracted, the left common iliac artery was found in the operating field. This could be explained because the left common iliac artery was close to the edge of left psoas muscle as Figure 1.

The retractor blades and stability pin were then removed. The psoas muscle was retracted and guide wire was replaced more posteriorly. The operation was performed as usual and MIS-OLIF PEEK cage (a 6° lordotic-angled CLYDESDALE®) 10 mm × 50 mm was inserted into the intervertebral disc space under fluoroscopic assistance. The final position from fluoroscopy revealed the tantalum marker of MIS-OLIF PEEK cage was pushed more to the right side of the vertebral body. Reposition of MIS-OLIF PEEK cage was not performed at that time. Posterior decompressive laminectomy at L4-5 and cortical bone trajectory screw fixation was then performed in the prone position.

Postoperatively, the preoperative pain on the left leg disappeared. However, she developed pain and numbness on her right leg corresponding to L4 dermatome. Plain films showed the position of MIS-OLIF PEEK cage was placed too deep over the edge of the right lateral vertebral body (Figure 2). She then was brought to the operating room to reposition the MIS-OLIF PEEK cage. CT and MRI were not performed before the second operation due to remarkable malposition of the MIS-OLIF PEEK cage with acquired pain and numbness of her right leg.

Intraoperatively, after general anesthesia, the patient was put in right lateral decubitus position. The MIS-OLIF PEEK cage was reached from left lateral approach. The removal tool and slap hammer were attached to MIS-OLIF PEEK cage. The slap hammer was impacted to remove MIS-OLIF PEEK cage. However, the MIS-OLIF PEEK cage could not be repositioned and was attached with vertebral bodies. The cause of this malposition might have been from the compression of posterior cortical bone trajectory screws

fixation. The posterior approach was then performed to remove rods from the cortical bone trajectory screws. The removal tool and slap hammer were then attached to the MIS-OLIF PEEK cage. Unfortunately, the MIS-OLIF PEEK cage became stuck and was unmovable.

The MIS-OLIF PEEK cage teeth might have locked with the right lateral end plates of vertebral bodies (Figure 3). The patient was then placed in reverse jack-knife position for opening of the right lateral intervertebral disc space. Retractor blade pins at L4 and L5 vertebral bodies were gradually distracted (Figure 4). The MIS-OLIF PEEK cage then was gently pulled back and adjusted to a more anterior trajectory to achieve an acceptable position (Figure 5).

Postoperatively, the pain on her right leg disappeared and the numbness was improved. She was able to walk without pain. At 3 months follow-up, her back and leg pain had significantly improved and her right leg numbness disappeared. The Oswestry Disability Index was 64.4 at preoperative time and was 26 and 20 at 2 weeks and 3 months postoperative, respectively.

3. Discussion

Minimally invasive lateral interbody fusion is an alternative procedure to the traditional approach for the treatment of degenerative disease of the lumbar spine. Outcome and fusion rate are comparable to traditional interbody fusion with short operating times, minimal blood loss, and few complications [20]. MIS-OLIF is an approach which reaches intervertebral disc through the retroperitoneal space between great vessels and psoas muscle. When we compare transpsoas approach, MIS-OLIF has several advantages such as less invasion of the psoas muscle and lumbar plexus, direct visualization of sensory nerves and important structures. Fujibayashi et al. concluded that MIS-OLIF can be safely performed without using neuromonitoring [21]. However, this novel approach needs more well-designed prospective studies with long-term follow-up. More outcomes and complications of ongoing studies will be published in near future. In this article, we reported the complication which was caused by inappropriate patient selection and inappropriate surgical technique for MIS-OLIF.

This patient might not be a good candidate for MIS-OLIF, because her prepsoas corridor at upper vertebral body of L5 was almost obliterated. Psoas muscle had to be strongly retracted and guide wire had to be placed more posteriorly which resulted in posterior position of MIS-OLIF peek cage. Additionally, her psoas muscle was rising away ventrally from the vertebral body which obstructed the pathway of the entry point to intervertebral disc (Figure 1(d)). Voyadzis et al. reported 3 cases of rising away psoas muscle from the vertebral body which could lead to aborted transpsoas lateral interbody fusion due to pervasive EMG responses throughout the disc space [22]. Currently, there is no report of such complication in MIS-OLIF procedure, but this can cause more difficulty in this situation.

According to the manufacturer, the proper size of the MIS-OLIF PEEK cage should span the entire ring apophysis in order to reach fully across the vertebral body end plate. If

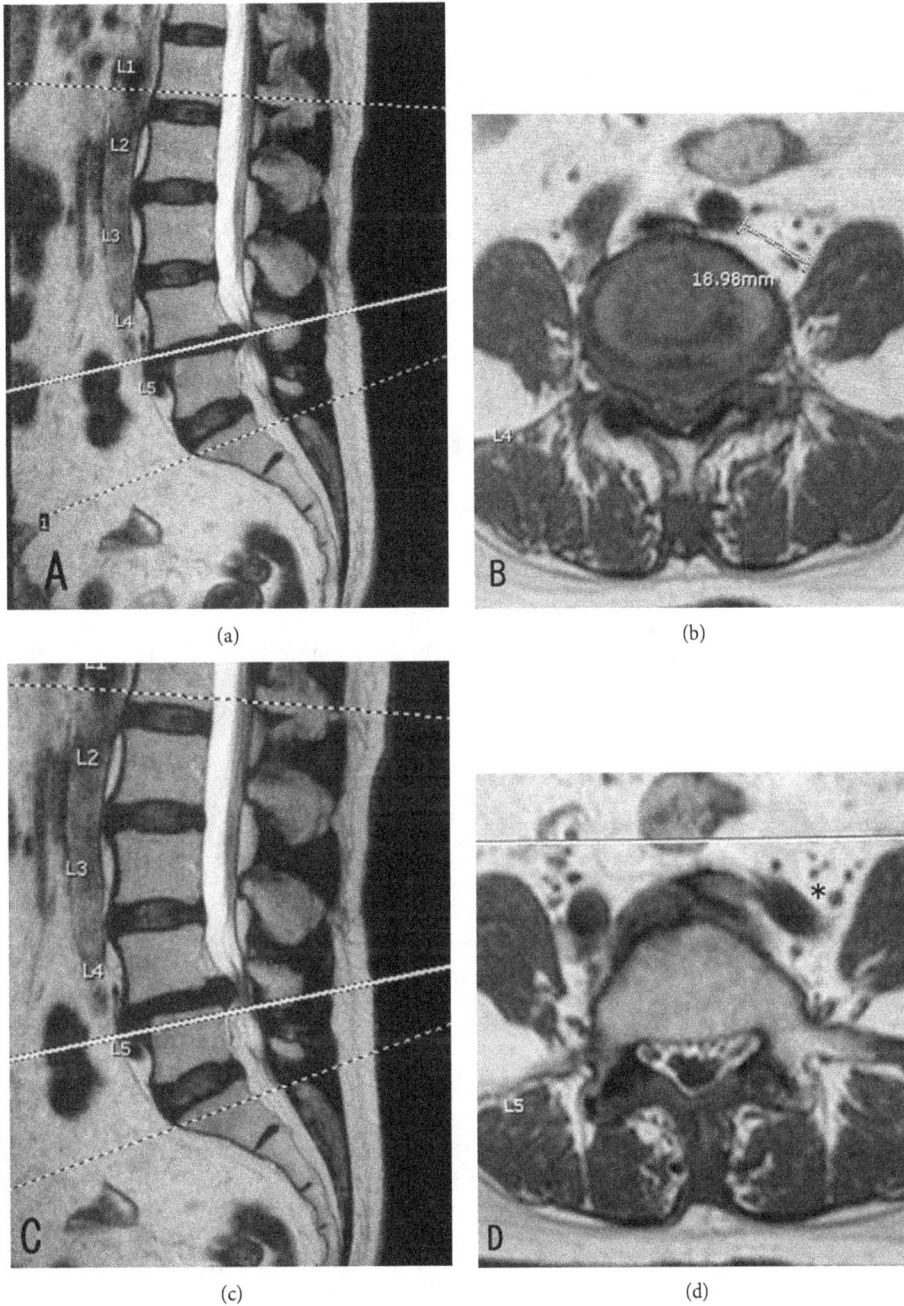

FIGURE 1: Preoperative MRI of lumbosacral spine T1W image showed prepsoas corridor at the level of intervertebral disc space L4-L5 (a and b) and at the level of upper vertebral body of L5 (c and d). Rising of psoas muscle was shown in (d). Left common iliac artery almost obliterates prepsoas space at level of upper vertebral body of L5 (black asterisk).

the position of MIS-OLIF PEEK cage is more posterior, this step is critical and overhang can create contralateral nerve root compression. Silvestre et al. reported outcomes and complications of OLIF with banana shape TLIF PEEK cage in 179 patients. They reported one case of right L4-5 paresthesia and weakness causing by a prominent of 36 mm long TLIF PEEK cage which compressed the dural sac contralaterally. Due to TLIF PEEK cage which is much smaller than MIS-OLIF PEEK cage, she successfully received revision with placement of shorter TLIF PEEK cage of 30 mm length, but

unfortunately she did not recover from her neurological injury [11]. In our case, we used a longer MIS-OLIF PEEK cage (50 mm in length) because this MIS-OLIF PEEK cage was placed more parallel to the posterior cortex of the vertebral body. Papanastassiou et al. reported two cases of contralateral femoral nerve compression after extreme lateral interbody fusion (XLIF). One of them was caused by a displaced endplate fracture fragment and another was caused by a far-lateral herniation. Nerve root decompressions were performed, and patients then experienced resolution of their

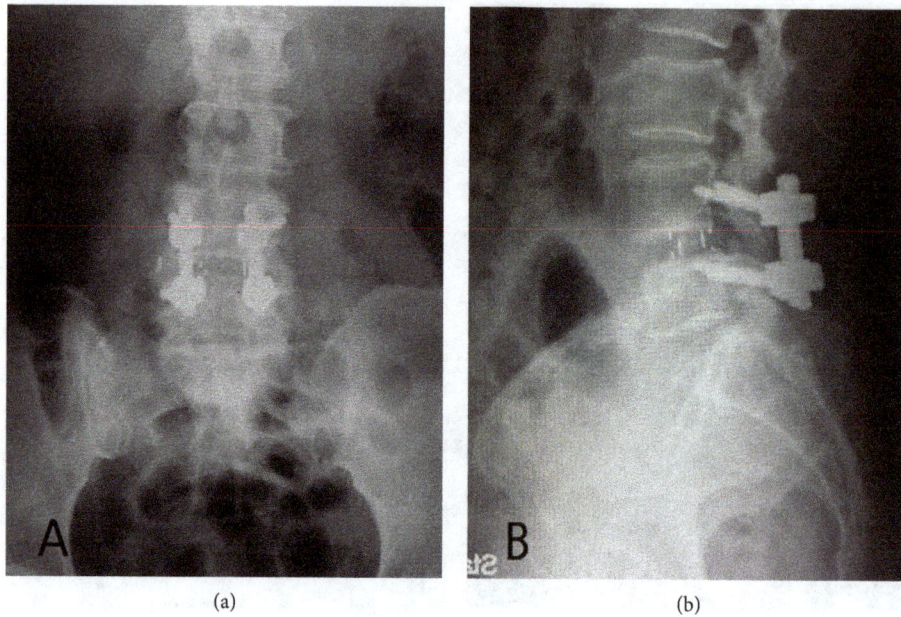

(a)   (b)

FIGURE 2: Postoperative plain films of lumbar spine AP and lateral (a and b) showed the MIS-OLIF PEEK cage was placed too deep over edge of right lateral of vertebral body.

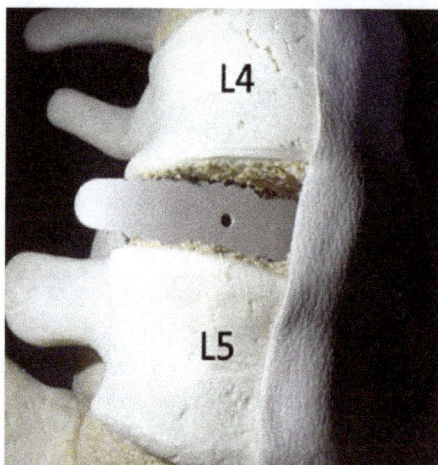

FIGURE 3: Model picture showed the possibility that MIS-OLIF PEEK cage locked with the vertebral endplates.

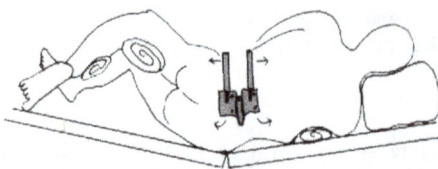

FIGURE 4: Drawing picture showed the reverse jack-knife position of the patient with distraction of retractor blade pins for loosening the MIS-OLIF PEEK cage form the vertebral endplates.

symptoms [23]. In our case, the deep and posterior MIS-OLIF PEEK cage position caused the compression of the nerve plexus, so we then tried to reposition the MIS-OLIF PEEK cage. When the reposition of the MIS-OLIF PEEK cage was performed, posterior instrumentation had to be removed as the first step for loosening of the intervertebral disc. Teeth on the surface of MIS-OLIF PEEK cage are designed for reducing the likelihood of expulsion. If the MIS-OLIF PEEK cage is inserted too deep, its teeth will lock with the edge of the vertebral body, preventing pull back of the MIS-OLIF PEEK cage. The surgical technique tips are important for complication, so to solve this problem, our technique should be considered. Reverse jack-knife position could open the contralateral disc space and the use of 2 retractor blade pins at upper and lower vertebral bodies should help to open the ipsilateral disc space. Longer retractor blade pins increase more distraction force. Bone removal may be required in case MIS-OLIF PEEK cage cannot be removed, but this may cause loosening of implant. Extraforaminal decompression of nerve root [23] as discussed above is the surgical option if we cannot directly reposition the MIS-OLIF PEEK cage. The disadvantages of this technique are more incision and more muscle dissection which need to be done. Another option of treatment is right side retroperitoneal approach and directly address to the MIS-OLIF PEEK cage. However, due to the MIS-OLIF PEEK cage was pointed to posterior of the right psoas muscle, where the nerve plexus is, so there is risk of nerve injury.

4. Conclusion

This study reported the complication from the deep and posterior position of PEEK cage in MIS-OLIF. The position and trajectory of MIS-OLIF PEEK cage are important during the insertion steps. It can cause contralateral nerve root compression and neurological complication. The surgical technique to proper pull the PEEK back into the acceptable position and relieve the pressure to the neural

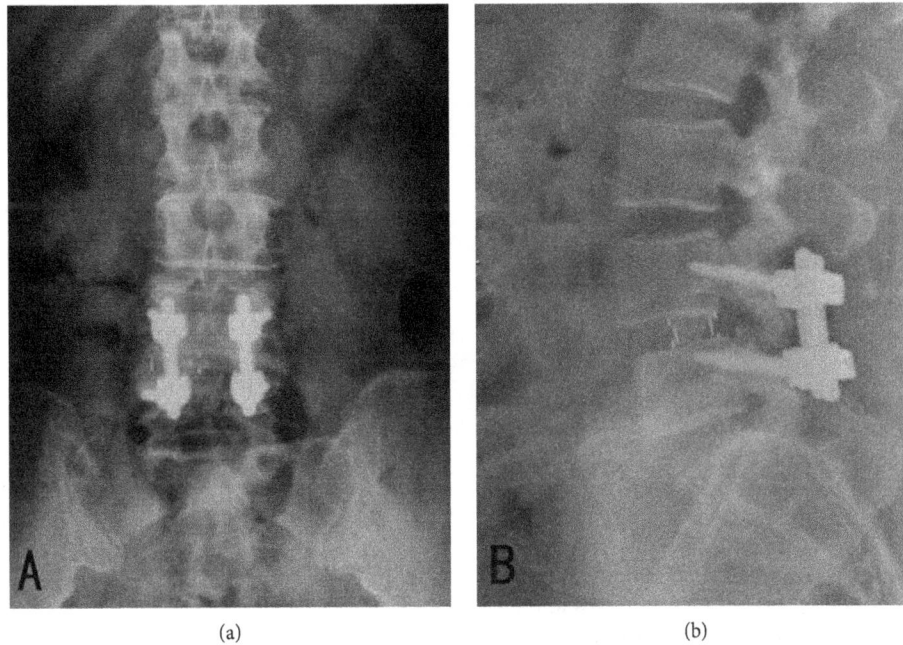

(a)   (b)

FIGURE 5: Three months postoperative plain films of lumbar spine AP and lateral (a and b) showed the acceptable position of MIS-OLIF PEEK cage.

structure should be considered and prepared, since the designed implant may cause difficulty of removal. We described and discussed possible techniques to correct this unusual complication.

Conflicts of Interest

The authors declare that they have no conflicts of interest.

References

[1] L. Pimenta, A. W. L. Turner, Z. A. Dooley, R. D. Parikh, and M. D. Peterson, "Biomechanics of lateral interbody spacers: going wider for going stiffer," *The Scientific World Journal*, vol. 2012, Article ID 381814, 6 pages, 2012.

[2] B. M. Ozgur, H. E. Aryan, L. Pimenta, and W. R. Taylor, "Extreme lateral interbody fusion (XLIF): a novel surgical technique for anterior lumbar interbody fusion," *The Spine Journal*, vol. 6, no. 4, pp. 435–443, 2006.

[3] A. Ahmadian, S. Verma, G. M. Mundis Jr., R. J. Oskouian Jr., D. A. Smith, and J. S. Uribe, "Minimally invasive lateral retroperitoneal transpsoas interbody fusion for L4-5 spondylolisthesis: clinical outcomes," *Journal of Neurosurgery: Spine*, vol. 19, no. 3, pp. 314–320, 2013.

[4] C. Castro, L. Oliveira, R. Amaral, L. Marchi, and L. Pimenta, "Is the lateral transpsoas approach feasible for the treatment of adult degenerative scoliosis?," *Clinical Orthopaedics and Related Research®*, vol. 472, no. 6, pp. 1776–1783, 2014.

[5] M. H. Mayer, "A new microsurgical technique for minimally invasive anterior lumbar interbody fusion," *Spine*, vol. 22, no. 6, pp. 691–699, 1997.

[6] T. T. Davis, R. A. Hynes, D. A. Fung et al., "Retroperitoneal oblique corridor to the L2-S1 intervertebral discs in the lateral

position: an anatomic study," *Journal of Neurosurgery: Spine*, vol. 21, no. 5, pp. 785–793, 2014.

[7] D. M. Molinares, T. T. Davis, and D. A. Fung, "Retroperitoneal oblique corridor to the L2-S1 intervertebral discs: an MRI study," *Journal of Neurosurgery: Spine*, vol. 24, no. 2, pp. 248–255, 2016.

[8] K. Abe, S. Orita, C. Mannoji et al., "Perioperative complications in 155 patients who underwent oblique lateral interbody fusion surgery: perspectives and indications from a retrospective, multicenter survey," *Spine*, vol. 42, no. 1, pp. 55–62, 2017.

[9] J. Jin, K. S. Ryu, J. W. Hur, J. H. Seong, J. S. Kim, and H. J. Cho, "Comparative study of the difference of perioperative complication and radiologic results: MIS-DLIF (minimally invasive direct lateral lumbar interbody fusion) versus MIS-OLIF (minimally invasive oblique lateral lumbar interbody fusion)," *Clinical Spine Surgery*, vol. 31, no. 1, pp. 31–36, 2018.

[10] S. Ohtori, S. Orita, K. Yamauchi et al., "Mini-open anterior retroperitoneal lumbar interbody fusion: oblique lateral interbody fusion for lumbar spinal degeneration disease," *Yonsei Medical Journal*, vol. 56, no. 4, pp. 1051–1059, 2015.

[11] C. Silvestre, J. M. Mac-Thiong, R. Hilmi, and P. Roussouly, "Complications and morbidities of mini-open anterior retroperitoneal lumbar interbody fusion: oblique lumbar interbody fusion in 179 patients," *Asian Spine Journal*, vol. 6, no. 2, pp. 89–97, 2012.

[12] J. Sato, S. Ohtori, S. Orita et al., "Radiographic evaluation of indirect decompression of mini-open anterior retroperitoneal lumbar interbody fusion: oblique lateral interbody fusion for degenerated lumbar spondylolisthesis," *European Spine Journal*, vol. 26, no. 3, pp. 671–678, 2017.

[13] K. Phan and R. J. Mobbs, "Oblique lumbar interbody fusion for revision of non-union following prior posterior

surgery: a case report," *Orthopaedic Surgery*, vol. 7, no. 4, pp. 364–367, 2015.

[14] J. Katzell, "Endoscopic foraminal decompression preceding oblique lateral lumbar interbody fusion to decrease the incidence of post operative dysaesthesia," *International Journal of Spine Surgery*, vol. 8, 2014.

[15] K. Kanno, S. Ohtori, S. Orita et al., "Miniopen oblique lateral L5-s1 interbody fusion: a report of 2 cases," *Case Reports in Orthopedics*, vol. 2014, Article ID 603531, 5 pages, 2014.

[16] C. Gragnaniello and K. Seex, "Anterior to psoas (ATP) fusion of the lumbar spine: evolution of a technique facilitated by changes in equipment," *Journal of Spine Surgery*, vol. 2, no. 4, pp. 256–265, 2016.

[17] J. Chang, J. S. Kim, and H. Jo, "Ventral dural injury after oblique lumbar interbody fusion," *World Neurosurgery*, vol. 98, pp. 881.e1–881.e4, 2017.

[18] G. Kubota, S. Orita, T. Umimura, K. Takahashi, and S. Ohtori, "Insidious intraoperative ureteral injury as a complication in oblique lumbar interbody fusion surgery: a case report," *BMC Research Notes*, vol. 10, no. 1, p. 193, 2017.

[19] H. J. Lee, J. S. Kim, K. S. Ryu, and C. K. Park, "Ureter injury as a complication of oblique lumbar interbody fusion," *World Neurosurgery*, vol. 102, pp. 693.e7–693.e14, 2017.

[20] J. A. Youssef, P. C. McAfee, C. A. Patty et al., "Minimally invasive surgery: lateral approach interbody fusion," *Spine*, vol. 35, no. 26S, pp. S302–S311, 2010.

[21] S. Fujibayashi, R. A. Hynes, B. Otsuki, H. Kimura, M. Takemoto, and S. Matsuda, "Effect of indirect neural decompression through oblique lateral interbody fusion for degenerative lumbar disease," *Spine*, vol. 40, no. 3, pp. E175–E182, 2015.

[22] J. M. Voyadzis, D. Felbaum, and J. Rhee, "The rising psoas sign: an analysis of preoperative imaging characteristics of aborted minimally invasive lateral interbody fusions at L4-5," *Journal of Neurosurgery: Spine*, vol. 20, no. 5, pp. 531–537, 2014.

[23] I. D. Papanastassiou, M. Eleraky, and F. D. Vrionis, "Contralateral femoral nerve compression: an unrecognized complication after extreme lateral interbody fusion (XLIF)," *Journal of Clinical Neuroscience*, vol. 18, no. 1, pp. 149–151, 2011.

35

Pyogenic Spondylitis Caused by Methicillin-Resistant *Staphylococcus aureus* Associated with Tracheostomy followed by Resection of Ossification of the Anterior Longitudinal Ligament

Michio Hongo , Naohisa Miyakoshi, Masashi Fujii, Yuji Kasukawa, Yoshinori Ishikawa, Daisuke Kudo, and Yoichi Shimada

Department of Orthopedic Surgery, Akita University Graduate School of Medicine, 1-1-1 Hondo, Akita 010-8543, Japan

Correspondence should be addressed to Michio Hongo; mhongo@doc.med.akita-u.ac.jp

Academic Editor: Johannes Mayr

Symptomatic ossification of the anterior longitudinal ligament (OALL) is rare. However, when the osteophyte enlarges and obstructive symptoms occur, the patient may require surgery. We present a case of pyogenic spondylitis caused by methicillin-resistant *Staphylococcus aureus* associated with tracheostomy followed by resection of OALL. A 69-year-old woman with OALL complained of dysphagia and suffocation, which was caused by prominent OALL at C4-5. Tracheostomy was performed, followed by osteophytectomy 6 weeks later. Two months after osteophytectomy, she complained of muscle weakness of the extremities, neck pain, and elevated temperature. Magnetic resonance imaging showed an intensity change at the C4-5 vertebrae and an epidural abscess that was causing cord compression requiring urgent decompression. Cultures identified methicillin-resistant *Staphylococcus aureus*. As osteolytic change and muscle weakness gradually progressed, she underwent anterior and posterior reconstruction with an autograft and instrumentation. Bone union was confirmed at 1 year postoperatively with improvement in neurological status. OALL has potentially the risk of airway obstruction. Therefore, appropriate diagnosis and prompt osteophytectomy are needed in cases of a large prominent ossification that puts the patient at risk of suffocation. However, it is noted that osteophytectomy following urgent tracheostomy carries the possible risk of infection.

1. Introduction

Ossification of the anterior longitudinal ligament (OALL) was first described by Forestier et al. [1, 2] as ankylosing hyperostosis of the spine. It is also known as diffuse idiopathic skeletal hyperostosis (DISH) [3]. OALL is usually asymptomatic and so is found incidentally. When the OALL is extraordinarily large, it can compress the pharyngoesophageal and laryngotracheal segments, resulting in several symptoms, including dysphagia, dyspnea, and hoarseness. The incidence of these symptoms, however, is relatively low. Airway obstruction is rare, but when it appears, it can be fatal. Here, we present a case of pyogenic spondylitis caused by Methicillin-resistant *Staphylococcus aureus* associated with tracheostomy followed by resection of OALL. It eventually was complicated with myelopathy caused by ossification of the posterior longitudinal ligament (OPLL).

2. Case Report

2.1. History and Examination. A 69-year-old woman who had had dysphagia for 3 years visited our hospital because of having difficulty drinking. She had a history of type 2 diabetes mellitus, angina, Basedow disease, gallstones, and a left femoral diaphyseal fracture. Firstly, she was suspicious of having neurological dysphagia. However, her neurological examination was within normal limits, according to the evaluation by neurology department. Plain radiographs of the cervical spine showed prominence of OALL at C4-5. Esophagography revealed barium retention at the laryngeal part of the pharynx (Figure 1) and anterior displacement of the esophagus and trachea at C4-5 due to OALL, although swallow motility otherwise appeared normal. Radiographs of the thoracic and lumbar spine were compatible with DISH. Computed tomography (CT) revealed the prominence of the

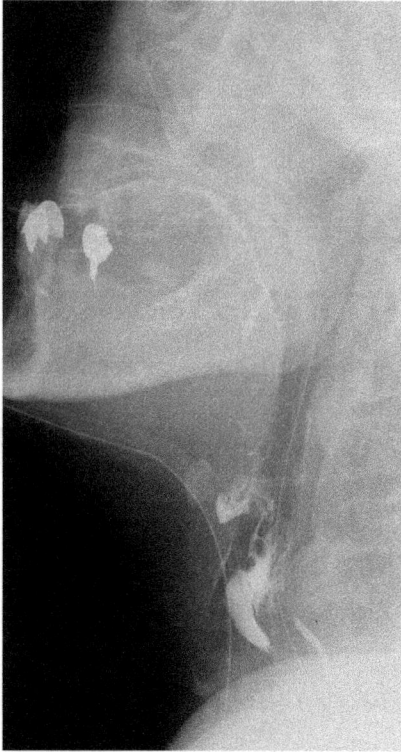

FIGURE 1: Esophagography showing prominent ossification of OALL compressing the esophagus and trachea.

OALL accompanied with displacement of the esophagus at C4-5 (Figures 2(a) and 2(b)).

2.2. First Treatment. We considered surgery to remove the prominent OALL, but the otolaryngologist warned of impending suffocation. Urgent tracheostomy was therefore performed to avoid that situation. Osteophytectomy immediately following tracheostomy offered a potentially high risk of infection because the two skin incisions would be close. Therefore, we waited for the soft tissues to recover. However, her swallowing function did not improve, so, unavoidably, we performed an osteophytectomy using a left anterolateral transcervical approach 6 weeks after the tracheostomy (Figure 3).

2.3. Second Treatment. Two months after the OALL resection, she complained of severe neck pain and an elevated temperature. Laboratory studies showed an increased C-reactive protein (CRP) of 7.97 mg/dL and a white blood cell count (WBC) of 11,300 cells/mm^3. Clinical examination revealed muscle weakness in the upper limbs (shoulder abduction, elbow flexion, and elbow extension of 2/5, 3/5, and 4/5, resp.). Cervical magnetic resonance imaging (MRI) showed spinal stenosis at C4-5 due to ossification of the posterior longitudinal ligament (OPLL) and a signal intensity change of the intervertebral disc of C5-6 (Figure 4).

Because her paralysis was progressive, we performed urgent decompression by laminectomy at C3-7. There was no abscess or granuloma caused by infection at the epidural

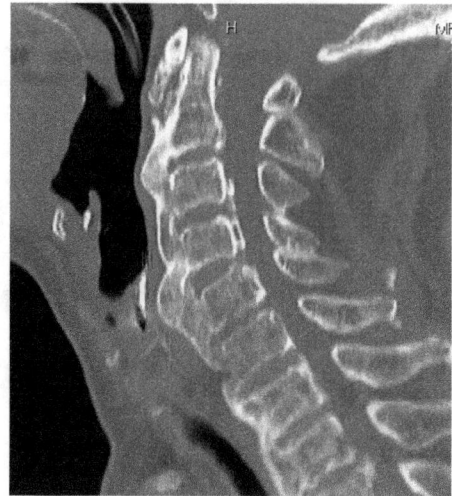

(a)

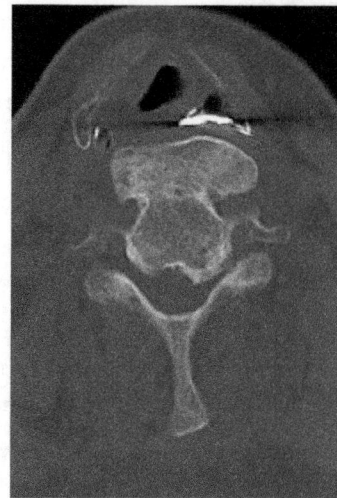

(b)

FIGURE 2: Sagittal (a) and axial (b) image of CT showing extensive OALL at C4-5.

space or posterior column of the cervical spine. After the decompression surgery, she wore a Philadelphia collar, and her muscle strength improved gradually (shoulder abduction, elbow flexion, and elbow extension were 4/5, 4/5, and 4/5, resp.). However, her high body temperature and laboratory evidence of an inflammatory reaction continued. The 6-week follow-up CT findings indicated an osteolytic change at the C4 and 5 vertebra and partial kyphosis at this level (Figure 5). The intensity change on the C4-5 vertebra and the epidural abscess were obvious on MRI with gadolinium contrast.

2.4. Third Treatment and Postoperative Course. We decided to reoperate to remove any infected tissue and reconstruct the cervical spine. She underwent debridement, anterior spinal fusion using iliac bone graft (C3-6), and posterior spinal fusion using lateral mass screws and pedicle screws (C2-7) (Figures 6(a) and 6(b)). She was fitted with a Philadelphia collar for postoperative immobilization.

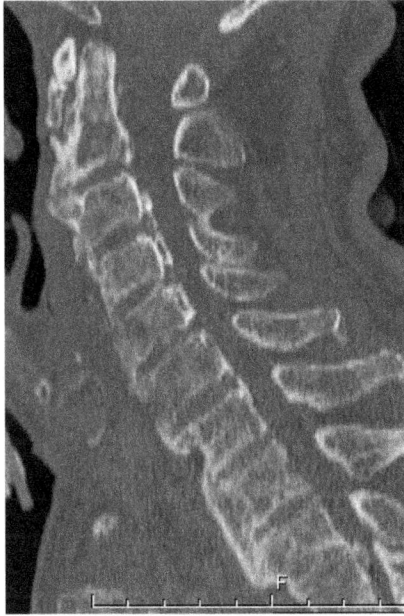

FIGURE 3: Sagittal CT image after removal of OALL.

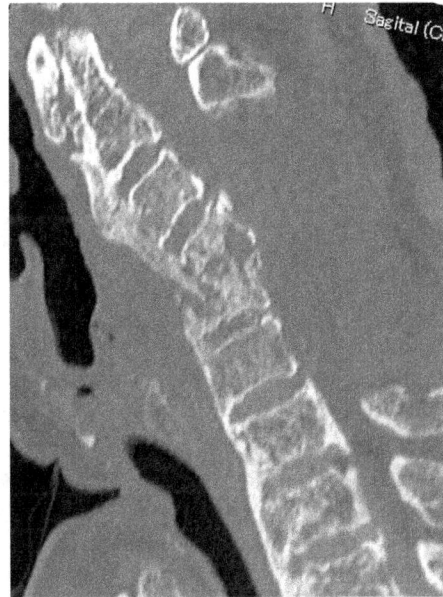

FIGURE 5: Sagittal CT showing an osteolytic and destructive change at the C4 and 5 vertebra and local kyphosis.

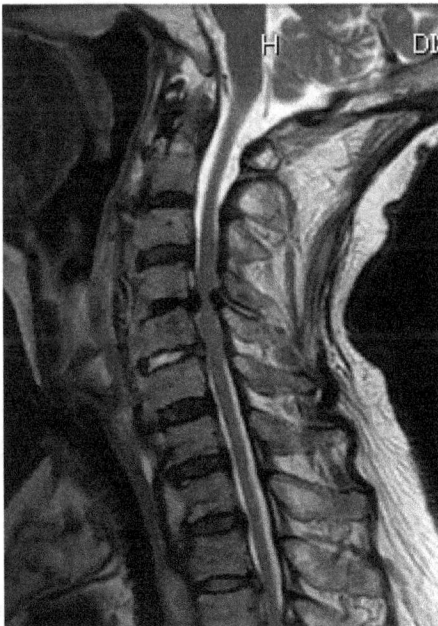

FIGURE 4: Magnetic resonance imaging after removal of OALL showing spinal canal stenosis due to ossification of the posterior longitudinal ligament at C4-5.

Intraoperative cultures identified methicillin-resistant *Staphylococcus aureus*. Antibiotic therapy comprised intravenous administration of vancomycin (0.5 g three times daily) and fosfomycin (1 g three times daily), as well as oral administration of rifampicin (150 mg three times daily). At 4 weeks postoperatively, she experienced a recovery of strength and was able to sit up by herself. The laboratory studies normalized, and she was discharged. Spinal stabilization was established one year after the surgery (Figure 6) with obvious bone union confirmed on CT. She showed no deterioration in neurological status.

3. Discussion

OALL has been described as a possible cause of dysphagia [4, 5]. The incidence of dysphagia in patients with OALL has been reported to be 17–28% [3, 6, 7]. The various mechanisms of dysphagia are mechanical compression causing esophageal obstruction, pharyngoesophageal irritation, and a local inflammatory response resulting in cricopharyngeal spasm and esophageal denervation [8]. In the present case, no underlying neurological disorders were identified, and the examination of her swallowing function revealed no abnormal movements. Eventually, a prominent OALL was diagnosed as the cause of dysphagia 3 years after the patient's initial complaint and 2 weeks after her presentation to our clinic.

Airway obstruction with or without dysphagia caused by hypertrophic anterior cervical osteophytes is an uncommon pathology, with few reported cases [9–11]. Giger et al. reported a case with progressive dysphagia and acute dyspnea, necessitating emergency tracheotomy [10]. The patient underwent surgical removal of all osteophytes, which led to resolution of the symptoms. Carlson et al. retrospectively investigated nine patients with complaints of dysphagia and who underwent osteophytectomy [11]. Two of the nine patients with dysphagia had simultaneous airway complaints, and one of them required concurrent tracheostomy. In addition to dysphagia and respiratory distress, aspiration pneumonia caused by diffuse cervical hyperostosis was reported [9]. Our patient underwent tracheostomy because of airway obstruction. Careful attention and prompt treatment for failing respiratory function are needed in patients who complain of dysphagia and who have a prominent OALL.

OPLL frequently coexists with OALL, possibly causing spinal cord compression and symptomatic myelopathy. Mizuno et al. reported seven patients with OALL, all of whom complained of dysphagia and underwent removal of

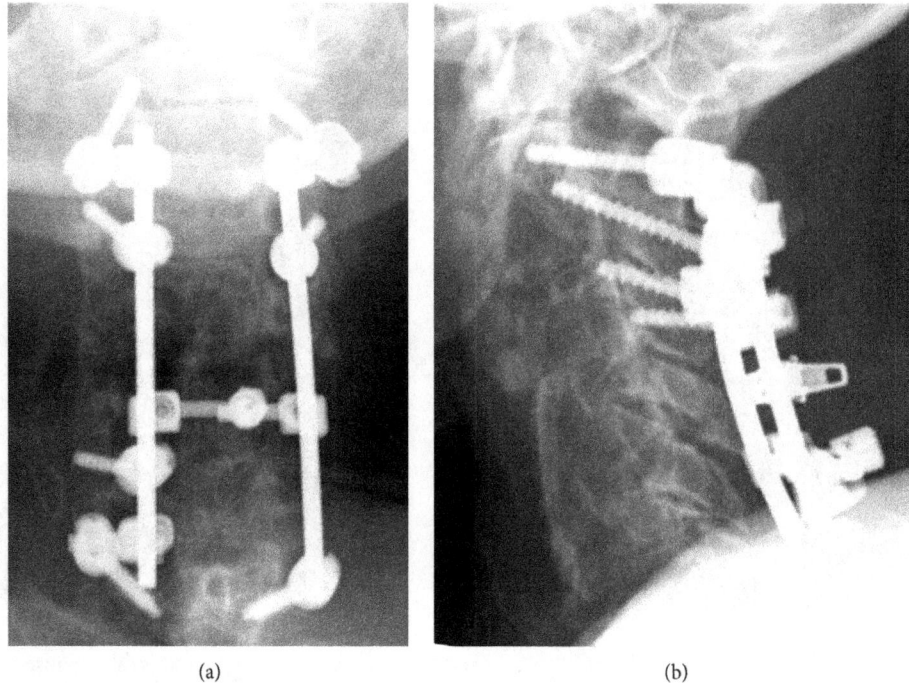

(a)   (b)

FIGURE 6: Plain radiography 1 year postoperatively. (a) AP view and (b) lateral view.

the OALL [12]. Five of the patients concurrently had OPLL that required decompression and fusion. Ando et al., although evaluating the surgical outcome of ossification of the thoracic ligamentum flavum (OLF), described the types of OALL that were strongly associated with the severe symptoms and surgical outcomes of OLF [13]. This association was considered to be caused by a mechanical stress shield arising from the OALL. Therefore, under the circumstance of asymptomatic spinal stenosis before the initial surgery in the current case, removal of the prominent ossification and the osteolytic change due to spondylitis increased segmental mobility, leading to worsening of the myelopathy.

Surgical intervention is indicated for patients with respiratory complaints and myelopathy and who failed conservative treatment. The simple removal of OALL through an anterolateral transcervical approach has been shown to alleviate dysphagia [5, 11, 14]. However, several reports recommended that a fusion procedure should accompany removal of OALL to prevent postoperative instability or osteophyte progression and to decompress the spinal cord [15]. Miyamoto et al. reported that surgical resection of osteophytes resulted in a high likelihood of osteophyte recurrence [16].

In the current case, the risk of infection at the surgical site through the anterior approach next to the location of the tracheostomy was still anticipated. Increased risk of postoperative infection in posterior instrumentation for DISH has been reported [17] although tracheostomy did not increase the risk of infection in subsequent anterior cervical surgery in patients with cervical cord injury [18]. Careful preparation of the skin and placement of the second surgical incision lateral to the tracheostomy site should have been prepared. Unavoidable osteophytectomy improved the swallowing function temporarily, but it caused pyogenic spondylitis, which induced

instability and resulted in the associated myelopathy. Finally, combined anterior and posterior decompression and fusion with anterior autograft successfully restored the neurological status and eliminated the dysphagia. Solid fusion was achieved once the infected tissues had healed. After reviewing the process of our case, we believe that we could have made an earlier diagnosis of prominent OALL that was likely to cause suffocation. We then would have performed osteophytectomy before tracheostomy.

Conflicts of Interest

The authors declare no conflicts of interest associated with this manuscript.

Authors' Contributions

Hongo and Miyakoshi conceived and designed the study. Miyakoshi and Kasukawa analysed and interpreted data. Hongo and Fujii drafted the manuscript. All authors reviewed the article. Miyakoshi and Hongo critically revised the article. Shimada supervised the study.

References

[1] J. Forestier and J. Rotes-Querol, "Senile ankylosing hyperostosis of the spine," *Annals of the Rheumatic Diseases*, vol. 9, no. 4, pp. 321–330, 1950.

[2] J. Forestier and R. Lagier, "Ankylosing hyperostosis of the spine," *Clinical Orthopaedics and Related Research*, vol. 74, no. 1, pp. 65–83, 1971.

[3] D. Resnick, S. R. Shaul, and J. M. Robins, "Diffuse idiopathic skeletal hyperostosis (DISH): Forestier's disease with extraspinal manifestations," *Radiology*, vol. 115, no. 3, pp. 513–524, 1975.

[4] F. W. Gamache Jr. and R. M. Voorhies, "Hypertrophic cervical osteophytes causing dysphagia. A review," *Journal of Neurosurgery*, vol. 53, no. 3, pp. 338–344, 1980.

[5] R. R. McCafferty, M. J. Harrison, L. B. Tamas, and M. V. Larkins, "Ossification of the anterior longitudinal ligament and Forestier's disease: an analysis of seven cases," *Journal of Neurosurgery*, vol. 83, no. 1, pp. 13–17, 1995.

[6] D. Resnick, "Diffuse idiopathic skeletal hyperostosis," *American Journal of Roentgenology*, vol. 130, no. 3, pp. 588-589, 1978.

[7] J. Song, J. Mizuno, and H. Nakagawa, "Clinical and radiological analysis of ossification of the anterior longitudinal ligament causing dysphagia and hoarseness," *Neurosurgery*, vol. 58, no. 5, pp. 913–919, 2006.

[8] J. J. Verlaan, P. F. Boswijk, J. A. de Ru, W. J. A. Dhert, and F. Cumhur Oner, "Diffuse idiopathic skeletal hyperostosis of the cervical spine: an underestimated cause of dysphagia and airway obstruction," *Spine Journal*, vol. 11, no. 11, pp. 1058–1067, 2011.

[9] C. Warnick, M. S. Sherman, and R. W. Lesser, "Aspiration pneumonia due to diffuse cervical hyperostosis," *Chest*, vol. 98, no. 3, pp. 763-764, 1990.

[10] R. Giger, P. Dulguerov, and M. Payer, "Anterior cervical osteophytes causing dysphagia and dyspnea: an uncommon entity revisited," *Dysphagia*, vol. 21, no. 4, pp. 259–263, 2006.

[11] M. L. Carlson, D. J. Archibald, D. E. Graner, and J. L. Kasperbauer, "Surgical management of dysphagia and airway obstruction in patients with prominent ventral cervical osteophytes," *Dysphagia*, vol. 26, no. 1, pp. 34–40, 2011.

[12] J. Mizuno, H. Nakagawa, and J. Song, "Symptomatic ossification of the anterior longitudinal ligament with stenosis of the cervical spine: a report of seven cases," *Journal of Bone and Joint Surgery, British Volume*, vol. 87, no. 10, pp. 1375–1379, 2005.

[13] K. Ando, S. Imagama, N. Wakao et al., "Examination of the influence of ossification of the anterior longitudinal ligament on symptom progression and surgical outcome of ossification of the thoracic ligamentum flavum: a multicenter study," *Journal of Neurosurgery: Spine*, vol. 16, no. 2, pp. 147–153, 2012.

[14] M. E. Oppenlander, D. A. Orringer, F. La Marca et al., "Dysphagia due to anterior cervical hyperosteophytosis," *Surgical Neurology*, vol. 72, no. 3, pp. 266–270, 2009.

[15] J. S. Hwang, C. K. Chough, and W. I. Joo, "Giant anterior cervical osteophyte leading to dysphagia," *Korean Journal of Spine*, vol. 10, no. 3, pp. 200–202, 2013.

[16] K. Miyamoto, S. Sugiyama, H. Hosoe, N. Iinuma, Y. Suzuki, and K. Shimizu, "Postsurgical recurrence of osteophytes causing dysphagia in patients with diffuse idiopathic skeletal hyperostosis," *European Spine Journal*, vol. 18, no. 11, pp. 1652–1658, 2009.

[17] Y. Robinson, A. L. Robinson, and C. Olerud, "Complications and survival after long posterior instrumentation of cervical and cervicothoracic fractures related to ankylosing spondylitis or diffuse idiopathic skeletal hyperostosis," *Spine*, vol. 40, no. 4, pp. E227–E233, 2015.

[18] B. E. Northrup, A. R. Vaccaro, J. E. Rosen, R. A. Balderston, and J. M. Cotler, "Occurrence of infection in anterior cervical fusion for spinal cord injury after tracheostomy," *Spine*, vol. 20, no. 22, pp. 2449–2453, 1995.

36

Total Hip Lithiasis: A Rare Sequelae of Spilled Gallstones

Vineet Tyagi ⓘD, Daniel H. Wiznia ⓘD, Adrian K. Wyllie, and Kristaps J. Keggi

Department of Orthopaedics and Rehabilitation, Yale University School of Medicine, 47 College Street, Second Floor, New Haven, CT 06510, USA

Correspondence should be addressed to Vineet Tyagi; vineet.tyagi@yale.edu

Academic Editor: George Mouzopoulos

Laparoscopic cholecystectomy is a surgical treatment for acute cholecystitis or symptomatic cholelithiasis. One potential complication, the spillage of gallstones into the peritoneal cavity, can form a nidus for infection and may be associated with hepatic, retroperitoneal, thoracic, and abdominal wall abscesses. We report a case of a patient presenting with a right iliopsoas abscess and an infected right hip prosthesis status postlaparoscopic cholecystectomy. A CT demonstrated that the acetabular shell was overmedialized and perforated through the medial wall. The patient was taken to the operating room for explantation of components. A collection of gallstones was identified deep to the acetabulum during the explantation. The case highlights the importance of avoiding overmedialization of the acetabular component, which can provide a direct route for infection into the hip joint.

1. Introduction

Laparoscopic cholecystectomy (LC) is the procedure of choice for routine gallbladder removal and is among one of the most frequently performed surgical procedures in the United States. One common complication of the laparoscopic technique is the spillage of gallstones. It is estimated that approximately 30% of stones are spilled into the intraperitoneal space owing to perforation of the gallbladder during dissection [1, 2]. It is reported that gallstones are dropped by surgeons in an additional 7% of cholecystectomies, and studies suggest that 16–50% of dropped stones are unrecovered [3, 4]. It is well recognized that retained stones can become niduses for infection that may result in complications. In their review of complications from dropped gallstones from 1987 to 2005, Zehetner et al. demonstrated that the most common complications were abscesses, fistulas, and sinus tracts, many of which can take weeks to years to present [2].

An iliopsoas abscess is a relatively uncommon condition, and diagnosis is often missed or delayed, resulting in subsequent increases in mortality and morbidity. An iliopsoas abscess is a purulent collection within the psoas muscle compartment [5]. The psoas muscle is a retroperitoneal muscle that originates from the lateral borders of the 12th thoracic to 5th lumbar vertebrae and inserts on the lesser trochanter of the femur [6]. The iliopsoas bursa is the largest bursa in the body and presents with several different anatomical variations. It may extend proximally into the iliac fossa and distally to the lesser trochanter. Communication between this bursa and the hip joint occurs in approximately 15% of adults. In patients with hip pathology, there is a 30–40% frequency of communication between the two structures [7]. Tracking infections from the retroperitoneal psoas to the hip region have been reported with cases of tuberculous vertebral disease. Infections may spread to adjacent tissues contiguous with the iliopsoas bursa and can potentially track into the hip joint. Dinç et al. reported a case series of 21 patients with tuberculous spondylitis who developed iliopsoas abscesses requiring percutaneous drainage [8]. These findings may also be seen in patients who have paraspinal abscesses secondary to tuberculosis, and drainage through a subinguinal approach may be necessary to evacuate the collection before it spreads to the hip joint [9, 10].

Prosthetic infection is a serious concern for all arthroplasty surgeons and can be a devastating complication. Excessive medialization of the acetabular component can lead to a perforation in the medial wall and a potential communication with the hip joint and intraperitoneal contents and can act as a potential track for infections. In the case report below, we describe how dropped gallstones seeded a hip periprosthetic infection because the acetabular component was overmedialized and breached the medial acetabulum cortex, which likely put the component in contact to the dropped gallstones.

Overmedialization or protrusio acetabuli can expose the metal surface of the acetabular prosthesis to pelvic organs such as the bladder, ureter, or colon which may cause serious injuries or infections. Grauer et al. reported a case of a bladder tear occurring intraoperatively during a revision total hip arthroplasty (THA) [11]. They postulated that previous hip procedures lead to adhesions of the bladder to the pelvic floor and could predispose the bladder to injury during THA revisions.

Furthermore, as more of these two stage revision procedures are performed, Huo et al. suggested that it may be useful to consider patient-specific, customized, temporary methyl methacrylate prosthesis used by the senior author since 1992 when performing two stage revisions to treat periprosthetic hip infections. These implants allow for improved femoral head offset and leg length symmetry and allow the patient to mobilize prior to their second stage revision [12, 13]. Here, we present the first reported case of spilled gallstones causing a periprosthetic total hip infection.

2. Case Report

The patient was a 70-year-old female whose past medical history was significant for arthritis and a right total hip arthroplasty approximately 9 years ago. A laparoscopic cholecystectomy (LC) for acute cholecystitis was performed approximately at another hospital approximately two months prior to presentation. She developed a surgical site infection with *Escherichia coli (E. coli)* bacteremia following her LC and was treated successfully with intravenous (IV) antibiotics. The postoperative course was also complicated by choledocholithiasis requiring an endoscopic retrograde cholangiopancreatography (ERCP) with stone pulverization and placement of two plastic 10F × 12 cm biliary stents. Two days prior to admission, she was hospitalized at an outside facility in septic shock with fevers, chills, lethargy, altered mental status, and blood and urine cultures positive for *E. coli*. At that time, she endorsed right hip pain and an inability to move her hip or leg. A computed tomography (CT) scan of her right hip revealed two partly calcified soft tissue masses associated with the right iliopsoas and obturator internus muscles (Figure 1). A CT-guided fine needle biopsy of the right hip and psoas locules aspirated 100 mL of frank pus notable for a nucleated cell count of 344,000 (98% PMNs) with growth of *E. coli*. As a result, the patient was transferred to our institution with concerns for an iliopsoas abscess and a periprosthetic infection.

On admission, she was febrile to 102.7 F without any significant distress. Her physical examination was remarkable for a well-healed, right lateral hip incision with no erythema or drainage. She experienced pain with right hip flexion and internal rotation. Laboratory studies showed WBC,

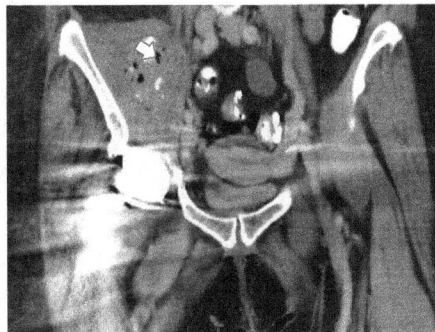

FIGURE 1: CT: right iliopsoas abscess with calcifications and air (arrowhead).

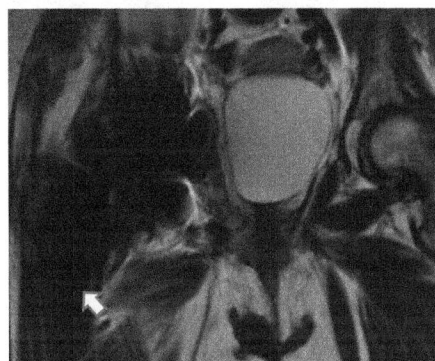

FIGURE 2: MRI right hip. Large air- and fluid-filled collection tracking along the iliopsoas bursa and psoas muscle (arrowhead).

hemoglobin and hematocrit, basic metabolic profile, and liver function tests all within normal limits. A 3 cm hepatic abscess was identified on CT scan of the abdomen and pelvis. An MRI of the right hip showed a large air- and fluid-filled collection tracking along the iliopsoas bursa and psoas musculature into the pelvis (Figure 2). This collection communicated with the hip prosthesis, and on CT imaging, the acetabulum component appeared to be medialized beyond the medial wall of the acetabulum as depicted in Figure 3. Regarding the hepatic abscess, the patient was managed with IV antibiotics and interventional radiology (IR) placed drainage catheter.

To address the hip periprosthetic infection, the patient was managed in multiple surgical stages. In the first stage, an irrigation and debridement of the right hip and explantation of components were performed through an anterior approach. The femoral and acetabular components were explanted. Purulent material was seen draining from the pelvis through a medial acetabular wall defect into the hip joint. Approximately 1 liter of pus was evacuated from the hip joint. Multiple irregularly shaped granulated pea-sized pieces of hard brown substance were found deep in the acetabulum. A handful of this material was removed which suggested that these were spilled gallstones from the patient's recent LC.

Temporary components were replanted with an antibiotic impregnated cement spacer system [13] (Figures 4 and 5). An

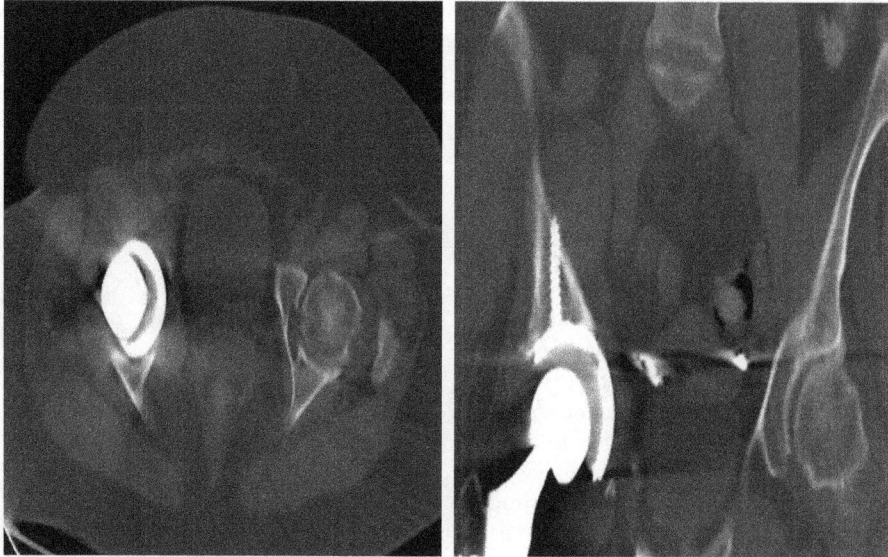

FIGURE 3: Axial and coronal CT scan showing excessive medialization of the acetabular component.

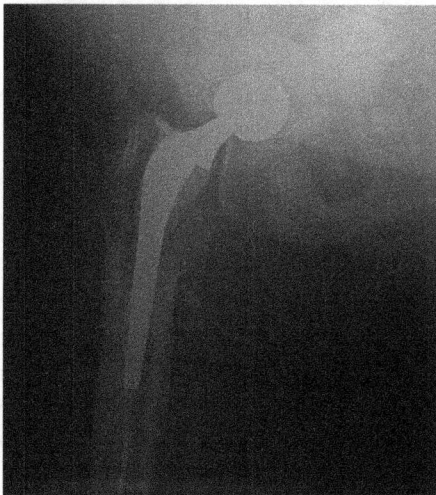

FIGURE 4: Stage 1: postoperative XR right hip.

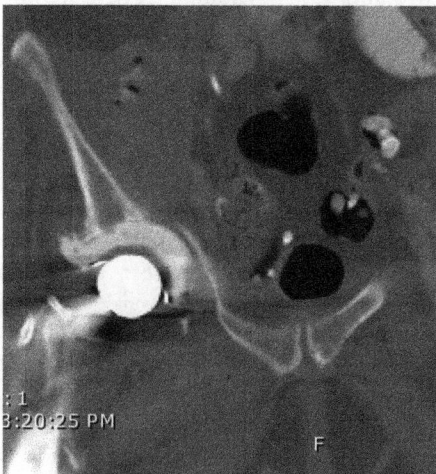

FIGURE 5: Stage 1: postoperative CT scan.

antibiotic cement spacer with gentamicin was placed in the acetabulum defect, and a loosely fitted antibiotic-cemented stem was placed in the proximal femur.

The intrapelvic iliopsoas collection could not be fully debrided through the anterior approach, and IR was consulted for drain placement and serial debridements, which were conducted with a rotating basket Trerotola device over the course of the next four weeks. In Figure 6, contrast dye can be seen tracking from within the iliopsoas abscess into the hip joint.

Four weeks following her explantation, the patient returned to the operating room for placement of a second temporary weight bearing custom-fitted prosthesis made from methyl methacrylate with gentamicin-impregnated antibiotics [13] (Figures 7 and 8). For the acetabulum, methyl methacrylate was molded in its doughy state into the cavities and deformities of the acetabulum, and a polyethylene acetabulum was pressed into the cement. The femur was reamed to size of a large diameter chest tube. A femoral stem and a reinforcing wire were cemented into the chest tube, and once the cement was hardened, the femoral stem encased in a solid cylinder of bone cement was removed from the chest tube and malleted into the proximal femur.

Postoperatively, the patient did well. She was made weight bearing as tolerated, ambulated with physical therapy and elected to delay placement of permanent components. She was eventually discharged to a short-term rehabilitation facility with a 6-week course of IV antibiotics.

Approximately 18 months later, she presented to our clinic complaining of hip and thigh pain with ambulation. She was followed by infectious disease as an outpatient with multiple hip aspirations which had negative cultures. X-rays revealed her temporary prosthesis to be stable, but with radiolucencies primarily around the femoral component (Figure 8). The patient was taken to the operating room, the temporary prosthesis was removed, and a long porous coated system was inserted (Figure 9). Intraoperative cultures

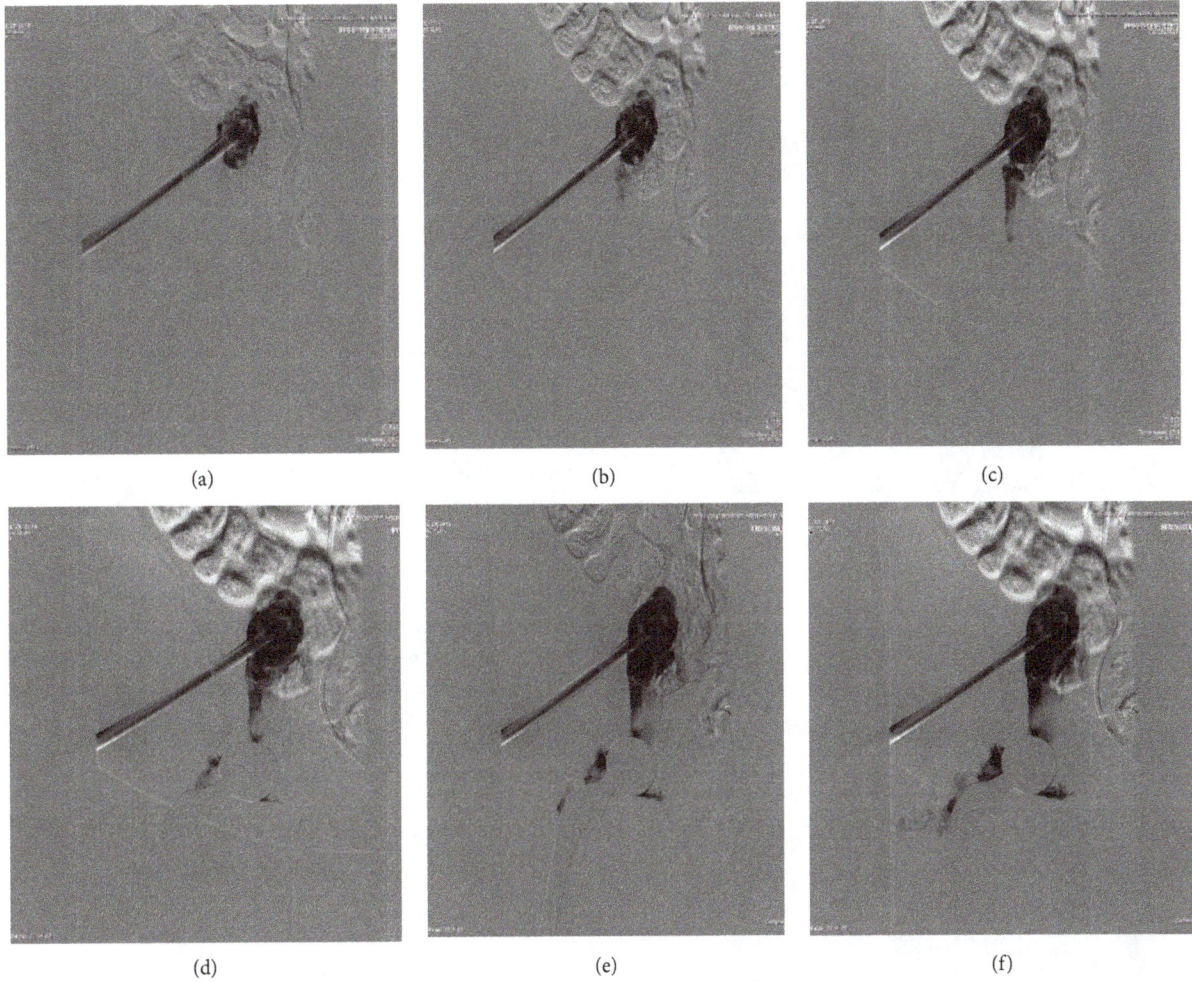

FIGURE 6: Flow of contrast dye tracking along the iliopsoas bursa into the hip joint.

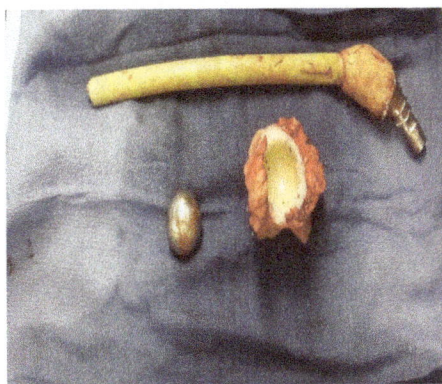

FIGURE 7: A custom-fitted temporary prosthesis.

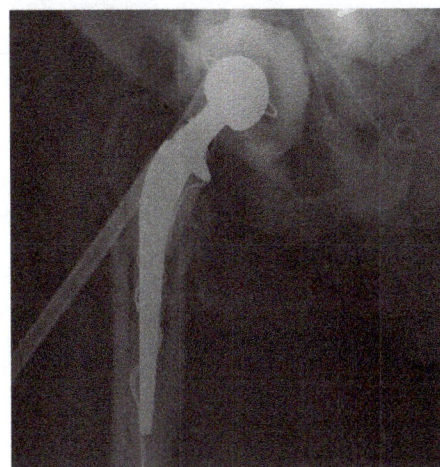

FIGURE 8: XR right hip. Stage 2: temporary prosthesis.

grew vancomycin-resistant enterococcus (VRE), and the patient was eventually discharged to home with a 12-week course of daptomycin and outpatient physical therapy. Now, two years from her initial explantation, she continues to follow up monthly in our clinic and states that she is doing well. Her final construct is shown in Figure 10. She continues to have a moderate limp but ambulates without assistive devices. Her pain is much improved and she is no longer on chronic antibiotic suppression with no clinical signs or symptoms of recurrent infection.

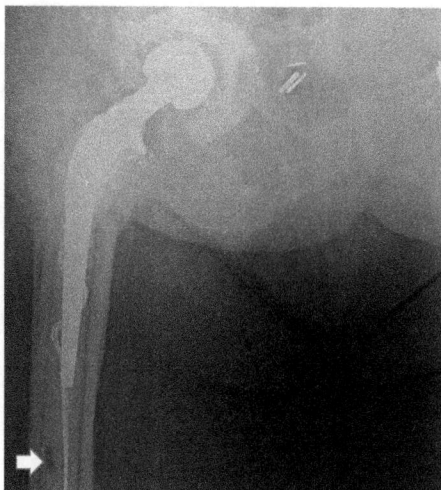

Figure 9: XR right hip. Radiolucencies around the femoral component (arrowhead).

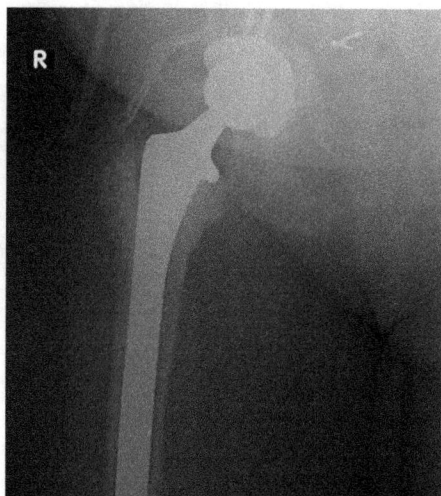

Figure 10: XR right hip. Long porous coated system.

3. Discussion

Our case demonstrates the unique consequence of spilled gallstones following LC. These stones can be spilled from manipulation during retraction, dissection, and removal of the gallbladder. In addition, abscesses are by far the most frequent complication [14]. They are usually located intraperitoneally (56%), either in the subhepatic region, abdominal wall (20%), thoracic (13%), and retroperitoneal space (11%) [15]. In a retrospective review, the median and mean times from LC to the first onset of symptoms were 3 and 5.5 months, respectively [16].

To our knowledge, this is the first reported case of dropped gallstones causing an iliopsoas abscess and a periprosthetic total hip infection. Chin et al. reports a case of a patient presenting 8 months after a laparoscopic cholecystectomy with a 6 × 4 cm firm mass superficial to the right hip joint in the iliopsoas bursa. The mass was excised, and an abscess cavity containing two large faceted gallstones was

found [17]. There was no connection to the peritoneal cavity or any reported involvement of the hip joint or muscle.

It is our belief that the medial wall defect of the acetabulum caused by overmedialization of the patient's primary acetabular component provided the principle path of infection into the hip joint. However, it is also possible that the abscess tracked along the iliopsoas bursa into the hip joint. The fluoroscopic IR images demonstrate the flow of contrast from the intrapelvic abscess along the iliopsoas bursa into the hip joint. As previously discussed, this anatomical connection has been well documented in patients with tuberculous infections of the spine which communicates with the hip.

This case demonstrates the potential deleterious effects of spilled gallstones and subsequent abscess formation in patients with total hip prosthetics. This case is unique as an extensive review of the literature failed to show an association between dropped gallstones and iliopsoas abscesses or periprosthetic total hip infections. Surgeons taking care of patients with total hip prostheses with an overmedialized acetabulum component which has breached the medial cortex should be aware of this potential complication with LC. Finally, we would like to highlight the importance of custom-fitted temporary prosthesis. They have greater mechanical stability since they can be fashioned to deal with individual variations of destroyed bone or acetabular cavities. This in turn allows for better postoperative function, decreases the incidence of dislocation and minimizes pain [18]. In addition to these mechanical advantages, the type and dose of antibiotics mixed in with the methyl methacrylate can be tailored to address the specific bacteria encountered in any one case.

Conflicts of Interest

The authors declare that they have no conflicts of interest.

References

[1] A. K. Singh, R. B. Levenson, D. A. Gervais, P. F. Hahn, K. Kandarpa, and P. R. Mueller, "Dropped gallstones and surgical clips after cholecystectomy: CT assessment," *Journal of Computer Assisted Tomography*, vol. 31, no. 5, pp. 758–762, 2007.

[2] J. Zehetner, A. Shamiyeh, and W. Wayand, "Lost gallstones in laparoscopic cholecystectomy: all possible complications," *American Journal of Surgery*, vol. 193, no. 1, pp. 73–78, 2007.

[3] J. Diez, C. Arozamena, L. Gutierrez et al., "Lost stones during laparoscopic cholecystectomy," *HPB Surgery*, vol. 11, no. 2, 109 pages, 1998.

[4] L. Sarli, N. Pietra, R. Costi, and M. Grattarola, "Gallbladder perforation during laparoscopic cholecystectomy," *World Journal of Surgery*, vol. 23, no. 11, pp. 1186–1190, 1999.

[5] I. H. Mallick, M. H. Thoufeeq, and T. P. Rajendran, "Iliopsoas abscesses," *Postgraduate Medical Journal*, vol. 80, no. 946, pp. 459–462, 2004.

[6] C. G. Cronin, D. G. Lohan, C. P. Meehan et al., "Anatomy, pathology, imaging and intervention of the iliopsoas muscle revisited," *Emergency Radiology*, vol. 15, no. 5, pp. 295–310, 2008.

[7] P. Wunderbaldinger, C. Bremer, E. Schellenberger, M. Cejna, K. Turetschek, and F. Kainberger, "Imaging features of iliopsoas bursitis," *European Radiology*, vol. 12, no. 2, pp. 409–415, 2002.

[8] H. Dinç, A. Ahmetoğlu, S. Baykal, A. Sari, Ö. Sayil, and H. R. Gümele, "Image-guided percutaneous drainage of tuberculous iliopsoas and spondylodiskitic abscesses: midterm results," *Radiology*, vol. 225, no. 2, pp. 353–358, 2002.

[9] V. K. Tang, H. L. Hsu, T. C. Hsieh, and W. S. Lee, "Vertebral tuberculosis complicated with retropharyngeal, parathoracic, and huge iliopsoas abscess, successfully treated with image-guided percutaneous drainage," *Journal of Microbiology, Immunology, and Infection*, vol. 50, no. 2, pp. 263-264, 2015.

[10] W. Tanomkiat and B. Buranapanitkit, "Percutaneous drainage of large tuberculous iliopsoas abscess via a subinguinal approach: a report of two cases," *Journal of Orthopaedic Science*, vol. 9, no. 2, pp. 157–161, 2004.

[11] J. N. Grauer, A. Halim, and K. J. Keggi, "Bladder tear during revision total hip arthroplasty," *The American Journal of Orthopedics*, vol. 43, no. 8, pp. E185–8, 2014.

[12] M. H. Huo, E. A. Salvati, J. R. Lieberman, A. H. Burstein, and P. D. Wilson Jr, "Custom-designed femoral prostheses in total hip arthroplasty done with cement for severe dysplasia of the hip," *The Journal of Bone & Joint Surgery*, vol. 75, no. 10, pp. 1497–1504, 1993.

[13] M. H. Huo, A. Elliott, and K. J. Keggi, "Periprosthetic infection in total hip replacement management with temporary prostheses and antibiotic-impregnated cement between stages," *Journal of Orthopaedic Techniques*, vol. 2, no. 3, pp. 93–101, 1994.

[14] M. Horton and M. G. Florence, "Unusual abscess patterns following dropped gallstones during laparoscopic cholecystectomy," *The American Journal of Surgery*, vol. 175, no. 5, pp. 375–379, 1998.

[15] T. Sathesh-Kumar, A. P. Saklani, R. Vinayagam, and R. L. Blackett, "Spilled gall stones during laparoscopic cholecystectomy: a review of the literature," *Postgraduate Medical Journal*, vol. 80, no. 940, pp. 77–79, 2004.

[16] J. C. Woodfield, M. Rodgers, and J. A. Windsor, "Peritoneal gallstones following laparoscopic cholecystectomy," *Surgical Endoscopy*, vol. 18, no. 8, pp. 1200–1207, 2004.

[17] P. T. Chin, S. Boland, and J. P. Percy, ""Gallstone hip" and other sequelae of retained gallstones," *HPB Surgery*, vol. 10, no. 3, 168 pages, 1997.

[18] E. Ginesty, C. Dromer, D. Galy-Fourcade et al., "Iliopsoas bursopathies. A review of twelve cases," *Revue du rhumatisme*, vol. 65, no. 3, pp. 181–186, 1998.

37

Iatrogenic Obturator Hip Dislocation with Intrapelvic Migration

Shachar Kenan ⓘ,[1] **Spencer Stein,**[1] **Robert Trasolini,**[2] **Daniel Kiridly,**[1]
and Bruce A. Seideman[3]

[1]*Department of Orthopaedics, Hofstra North Shore Long Island Jewish, Northwell Health Medical Center, New Hyde Park, NY, USA*
[2]*Department of Orthopaedics, New England Baptist Hospital, Boston, MA, USA*
[3]*Department of Orthopaedics, Hofstra North Shore Long Island Jewish, Northwell Health Medical Center, St. Francis Hospital, Roslyn, NY, USA*

Correspondence should be addressed to Shachar Kenan; shachar.kenan@gmail.com

Academic Editor: Elke R. Ahlmann

Obturator hip dislocations are rare, typically resulting from high-energy trauma in native hips. These types of dislocations are treated with closed reduction under sedation. Open reduction and internal fixation may be performed in the presence of associated fractures. Still rarer are obturator hip dislocations that penetrate through the obturator foramen itself. These types of dislocations have only been reported three other times in the literature, all within native hips. To date, there have been no reports of foraminal obturator dislocations after total hip arthroplasty. We report of the first periprosthetic foraminal obturator hip dislocation, which was caused iatrogenically during attempts at closed reduction of a posterior hip dislocation in the setting of a chronic greater trochanter fracture. Altered joint biomechanics stemming from a weak hip abductor mechanism rendered the patient vulnerable to this specific dislocation subtype, which ultimately required open surgical intervention. An early assessment and identification of this dislocation prevented excessive closed reduction maneuvers, which otherwise could have had detrimental consequences including damage to vital intrapelvic structures. This case report raises awareness to this very rare, yet potential complication after total hip arthroplasty.

1. Introduction

Total hip arthroplasty (THA) has been the treatment of choice for patients with end stage femoroacetabular joint degeneration with the goals of relieving pain, restoring function, and improving quality of life. Possible complications include infection, neurovascular damage, dislocation, periprosthetic fracture, aseptic loosening, and leg length discrepancy. Dislocation, one of the most common complications after THA, occurs in approximately 0.3% to 10% of primary THAs and up to 28% for revision THA [1–9]. A meta-analysis of 260 clinical studies, which included 13,203 primary total hip arthroplasties, noted dislocation rates of 3.23%, 2.18%, and 0.55% for posterior, anterolateral, and direct lateral approaches, respectively [10]. Patient risk factors include older age, female gender, prior surgery, neuromuscular disorders, dementia, and alcohol abuse [11]. Surgical risk factors include component malpositioning, failure to restore

leg length or offset, posterior approach, and implants which decrease the head to neck ratio [11]. Anatomically, hip dislocations are described as anterior or posterior to the acetabulum. Anterior hip dislocations are further subclassified as superior, inferior, luxation erecta of hip, obturator, or pubic type [12].

Inferior obturator dislocations tend to be traumatic, occurring with hip flexion, external rotation, and forced abduction. Due to the rarity of this type of dislocation, it is difficult to assess its true incidence. To our knowledge, only 29 cases of obturator hip dislocation have been reported in the literature [12–36]. Dislocations of this nature typically occurred in native hips in the setting of trauma, with a majority being associated with femoral neck, head, or acetabular fractures. Three of these documented dislocations described the displacement of the femoral head with penetration through the obturator foramen; however, those cases were all within native hips, and none were periprosthetic [13, 14, 18].

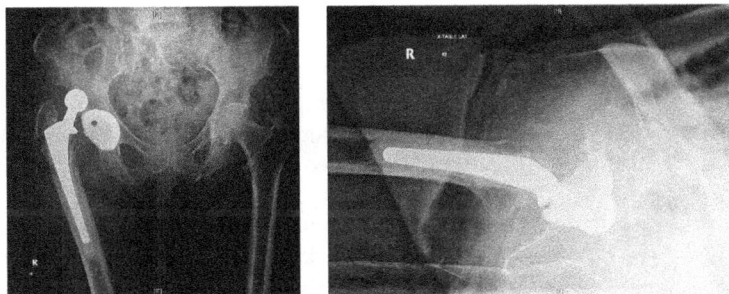

FIGURE 1: Anteroposterior (AP) pelvis and lateral right hip radiographs showing a posterosuperior dislocation of the right cemented femoral component with associated chronic greater trochanteric periprosthetic fracture and chronic left inferior pubic rami fracture.

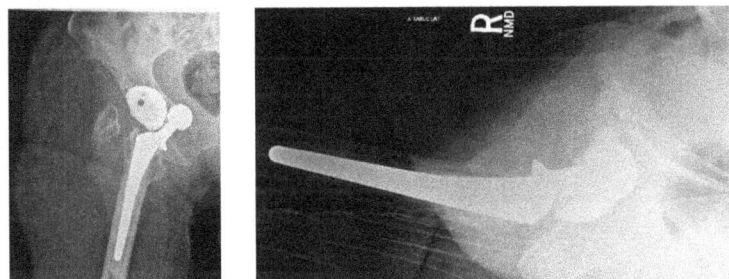

FIGURE 2: Anteroposterior (AP) and lateral right hip radiographs, status post attempted closed reduction revealing right iatrogenic obturator hip dislocation with femoral component intrapelvic migration.

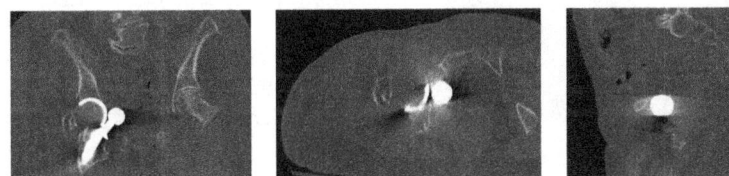

FIGURE 3: Coronal, axial, and sagittal computed tomography (CT) images showing femoral component dislocation through the right obturator canal and abutting the urinary bladder.

This case report is the first documented description of a periprosthetic foraminal obturator hip dislocation. The patient is an 83-year-old female, sixteen years status post right posterior total hip arthroplasty, who sustained an iatrogenic obturator hip dislocation with femoral head component penetration through the obturator canal resulting from an attempt at closed reduction of a posterior hip dislocation. The authors have obtained the patient's informed written consent for print and electronic publication of the case report.

2. Case Presentation

2.1. Clinical. An 83-year-old female with a past medical history of rheumatoid arthritis (on DMARD's), asthma, depression, gastroesophageal reflux disease (GERD), and lumbar spondylosis, as well as a past surgical history of right posterior total hip arthroplasty (1999), bilateral total knee arthroplasties (2003, 2012), and right shoulder hemiarthroplasty (2010), presented with five days of right hip pain and inability to ambulate after bending down. In the emergency department, initial radiographs revealed a right posterior hip dislocation, as well as chronic appearing fractures of the right greater trochanter and left inferior public rami (Figure 1). Her right lower extremity was shortened, internally rotated, and adducted. A propofol-induced conscious sedation was performed by the emergency physician and closed reduction was attempted by an experienced orthopaedic resident. The reduction maneuver involved hip flexion, traction, adduction, and internal rotation followed by external rotation and abduction. After three attempts, post reduction radiographs were significant for a right inferior obturator hip dislocation (Figure 2). The patient tolerated the procedure and was neurovascularly intact distal to her hip. Computed tomography (CT) was performed, which confirmed a persistently dislocated femoral head with intrapelvic migration through the right obturator foramen (Figures 3 and 4). Having failed three attempts at closed reduction, the patient was taken to the operating room for open reduction and revision arthroplasty.

Using a posterolateral approach, the femoral head was found to be locked inferior and posterior to the acetabulum.

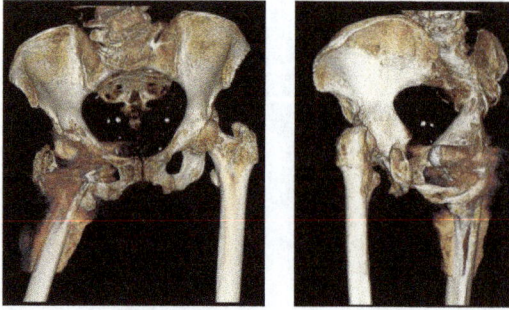

FIGURE 4: Three-dimensional reformatted computed tomography (CT) images showing femoral component dislocation through the right obturator canal.

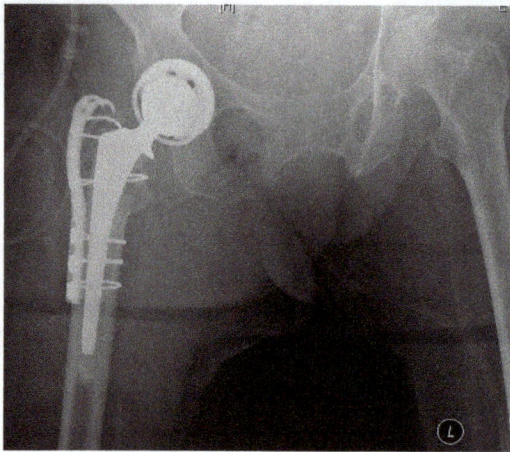

FIGURE 5: Anteroposterior (AP) pelvis radiograph, status post right hip open reduction, revision total hip arthroplasty with constrained liner and greater trochanteric hook plate with cerclage cables.

Manual traction was utilized to successfully extricate the femoral component from within the obturator ring. Both the femoral and acetabular components were stable; however, a large amount of posterior wear was noted on the liner, which was exchanged for a constrained component. A greater trochanteric hook plate with cerclage cables was then utilized for the fixation of the greater trochanteric fragment (Figure 5). Excellent stability with a full range of motion was noted.

Postoperatively, the patient was weight bearing as tolerated, with standard posterior hip precautions including an abduction pillow. Aspirin 325 mg BID was used for deep vein thrombosis (DVT) prophylaxis. Although the patient initially did very well, she developed urosepsis six months after the index procedure, leading to an acute right periprosthetic septic hip with *Proteus mirabilis*. Radiographs showed greater trochanteric escape from the hook plate (Figure 6). She then underwent irrigation and debridement with greater trochanter excision and hook plate removal (Figure 7). The patient was discharged with 6 weeks of ceftriaxone antibiotics via a peripherally inserted central catheter and has since been doing well with no further dislocations.

3. Discussion

Obturator hip dislocation after total hip arthroplasty is a rare complication. The nature of dislocation is dependent on a multitude of factors, with trauma being the most common predisposing factor. In the setting of trauma, patients may present with associated injuries such as external iliac artery occlusion, ipsilateral fractures of the acetabulum, femoral neck, greater trochanter, or femoral shaft, as well as long-term sequelae such as myositis ossificans [37]. Unlike periprosthetic hips, native hip dislocations may additionally present with femoral head impaction fractures resulting from impaction of the femoral head on the anteroinferior rim of the acetabulum [37]. Such impaction fractures lead to femoral head defects, similar to Hill-Sachs lesions of the proximal humerus after anterior shoulder dislocations.

We described an iatrogenic obturator anterior hip dislocation in a patient who had sustained a subacute posterior hip dislocation in association with a chronic greater trochanteric fracture. The patient was treated with revision arthroplasty and greater trochanteric open reduction internal fixation (ORIF). A fracture of the greater trochanter after total hip arthroplasty is classified as a Vancouver AG periprosthetic fracture [38]. According to a study of 32,644 primary total hip arthroplasties, a Vancouver AG fracture was the most common subtype of fracture, occurring in 32% of patients who sustained a postoperative periprosthetic hip fracture [39]. The overall rate of periprosthetic hip fractures was 3.5% in this same study group. The treatment of these fractures depends on the amount of displacement. For minimally displaced Vancouver AG fractures, patients are treated conservatively, with protected weight bearing and abductor hip precautions [40]. Displaced greater trochanter fractures require surgical fixation using wires, screws, cables, or specialized plates [40]. In our case, ORIF was performed due to the associated hip dislocation and fragment instability.

There is a paucity of literature describing obturator anterior hip dislocations after total hip arthroplasty. Most cases report native hip obturator dislocation following significant trauma with only three confirmed cases of femoral head penetration through the obturator foramen. These patients included a 24-year-old female with Ehlers-Danlos syndrome, a 33-year-old who presented with a neglected obturator dislocation six months after injury, and a 40-year-old female after a horse riding accident [13, 14, 18].

We believe that our patient's subacute presentation coupled with a preexisting greater trochanteric fracture contributed to an obturator hip dislocation after standard hip reduction attempts. Decreased abductor forces due to the greater trochanteric fracture led to hip instability, allowing the femoral prosthesis to migrate anteriorly and inferiorly. Post reduction three-dimensional reformatted CT scans (Figure 4) excellently illustrate this rare anatomic deformity.

4. Conclusion

This case serves as an example of anterior obturator hip dislocation after an attempt at closed reduction. It is important to understand that the mechanism of abduction and external

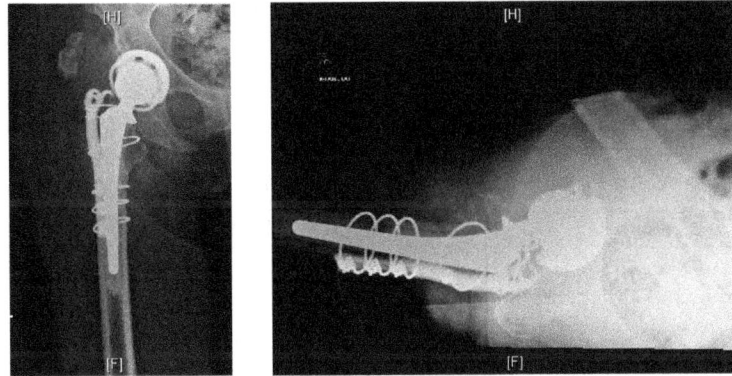

FIGURE 6: Anteroposterior (AP) and lateral right hip radiographs, seven months status post revision total hip arthroplasty with greater trochanter escape from hook plate.

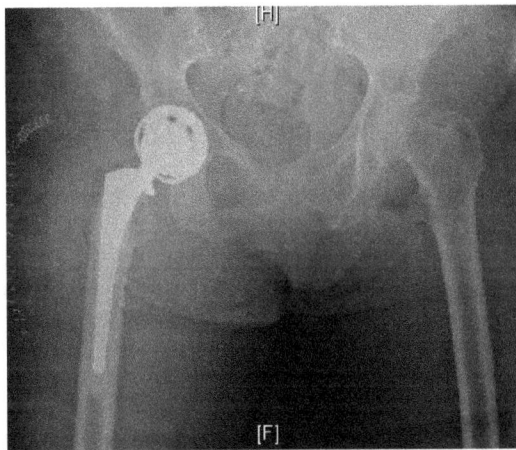

FIGURE 7: Anteroposterior (AP) pelvis radiograph, status post right hip irrigation and debridement, greater trochanter excision, hook plate, and cable removal of hardware.

rotation resulting in obturator hip dislocation is the same maneuver that is used during standard hip dislocation reduction attempts. Great care should therefore be taken when attempting a closed reduction in the presence of an ipsilateral greater trochanteric fracture, with radiographs performed after each attempt. Multiple failed attempts in this setting may eventually lead to incarceration of the femoral head through the obturator foramen, which should be confirmed by radiographs and computed tomographic (CT) scans.

In the setting of a confirmed foraminal obturator hip dislocation, there should be a low threshold for open reduction to avoid damage to neighboring critical intrapelvic structures from excessive closed reduction attempts. Furthermore, this case highlights the importance of close follow-up, especially in patients who are immunosuppressed and are at a high risk of periprosthetic infection. Early detection and treatment of potential sources of infection such as open wounds and ulcers, urinary tract infections (UTIs), and respiratory infections are critical to preventing hematogenous spread. Awareness of patient-specific factors that alter hip biomechanics, such as abductor mechanism disruption, should prompt

added care and precaution during traditional closed reduction maneuvers, helping the treating orthopaedist avoid this type of dislocation.

Conflicts of Interest

The authors declare that they have no conflicts of interest.

References

[1] D. D. Goetz, B. R. Bremner, J. J. Callaghan, W. N. Capello, and R. C. Johnston, "Salvage of a recurrently dislocating total hip prosthesis with use of a constrained acetabular component. A concise follow-up of a previous report," *The Journal of Bone and Joint Surgery American Volume*, vol. 86-A, no. 11, pp. 2419–2423, 2004.

[2] A. Ekelund, "Trochanteric osteotomy for recurrent dislocation of total hip arthroplasty," *The Journal of Arthroplasty*, vol. 8, no. 6, pp. 629–632, 1993.

[3] K. F. Baldwin and L. D. Dorr, "The unstable total hip arthroplasty: the role of postoperative bracing," *Instructional Course Lectures*, vol. 50, pp. 289–293, 2001.

[4] M. J. Anderson, W. R. Murray, and H. B. Skinner, "Constrained acetabular components," *The Journal of Arthroplasty*, vol. 9, no. 1, pp. 17–23, 1994.

[5] M. A. Ritter, "Dislocation and subluxation of the total hip replacement," *Clinical Orthopaedics and Related Research*, no. 121, pp. 92–94, 1976.

[6] J. P. Rao and R. Bronstein, "Dislocations following arthroplasties of the hip. Incidence, prevention, and treatment," *Orthopaedic Review*, vol. 20, no. 3, pp. 261–264, 1991.

[7] B. F. Morrey, "Instability after total hip arthroplasty," *The Orthopedic Clinics of North America*, vol. 23, no. 2, pp. 237–248, 1992.

[8] C. D. Fackler and R. Poss, "Dislocation in total hip arthroplasties," *Clinical orthopaedics and related research*, vol. 151, article 169, 178 pages, 1980.

[9] N. S. Eftekhar, "Dislocation and instability complicating low friction arthroplasty of the hip joint," *Clinical Orthopaedics and Related Research*, no. 121, pp. 120–125, 1976.

[10] J. L. Masonis and R. B. Bourne, "Surgical approach, abductor function, and total hip arthroplasty dislocation," *Clinical Orthopaedics and Related Research*, vol. 405, pp. 46–53, 2002.

[11] R. B. Bourne and R. Mehin, "The dislocating hip: what to do, what to do," *The Journal of Arthroplasty*, vol. 19, no. 4, pp. 111–114, 2004.

[12] A. Sultan, T. A. Dar, M. I. Wani, M. M. Wani, and S. Shafi, "Bilateral simultaneous anterior obturator dislocation of the hip by an unusual mechanism—a case report," *Turkish Journal of Trauma and Emergency Surgery*, vol. 18, no. 5, pp. 455–457, 2012.

[13] A. Pankaj, M. Sharma, V. Kochar, and V. A. Naik, "Neglected, locked, obturator type of inferior hip dislocation treated by total hip arthroplasty," *Archives of Orthopaedic and Trauma Surgery*, vol. 131, no. 4, pp. 443–446, 2011.

[14] J. D. Chang, J. H. Yoo, G. S. Umarani, and Y. S. Kim, "Obturator hip dislocation with intrapelvic migration of the femoral head in Ehlers-Danlos syndrome," *Journal of Orthopaedic science*, vol. 17, no. 1, pp. 87–89, 2012.

[15] D. M. Avery 3rd and G. F. Carolan, "Traumatic obturator hip dislocation in a 9-year-old boy," *The American Journal of Orthopedics*, vol. 42, no. 9, pp. E81–E83, 2013.

[16] R. Hani, M. Kharmaz, and M. S. Berrada, "Traumatic obturator dislocation of the hip joint: a case report and review of the literature," *The Pan African Medical Journal*, vol. 21, p. 55, 2015.

[17] A. D. Toms, S. Williams, and S. H. White, "Obturator dislocation of the hip," *The Journal of Bone and Joint Surgery British Volume*, vol. 83, no. 1, pp. 113–115, 2001.

[18] M. Rancan, M. P. Esser, and T. Kossmann, "Irreducible traumatic obturator hip dislocation with subcapital indentation fracture of the femoral neck: a case report," *The Journal of Trauma*, vol. 62, no. 6, pp. E4–E6, 2007.

[19] M. Allagui, B. Touati, I. Aloui, M. F. Hamdi, M. Koubaa, and A. Abid, "Obturator dislocation of the hip with ipsilateral femoral neck fracture: a case report," *Journal of Clinical Orthopaedics and Trauma*, vol. 4, no. 3, pp. 143–146, 2013.

[20] R. Arjun, V. Kumar, B. Saibaba, R. John, U. Guled, and S. Aggarwal, "Ipsilateral obturator type of hip dislocation with fracture shaft femur in a child: a case report and literature review," *Journal of Pediatric Orthopedics Part B*, vol. 25, no. 5, pp. 484–488, 2016.

[21] A. A. Karaarslan, N. Acar, T. Karci, and E. Sesli, "A bilateral traumatic hip obturator dislocation," *Case Reports in Orthopedics*, vol. 2016, Article ID 3145343, 2 pages, 2016.

[22] P. Boyer, M. Bassaine, and D. Huten, "Traumatic obturator foramen hip dislocation: a case report and review of the literature," *Revue de chirurgie orthopedique et reparatrice de l'appareil moteur*, vol. 90, no. 7, pp. 673–677, 2004.

[23] F. Duygulu, S. Karaoglu, S. Kabak, and O. I. Karahan, "Bilateral obturator dislocation of the hip," *Archives of Orthopaedic and Trauma Surgery*, vol. 123, no. 1, pp. 36–38, 2003.

[24] S. Endo, S. Hoshi, H. Takayama, and E. Kan, "Traumatic bilateral obturator dislocation of the hip joint," *Injury*, vol. 22, no. 3, pp. 232-233, 1991.

[25] A. Gibbs, "Bilateral obturator dislocation of the hip joint," *Injury*, vol. 12, no. 3, pp. 250-251, 1980.

[26] R. J. Izquierdo and D. Harris, "Obturator hip dislocation with subcapital fracture of the femoral neck," *Injury*, vol. 25, no. 2, pp. 108–110, 1994.

[27] R. L. Leyshon, "Obturator dislocation of the hip," *Injury*, vol. 13, no. 3, pp. 263-264, 1981.

[28] S. J. McClelland, P. A. Bauman, C. F. Medley Jr., and M. L. Shelton, "Obturator hip dislocation with ipsilateral fractures of the femoral head and femoral neck. A case report," *Clinical Orthopaedics and Related Research*, vol. 224, pp. 164–168, 1987.

[29] A. A. Mendez, D. Keret, and G. D. MacEwen, "Obturator dislocation as a complication of closed reduction of the congenitally dislocated hip: a report of two cases," *Journal of Pediatric Orthopedics*, vol. 10, no. 2, pp. 265–268, 1990.

[30] S. Sambandan, "Obturator dislocation of the hip associated with fracture shaft of femur: a case report," *Singapore Medical Journal*, vol. 27, no. 5, pp. 442–445, 1986.

[31] M. R. Sarkar, N. Mastragelopulos, and U. Pfister, "Obturator dislocation of the hip joint," *Unfallchirurgie*, vol. 16, no. 1, pp. 3–7, 1990.

[32] W. J. Scadden and W. G. Dennyson, "Unreduced obturator dislocation of the hip—a case report," *South African Medical Journal*, vol. 53, no. 15, pp. 601-602, 1978.

[33] D. J. Church, H. M. Merrill, S. Kotwal, and J. R. Dubin, "Novel technique for femoral head reconstruction using allograft following obturator hip dislocation," *Journal of Orthopaedic Case Reports*, vol. 6, no. 1, pp. 48–51, 2016.

[34] I. Elouakili, Y. Ouchrif, R. Ouakrim et al., "Luxation obturatrice de la hanche: un traumatisme rare en pratique sportive," *The Pan African Medical Journal*, vol. 21, p. 230, 2015.

[35] E. Argintar, B. Whitfield, and J. DeBritz, "Missed obturator hip dislocation in a 19-year-old man," *American Journal of Orthopedics*, vol. 41, no. 3, pp. E43–E45, 2012.

[36] K. Niciejewski, W. Banachowski, and A. Kowalczyk, "Obturator dislocation—a rare complication of the total hip prosthesis. Case study," *Chirurgia narzadow ruchu i ortopedia polska*, vol. 76, no. 5, pp. 295–297, 2011.

[37] R. E. Erb, J. R. Steele, E. P. Nance Jr., and J. R. Edwards, "Traumatic anterior dislocation of the hip: spectrum of plain film and CT findings," *American Journal of Roentgenology*, vol. 165, no. 5, pp. 1215–1219, 1995.

[38] C. P. Duncan and B. A. Masri, "Fractures of the femur after hip replacement," *Instructional Course Lectures*, vol. 44, pp. 293–304, 1995.

[39] M. P. Abdel, C. D. Watts, M. T. Houdek, D. G. Lewallen, and D. J. Berry, "Epidemiology of periprosthetic fracture of the femur in 32,644 primary total hip arthroplasties: a 40-year experience," *The Bone & Joint Journal*, vol. 98-B, no. 4, pp. 461–467, 2016.

[40] D. Marsland and S. C. Mears, "A review of periprosthetic femoral fractures associated with total hip arthroplasty," *Geriatric Orthopaedic Surgery & Rehabilitation*, vol. 3, no. 3, pp. 107–120, 2012.

Permissions

List of Contributors

C. Siebenmann, F. Ramadani, G. Barbier, E. Gautier
and P.Vial
Department of Orthopedic Surgery, HFR Fribourg-
Hôpital Cantonal, Switzerland

Rohan Bhimani
Department of Orthopaedics, 11th Road, Khar (West),
Hinduja Healthcare Surgical, Mumbai 400052, India

Preeti Singh
Department of Orthopaedics, Osmania General
Hospital, Hyderabad 500012, India

Fardeen Bhimani
Department of Orthopaedics, Bharati Hospital, Pune
411043, India

Richard N. Puzzitiello, Avinesh Agarwalla, Austin
Stone and Brian Forsythe
Midwest Orthopaedics at Rush, Rush University
Medical Center, Chicago, IL, USA

Juan Martín Patiño, Alejandro Rullan Corna,
Alejandro Michelini, Ignacio Abdon and Alejandro
José Ramos Vertiz
Hospital Militar Central, Buenos Aires, Argentina

Takeshi Inoue, Makoto Kubota, and Keishi Marumo
Department of Orthopaedic Surgery, Jikei University
School of Medicine, 3-25-8 Nishishinnbashi, Minato-
ku, Tokyo 105-8461, Japan

Kazuhiko Udagawa, Yasuo Niki, Kengo Harato and
Shu Kobayashi
Department of Orthopaedic Surgery, Keio University
School of Medicine, Tokyo, Japan

So Nomoto
Department of Orthopaedic Surgery, Yokohama-City
Tobu Hospital, Yokohama, Japan

Sanjum P. Samagh, Fernando A. Huyke, Lucas
Buchler, Michael A. Terry and Vehniah K. Tjong
Department of Orthopaedic Surgery, Northwestern
University Feinberg School of Medicine, 259 East Erie
Street, Suite 1350, Chicago, IL 60611, USA

John G. Skedros, James S. Smith, Marshall K. Henrie,
and Ethan D. Finlinson
Department of Orthopaedic Surgery and Utah
Orthopaedic Specialists, e University of Utah, 5323
South Woodrow Street, Salt Lake City, UT 84107, USA

Joel D. Trachtenberg
St. Marks Hospital, Salt Lake City, UT, USA

Malynda S. Messer, Brendan Southam and Brian M.
Grawe
Department of Orthopaedic Surgery, University of
Cincinnati Medical Center, 231 Albert Sabin Way,
Cincinnati, OH 45267-0212, USA

M. O. Abrego, F. L. De Cicco, N. E. Gimenez, P.
Sotelano, M. N. Carrasco and M. G. Santini Araujo
Trauma and Orthopaedics Institute "Carlos
Ottolenghi", Italian Hospital of Buenos Aires, Peron
4190, C11000ABD CABA, Argentina

M. O. Marquesini
Center for Diagnostic Imaging, Italian Hospital
of Buenos Aires, Peron 4190, C11000ABD CABA,
Argentina

Cristian Barrientos and Maximiliano Barahona
Orthopaedic Department at Hospital Clinico
Universidad de Chile, Santos Dumontt 999, Santiago,
Chile
Hospital Clinico Universidad de Chile, 999 Santos
Dumont av., Independencia, Santiago 8380456, Chile

Julian Brañes and Alvaro Martinez
Orthopaedic Department at Hospital San José, 1196
San Jose av. Independencia, Santiago 8380419, Chile

José-Luis Llanos
Coloproctology Surgery at Hospital Clinico
Universidad de Chile, Santos Dumontt 999, Santiago,
Chile

Kenichi Mishima, Hiroshi Kitoh, Masaki Matsushita,
Tadashi Nagata, Yasunari Kamiya and Naoki
Ishiguro
Department of Orthopaedic Surgery, Nagoya
University Graduate School of Medicine, 65 Tsurumai,
Showa-ku, Nagoya, Aichi 466-8550, Japan

Gilber Kask, Toni-Karri Pakarinen and Minna K.
Laitinen
Department of Orthopaedics and Traumatology, Unit
of Musculoskeletal Surgery, Tampere University
Hospital, Teiskontie 35, 33521 Tampere, Finland

Jyrki Parkkinen
Fimlab Laboratories, Arvo Ylpön katu 4, 33520
Tampere, Finland

Hannu Kuokkanen
Division of Plastic Surgery, Helsinki University Central Hospital, Topeliuksenkatu 5, 00260 Helsinki, Finland

Jyrki Nieminen
Coxa Hospital for Joint Replacement, Biokatu 6, 33520 Tampere, Finland

Mehmet Bülent Balioğlu
Department of Orthopaedics, Istinye University Liv Hospital, Istanbul, Turkey

Deniz Kargın and Akif Albayrak
Department of Orthopedics, Health Science University Baltalimani Bone Diseases Education and Research Hospital, Istanbul, Turkey

Yunus Atıcı
Department of Orthopaedics, Okan University Hospital, Istanbul, Turkey

Raja Bhaskara Rajasekaran, Dheenadhayalan Jayaramaraju, Dhanasekara Raja Palanisami, Ramesh Perumal and Rajasekaran Shanmuganathan
Department of Orthopaedics and Trauma, 313 Mettupalayam Road, Ganga Medical Centre and Hospitals Pvt. Ltd., Coimbatore, India

Jiro Ichikawa, Tetsuro Ohba, Koji Fujita, Shigeto Ebata and Hirotaka Haro
Department of Orthopaedic Surgery, Graduate School of Medicine, University of Yamanashi, 1110 Shimokato, Chuo, Yamanashi 409-3898, Japan

Hiroaki Kanda
Department of Pathology, The Cancer Institute of the Japanese Foundation for Cancer Research (JFCR), 3-8-31 Ariake, Koto-ku, Tokyo 135-8550, Japan

Souichi Ohta, Ryosuke Ikeguchi, Hiroki Oda, Hirofumi Yurie, Hisataka Takeuchi and Shuichi Matsuda
Department of Orthopaedic Surgery, Kyoto University, Kyoto, Japan

Kiyohisa Ogawa and Wataru Inokuchi
Department of Orthopedic Surgery, Eiju General Hospital, 2-3-23 Higashiueno, Taito-ku, Tokyo 110-8645, Japan

Patrick R. Keller and Heather A. Cole
Department of Orthopaedics and Rehabilitation, Vanderbilt University Medical Center, 4202 Doctors' Office Tower, 2200 Children's Way, Nashville, TN 37232-9565, USA

Jonathan G. Schoenecker
Department of Orthopaedics and Rehabilitation, Vanderbilt University Medical Center, 4202 Doctors' Office Tower, 2200 Children's Way, Nashville, TN 37232-9565, USA
Department of Pathology, Vanderbilt University Medical Center, 4202 Doctors' Office Tower, 2200 Children's Way, Nashville, TN 37232-9565, USA
Department of Pharmacology, Vanderbilt University Medical Center, 4202 Doctors' Office Tower, 2200 Children's Way, Nashville, TN 37232-9565, USA
Department of Pediatrics, Vanderbilt University Medical Center, 4202 Doctors' Office Tower, 2200 Children's Way, Nashville, TN 37232-9565, USA
Vanderbilt Center for Bone Biology, Vanderbilt University Medical Center, 4202 Doctors' Office Tower, 2200 Children's Way, Nashville, TN 37232-9565, USA

Christopher M. Stutz
Texas Scottish-Rite Children's Hospital for Children, 2222 Welborn Ave., Dallas, TX 75219, USA

Keizo Wada, Tomohiro Goto, Tomoya Takasago, Takahiko Tsutsui and Koichi Sairyo
Department of Orthopaedics, Institute of Biomedical Sciences, Tokushima University Graduate School, Tokushima, Japan

Hicham G. Abdel Nour, George S. El Rassi, Jack C. Daoud, Youssef G. Hassan, Rami A. Ayoubi and Nabih I. Joukhadar
Department of Orthopedic Surgery and Traumatology, Saint Georges University Medical Center, Balamand University, , Achrafieh, Beirut 1100 2807, Lebanon

Brendan R. Southam and Adam P. Schumaier
Department of Orthopaedics and Sports Medicine, University of Cincinnati, Cincinnati, OH 45220, USA

Alvin H. Crawford
Department of Orthopaedics, Cincinnati Children's Hospital Medical Center, Cincinnati, OH 45229, USA

David A. Billmire
Department of Plastic Surgery, Cincinnati Children's Hospital Medical Center, Cincinnati, OH 45229, USA

James Geller
Department of Oncology, Cincinnati Children's Hospital Medical Center, Cincinnati, OH 45229, USA

Daniel Von Allmen
Department of Surgery, Cincinnati Children's Hospital Medical Center, Cincinnati, OH 45229, USA

Sara Szabo
Department of Pathology, Cincinnati Children's Hospital Medical Center, Cincinnati, OH 45229, USA

Yusuke Minami, Seiichi Matsumoto, Keisuke Ae, Taisuke Tanizawa, Keiko Hayakawa and Yuki Funauchi
Department of Orthopedic Surgery, e Cancer Institute Hospital of the Japanese Foundation for Cancer Research, Tokyo, Japan

Sakae Okumura
Department of oracic Surgery, e Cancer Institute Hospital of the Japanese Foundation for Cancer Research, Tokyo, Japan

Yutaka Takazawa
Department of Pathology, e Cancer Institute Hospital of the Japanese Foundation for Cancer Research, Tokyo, Japan

Neal Singleton, Matthew Bowman, and David Bartle
Orthopaedic Department, Tauranga Hospital, Cameron Road, Tauranga, New Zealand

Hiroaki Tagomori, Nobuhiro Kaku, Tomonori Tabata and Hiroshi Tsumura
Department of Orthopaedic Surgery, Oita University, Oita, Japan

John W. Stelzer
Department of Orthopaedic Surgery, Massachusetts General Hospital, Harvard Medical School, Boston, MA, USA

Miguel A. Flores and Christopher Wasyliw
Department of Diagnostic Radiology, Florida Hospital, Orlando, FL, USA

Waleed Mohammad, Nathan Esplin and Jonathan J. Mayl
University of Central Florida College of Medicine, Orlando, FL, USA

Kenjiro Fujimura, Koji Sakuraba, Satoshi Kamura, Kiyoshi Miyazaki, Nobuo Kobara, Kazumasa Terada and Hisaaki Miyahara
Clinical Research Institute, National Hospital Organization, Kyushu Medical Center, Fukuoka, Japan
Department of Orthopaedic Surgery, National Hospital Organization, Kyushu Medical Center, Fukuoka, Japan

M. Prod'homme, S. Pour Jafar, P. Zogakis and P. Stutz
Orthopedic Surgery Department, Riviera-Chablais Hospital, Montreux, Switzerland

Kiyohito Naito, Yoichi Sugiyama, Mayuko Kinoshita and Kazuo Kaneko
Department of Orthopaedics, Juntendo University School of Medicine, Tokyo, Japan

Thitinut Dilokhuttakarn
Department of Orthopaedics, Juntendo University School of Medicine, Tokyo, Japan
Department of Orthopedics, Srinakharinwirot University, Nakhon Nayok, Thailand

Ahmed Zemirline
Centre de la Main de Bretagne, Centre Hospitalier de Saint Grégoire, Saint-Grégoire, France

Chihab Taleb
Unité de Chirurgie de la Main et du Poignet, Groupe Hospitalier de Mulhouse, Mulhouse, France

Philippe Liverneaux
Department of Hand Surgery, SOS Main, CCOM, University Hospital of Strasbourg, FMTS, University of Strasbourg, Icube CNRS 7357, 10 Avenue Baumann, 67400 Illkirch, France

Meni Mundama, Serge Ayong and Renaud Rossillon
Department of Orthopaedic Surgery, Clinique Saint-Pierre Ottignies, Avenue Reine Fabiola 9, 1340 Ottignies, Belgium

M. O. Abrego, F. L. De Cicco, J. G. Boretto, G. L. Gallucci and P. De Carli
Trauma and Orthopedics Institute "Carlos E. Ottolenghi", Italian Hospital of Buenos Aires, Buenos Aires, Argentina

Graeme Matthewson and Samuel Larrivee
University of Manitoba, S013-750 Bannatyne Avenue, Winnipeg, MB, Canada R3E 0W2

Tod Clark
Pan Am Clinic Foundation, 75 Poseidon Bay, Winnipeg, MB, Canada R3M 3E4

Giuseppe Rollo, Paolo Pichierri and Luigi Meccariello
Department of Orthopedics and Traumatology, Vito Fazzi Hospital, Lecce, Italy

Roberto Rotini
Shoulder and Elbow Unit, Rizzoli Orthopedic Institute, Bologna, Italy

Ante Prkic
Upper Limb Unit, Department of Orthopedic Surgery, Amphia Hospital, Breda, Netherlands

Denise Eygendaal
Upper Limb Unit, Department of Orthopedic Surgery, Amphia Hospital, Breda, Netherlands

Department of Orthopedic Surgery, AMC, Amsterdam, Netherlands

Michele Bisaccia and Riccardo Maria Lanzetti
Orthopedics and Traumatology Unit, SM Misericordia Hospital, University of Perugia, Perugia, Italy

Domenico Lupariello
Orthopedics and Traumatology Unit, Univerisity of Rome La Sapienza, Rome, Italy

Chaiwat Kraiwattanapong, Gun Keorochana, Thamrong Lertudomphonwanit, Pakkanut Sirijaturaporn and Methawut Thonginta
Department of Orthopaedics, Ramathibodi Hospital, Mahidol University, Bangkok, Thailand

Vanlapa Arnuntasupakul
Department of Anesthesiology, Ramathibodi Hospital, Mahidol University, Bangkok, Thailand

Rungthiwa Kantawan
Department of Nursing, Ramathibodi Hospital, Mahidol University, Bangkok, Thailand

Michio Hongo, Naohisa Miyakoshi, Masashi Fujii, Yuji Kasukawa, Yoshinori Ishikawa, Daisuke Kudo and Yoichi Shimada
Department of Orthopedic Surgery, Akita University Graduate School of Medicine, 1-1-1 Hondo, Akita 010-8543, Japan

Vineet Tyagi, Daniel H. Wiznia, Adrian K. Wyllie and Kristaps J. Keggi
Department of Orthopaedics and Rehabilitation, Yale University School of Medicine, 47 College Street, Second Floor, New Haven, CT 06510, USA

Shachar Kenan, Spencer Stein and Daniel Kiridly
Department of Orthopaedics, Hofstra North Shore Long Island Jewish, Northwell Health Medical Center, New Hyde Park, NY, USA

Robert Trasolini
Department of Orthopaedics, New England Baptist Hospital, Boston, MA, USA

Bruce A. Seideman
Department of Orthopaedics, Hofstra North Shore Long Island Jewish, Northwell Health Medical Center, St. Francis Hospital, Roslyn, NY, USA

Index